BIOLOGY OF AGING

For Medical and Life Sciences: A Biogerontology Perspective on the Hallmarks of Aging

S. PRAKASH

From Centenarians to Artificial Intelligence: Redefining the Future of Human Aging

notionpress.com

INDIA • SINGAPORE • MALAYSIA

ISBN
Hardcase 979-8-90540-984-4
Paperback 979-8-90510-907-2

First Edition: June 2026

वक्रतुण्ड महाकाय सूर्यकोटि समप्रभ।
निर्विघ्नं कुरु मे देव सर्वकार्येषु सर्वदा

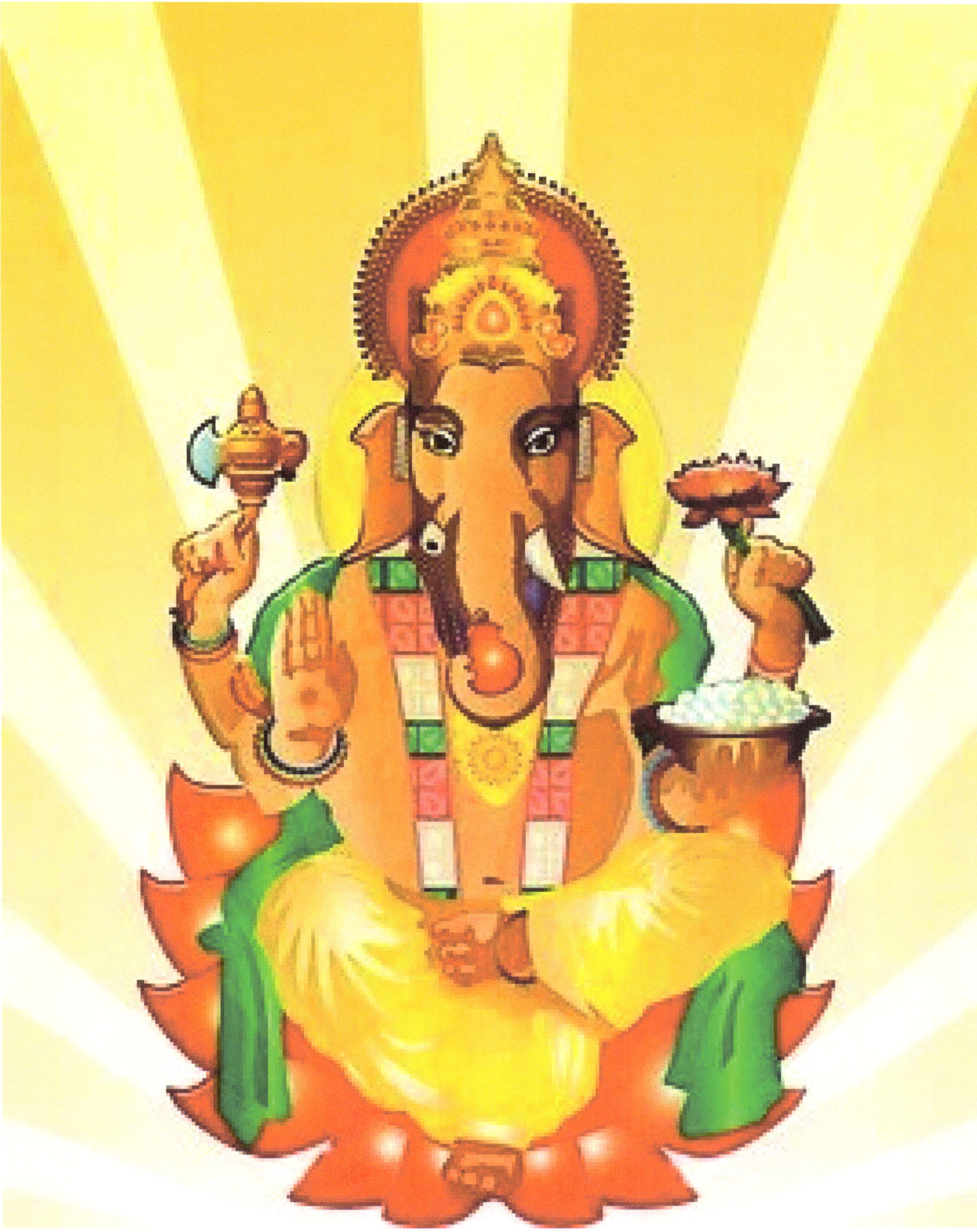

Contents

Disclaimer 9
About the Author 10
Dedication 11
Acknowledgement 12
Preface 13
Previous Books Written by Author 15

Chapter-1 .... **17**
Age-Related Decline in Key Molecules and Cellular Functions 17
Lysosomal Pathways in Aging: From Dysfunction to Cellular Rejuvenation 33
Cell Turnover, Regeneration, and the Hallmarks of Aging: A Dynamic View of Biological Renewal 35

Chapter-2 .... **47**
The NAD+ – CD38 – Sirtuin Pathway Linking Mitochondrial Dysfunction to Aging 47
NMN, NAMPT, PNC1 and the NAD+ Salvage Pathway: Central Regulators of Cellular Metabolism and Aging 53
Assessing and Modulating Mitochondrial Dysfunction in Aging Biology 59

Chapter-3 .... **70**
Metabolic Syndrome 70
Insulin Resistance 75

Chapter-4 .... **80**
Genomic instability – Hallmark of aging 80
What is p53? 84

Chapter-5 .... **92**
Mitochondria and Their Functional Role in Health and Disease 92
Mitochondrial Dysfunction – Hallmark of Aging 94

Chapter-6 .... **101**
What is Telomere? 101
Telomeres Shortening with Age – Hallmark of Aging 105

Chapter-7 .... **110**

Cell Injury - Apoptosis, Necrosis, Autophagy, and Senescence 110

Cellular Senescence – Hallmark of aging 114

Senolytics, Senescent Cell Clearance, and Their Role in Aging 117

Chapter-8 .... **123**

Autophagy and Clearance of Pathogens 123

Autophagy, Fasting, and Ketosis in Aging — Mechanisms and Therapeutic Implications 129

Glycation, Advanced Glycation End Products (AGEs), and Impaired Autophagy in Aging 132

Disabled Autophagy – Hallmark of Aging 135

mTOR vs Autophagy: Mutual Inhibition 138

Chapter-9 .... **141**

What is Epigenetics? 141

Epigenetic Alterations – Hallmark of Aging 149

The "Backup Copy" Theory of Aging and Epigenetic Information Loss 152

DNA Methylation and the Methylation Cycle in Health and Disease 159

What Is Methylation? 162

What Is MTHFR? 163

Methylation Balance and DNA Methylation in Health and Disease 172

Under vs Over Methylation 176

Digital Genome and Analog Epigenome: A Systems View of Biological Information 179

Chapter-10 .... **185**

Dysbiosis - Hallmark of Aging: Role of the Gut Microbiome in Epigenetic Regulation 185

Chapter-11 .... **199**

Loss of Proteostasis as a Hallmark of Aging 199

Loss of Proteostasis in Oral Tissues and Dental Regeneration 211

Chapter-12 .... **214**

Antagonistic Responses & Nutrient-Sensing Deregulation - Hallmark of Aging 214

mTOR–AMPK Axis in Aging and Longevity 218

Chapter-13 .... **224**

Stem Cell Exhaustion as an Integrative Hallmark of Aging 224

Regenerative Dentistry and Stem Cell-Based Therapies in Aging 231

Chapter-14 .... **234**

Altered Intercellular Communication - Hallmark of Aging 234

Altered Intercellular Communication in Aging: with Special Reference to IGF-1 Signaling, Nutrient Sensing, and Protein Intake 238

Altered Intercellular Communication in Oral Aging and Regenerative Dentistry 246

Chapter-15 .... **249**

Chronic Inflammation (Inflammaging) - Hallmark of Aging 249

Adipose Tissue Dysfunction as an Endocrine Driver of Inflammaging 254

Metabolic Overflow, Chronic Inflammation, and Protein-Driven Oncogenic Pathways in Aging 257

Chapter-16 .... **263**

What could be the other probable causes of Hallmarks of aging 263

Endocrine disruptors 263

Autoimmunity 266

Ferroptosis 270

Stress and Cortisol 274

Hormesis, Cortisol Dynamics, and the Hallmarks of Aging: Adaptive vs Maladaptive Stress in Human Biology 277

Chapter-17 .... **283**

From Biology to Algorithms: How AI is Transforming the Science of Aging 283

Chapter-18 .... **287**

Bioinformatics and the Systems-Level Decoding of the Hallmarks of Aging 287

Chapter-19 .... **290**

Biotechnology and the Therapeutic Modulation of the Hallmarks of Aging 290

CRISPR Technology/Tool 293

Chapter-20 .... **301**

Is Aging a Disease? A Critical Medical Perspective 301

Chapter-21 .... **306**

An Integrative Biology of Aging 306

The City Inside You - A Storybook Guide to the Hallmarks of Aging 314

The Forgetful Librarian - When the Instructions Go Wrong 319

"The Messengers of Cell City" - Hormones: Neuroendocrine Control in the Hallmarks of Aging 325

Lifestyle, Diet, and Epigenetic Regulation of Aging: From Nutrients to Gene Expression.............................. 337
Assessing the Hallmarks of Aging: Role of Genetic and Biochemical Testing.. 350
Epigenetic Reprogramming and OSK — Resetting the Biology of Aging 362
ORAC, Free Radicals, Antioxidants, and Aging 370
Biochemical Decline in Aging: From Mitochondrial Dysfunction to Targeted Nutritional Support 378
Energy Metabolism in Humans: Fuel Selection, Tissue Specificity, and Homeostatic Regulation 382
Fasting burns fat, starvation burns muscle - Fuel Switching in Fasting vs Starvation...................................... 390
IGF1 - The Paradox of Growth vs Longevity.. 397
Integration of Hallmarks of Aging in Cancer Biology: Pathways, Mechanisms, and Clinical Relevance............... 403
Loss of Cellular Identity 409

Chapter-22 411

Homeostasis - The Biology of Balance 411
The Metabolic Factory — Cholesterol Transport, Hormone Production,
Aging & The Sugar Overload Effect 423
The Digital Blueprint of Aging: From Centenarians to Algorithms 430
Can AI Predict and Delay Aging? The Science of Personalized Longevity 434
Machine Learning in Aging Biology: From Pathway Networks to Predictive Longevity Modeling 438

Disclaimer

This book is intended for educational purposes only and does not provide medical advice, diagnosis, or treatment recommendations.

Whether you are a student exploring aging biology or a reader interested in understanding how the human body changes over time, this book provides a thoughtful and structured introduction to one of the most important areas of modern science.

Rather than offering prescriptive solutions or speculative claims, this work focuses on evidence-based scientific understanding—encouraging readers to explore the biology of aging with critical thinking and academic rigor.

Designed primarily for students and learners in life sciences, this book serves as a conceptual guide rather than a clinical manual. It emphasizes understanding over intervention and focuses on the biological foundations of aging rather than claims of age reversal or therapeutic outcomes.

The content presented in this book is based on information derived from reputable scientific and medical sources, including peer-reviewed research and established institutions such as **PubMed, the National Library of Medicine (NIH), ScienceDirect, Frontiers journals, MDPI publications, and clinical resources like the Cleveland Clinic and Mayo Clinic.**

The author is not a licensed healthcare provider, and the material presented should not be used for self-diagnosis or self-treatment. Readers are strongly advised to consult a qualified healthcare professional or physician for any medical concerns, before making changes to diet, lifestyle, supplementation, or exercise routines.

While every effort has been made to ensure the accuracy and relevance of the information, scientific knowledge is continually evolving. The author does not guarantee completeness or absolute accuracy and shall not be held responsible for any outcomes resulting from the use or interpretation of the content.

By using this book, the reader acknowledges and agrees that the information is used at their own discretion and responsibility.

About the Author

S. Prakash is a science graduate and a project management–certified professional with a strong foundation in the **information technology (IT) industry**. Alongside his technical career, he has cultivated a deep and sustained interest in the study of classical Indian knowledge systems, including Vedanta, Darshan Shastra, and the Puranas.

His work is centered on bridging the gap between **modern biomedical science and traditional philosophical insights**, with a particular focus on understanding the mechanisms of human health, longevity, and aging. Through interdisciplinary exploration, he seeks to integrate scientific reasoning with time-tested knowledge to provide a broader perspective on life sciences.

Prakash is dedicated to research and education, aiming to make complex concepts accessible to a wide audience—including students, professionals, and general readers. His work emphasizes practical understanding and application, with the goal of improving quality of life and promoting healthy aging.

Driven by a strong sense of purpose and service, he strives to contribute meaningfully to society by sharing knowledge that supports well-being, awareness, and informed living.

S. Prakash is an author, researcher, and thinker committed to exploring the intersection of science, philosophy, and human health.

Dedication

This book is a humble offering of gratitude to my teacher and guru, whose unwavering inspiration has shaped my journey. With deep respect, I dedicate this work to **My Guru, Late Shree J.N Sharma Ji**.

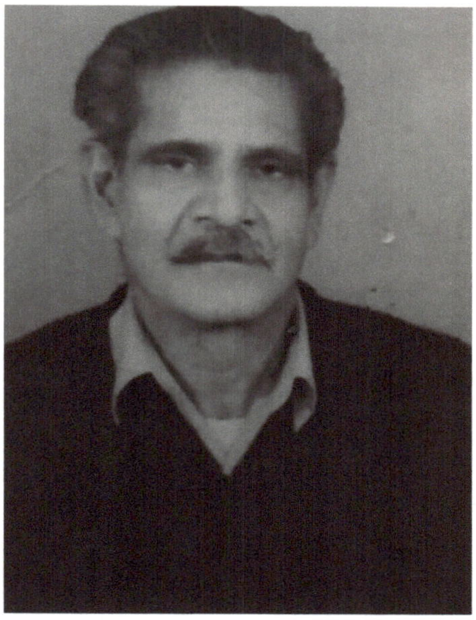

My book is published with Guruji's blessings, which I seek at his lotus feet

Acknowledgement

With deepest gratitude, I dedicate this book to my cherished parents, **Shri Satya Prakash Gupta and Mrs. Vijay Gupta,** whose endless blessings, steadfast guidance, and constant support have shaped my journey.

I bow in humble reverence to the everlasting blessings of my late grandparents, the Late Shri Devaki Nandan Varshney and the **Late Smt. Ramkali Devi**.

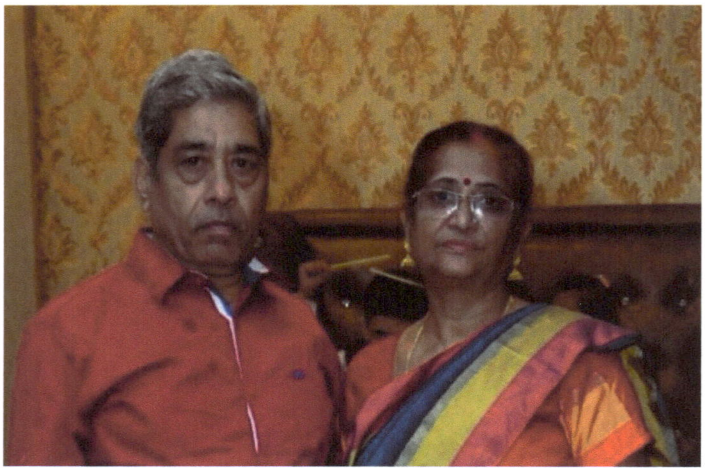

A special acknowledgment goes to my wife's grandmother, **Smt. Maya Devi**, whose diligent reading of my works and insightful encouragement constantly inspires me to contribute further to the field of authorship.

My work as a writer has been truly inspired by my dear wife, **Mrs. Lavi Gupta (Shivani), and my wonderful daughter, Gauri (Gunika Gupta)**, whose love and patience keep me going.

Finally, I am deeply grateful to my brother-in-law, **Hemant Kumar Gupta, and Gourav Gupta.** Their fascinating conversations about Medical Science, the Ramayana, Mahabharat, Puranas, and Vedas have sparked countless ideas and inspired my writing journey.

I am always grateful for my sister, **Akanksha Gupta, and my brother, Ajay Gupta**, who have always been a big support in my life.

Preface

Aging is one of the most complex and fundamental biological processes, influencing every system of the human body. Understanding its mechanisms is not confined to a single discipline; rather, it lies at the intersection of biochemistry, molecular biology, physiology, and emerging fields such as biotechnology, systems biology, and bioinformatics.

The concept of the *hallmarks of aging*, first proposed by Carlos López-Otín and colleagues, provides a unifying framework to understand how interconnected cellular and molecular processes drive aging and age-related diseases. From genomic instability and epigenetic alterations to mitochondrial dysfunction, cellular senescence, and chronic inflammation, these hallmarks offer a structured way to study aging biology.

In recent years, "longevity" has gained widespread attention. However, this book does not aim to promote the idea of reversing aging or offering simplistic solutions. Instead, it focuses on presenting evidence-based scientific concepts that explain how aging occurs at the cellular and systemic levels.

Aging biology is most rigorously studied within the field of biogerontology, which integrates knowledge across multiple core disciplines, including:

- **Biochemistry (metabolic pathways, oxidative stress, cellular energetics)**
- **Molecular biology (DNA damage, gene regulation, epigenetics)**
- **Cell biology (cellular senescence, stem cells, signaling pathways)**

While below areas are not the central focus of this book, they are included to provide a broader perspective on how contemporary aging research is conducted and translated into potential applications.

- **Biotechnology (therapeutic strategies and research tools)**
- **Microbiology (microbiome and host interactions)**
- **Bioinformatics (genomic and transcriptomic analysis)**

This book has been developed out of a strong academic interest in aging biology and a desire to make complex scientific concepts more accessible. The aim is not to replace standard medical or scientific textbooks, but to serve as a supplementary resource that helps learners build conceptual clarity and integrate knowledge across disciplines.

It is intended for students, researchers, and readers in life sciences who wish to explore the biological basis of aging in a structured and simplified manner. Readers are encouraged to use this book as a starting point for deeper study and to consult primary scientific literature for advanced understanding.

The author of this book is not a licensed medical practitioner, dietitian, or healthcare professional. This work is based on independent study, academic interest, and a synthesis of publicly available scientific literature in the fields of aging biology and life sciences.

The content presented in this book is intended solely for educational and informational purposes. It is designed to support learning and enhance understanding of biological processes related to aging and should not be interpreted as medical advice.

This book does not provide, and is not intended to provide, diagnosis, treatment, or therapeutic recommendations for any medical condition. Readers are strongly advised not to undertake self-diagnosis or self-treatment based on the information contained herein.

For any health-related concerns, decisions, or interventions, consultation with a qualified healthcare professional is essential. The author and publisher disclaim any responsibility for adverse effects resulting from the use or application of the information presented in this book.

By reading this book, the reader acknowledges and accepts that the material is informational in nature and does not substitute professional medical consultation or clinical judgment.

Key Features:

- Clear explanation of the 12+ hallmarks of aging
- Interdisciplinary approach across life sciences
- Simplified diagrams and structured content
- Focus on evidence-based scientific concepts
- Ideal for students, researchers, and curious learners

Previous Books Written by Author

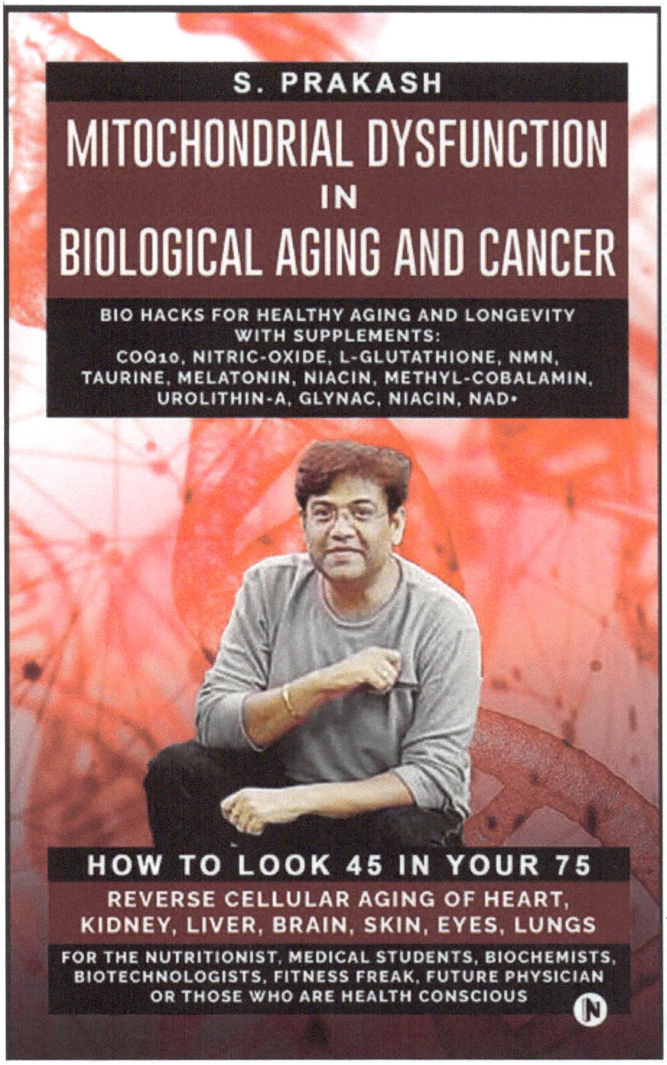

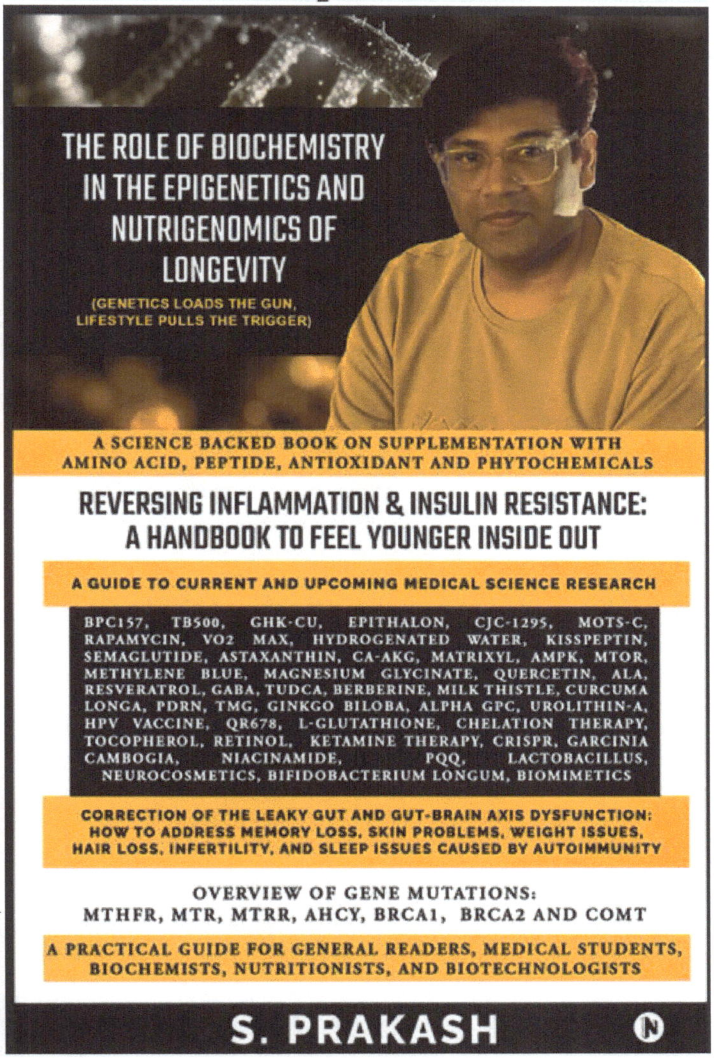

Chapter-1

Age-Related Decline in Key Molecules and Cellular Functions

Aging is a multifactorial biological process characterized by the progressive decline of molecular integrity, cellular function, and tissue homeostasis. As the human body ages, numerous biochemical molecules, signaling pathways, and regenerative mechanisms gradually deteriorate, contributing to functional decline and increased susceptibility to chronic diseases. These changes influence cellular energy production, genomic stability, immune regulation, tissue repair, and metabolic balance.

Understanding the molecular basis of aging is essential for students of biochemistry, molecular biology, biotechnology, microbiology, and biomedical sciences, as these mechanisms form the foundation of many age-related disorders, including cardiovascular disease, neurodegeneration, metabolic dysfunction, frailty, and cancer. This chapter explores the major molecules, cellular systems, and physiological processes that decline with age, their biological significance, and their implications for human health.

1. Decline in Energy and Metabolic Molecules

NAD^+ (Nicotinamide Adenine Dinucleotide)

NAD^+ is a critical coenzyme involved in mitochondrial ATP production, cellular metabolism, DNA repair, and regulation of sirtuin proteins. Aging is associated with progressive depletion of intracellular NAD^+ levels due to increased consumption during chronic inflammation and DNA damage repair, along with reduced biosynthesis.

Functional Impact

- Reduced mitochondrial energy production
- Impaired sirtuin-mediated cellular repair
- Increased oxidative stress
- Reduced metabolic efficiency
- **Decline reason:** Increased consumption (DNA repair, inflammation) and reduced synthesis
- **Impact:** Reduced energy, impaired sirtuin activity, aging

Mechanisms and Implications for Health

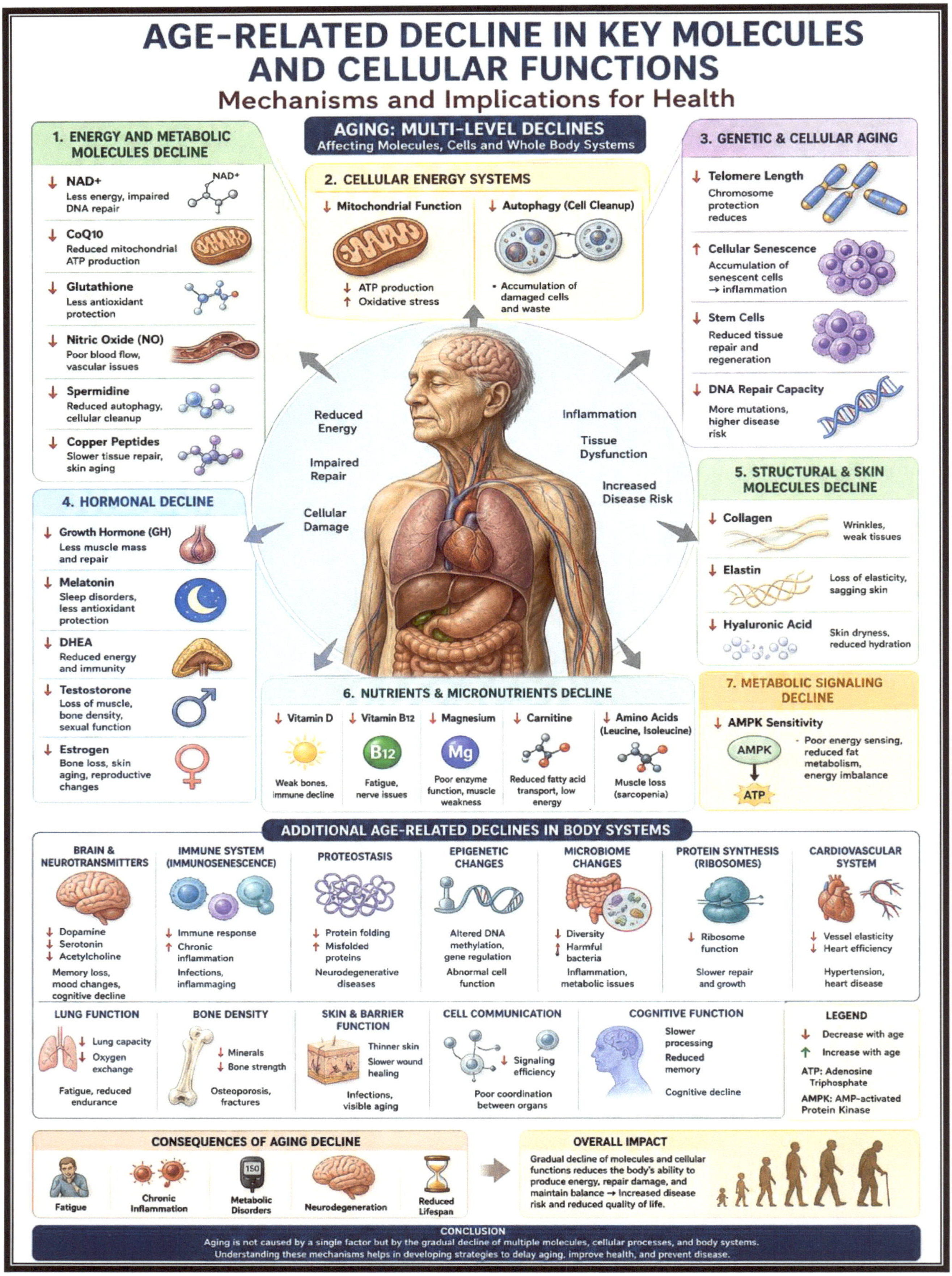

Declining NAD$^+$ levels are strongly associated with mitochondrial dysfunction and age-related metabolic decline.

- **Function:** Essential for energy production and cellular repair

Coenzyme Q10 (CoQ10)

CoQ10 is an essential component of the mitochondrial electron transport chain and plays a central role in ATP synthesis and antioxidant defence.

Age-Related Changes

- Reduced endogenous synthesis
- Increased oxidative stress
- Decline exacerbated by statin therapy

Functional Impact

- Reduced cellular energy production
- Fatigue and decreased muscle function
- Impaired mitochondrial efficiency
- **Function:** Helps mitochondria produce ATP
- **Decline reason:** Aging, statin use, oxidative stress
- **Impact:** Fatigue, reduced cellular energy

Glutathione

Glutathione is one of the body's major intracellular antioxidants and plays a key role in detoxification and protection against reactive oxygen species (ROS).

Causes of Decline

- Increased oxidative stress
- Reduced nutritional support
- Declining mitochondrial function

Functional Impact

- Cellular oxidative damage
- Impaired detoxification
- Increased inflammatory stress
- **Function:** Major antioxidant
- **Decline reason:** Increased oxidative stress, poor nutrition
- **Impact:** Cellular damage, weakened detoxification

Nitric Oxide (NO)

Nitric oxide is a signaling molecule essential for vascular function, endothelial health, and blood flow regulation.

Causes of Decline

- Endothelial dysfunction
- Oxidative stress
- Reduced nitric oxide synthase activity

Functional Impact

- Impaired circulation
- Vascular stiffness
- Increased cardiovascular risk
- **Function:** Improves blood flow and vascular health
- **Decline reason:** Endothelial dysfunction, aging
- **Impact:** Poor circulation, cardiovascular issues

Taurine

Taurine is a sulphur-containing amino acid synthesized primarily in the liver from cysteine and methionine. It is involved in mitochondrial function, calcium homeostasis, antioxidant defence, membrane stabilization, and cellular metabolism.

Recent research suggests that taurine levels decline with age and may contribute to several aging-related physiological alterations.

Functional Impact

- Reduced mitochondrial efficiency
- Increased oxidative stress
- Impaired muscle and neurological function
- Reduced cellular resilience

Taurine deficiency has been associated with impaired energy metabolism, inflammation, and age-related tissue dysfunction.

Spermidine

Spermidine is a naturally occurring polyamine involved in autophagy, cellular maintenance, and stress resistance.

Age-Related Decline

Reduced endogenous synthesis and altered metabolic regulation contribute to declining spermidine levels during aging.

Functional Impact

- Impaired autophagy
- Accumulation of damaged cellular components
- Reduced cellular renewal
- **Function:** Promotes autophagy (cell cleanup)
- **Decline reason:** Reduced synthesis with age
- **Impact:** Accumulation of damaged cells

Copper Peptides

Copper peptides contribute to tissue repair, collagen synthesis, angiogenesis, and skin regeneration.

Functional Impact

- Slower wound healing
- Reduced tissue regeneration
- Increased skin aging
- **Function:** Tissue repair, skin regeneration
- **Decline reason:** Reduced production with age
- **Impact:** Slower healing, skin aging

2. Decline in Cellular Energy Systems

Mitochondrial Dysfunction

Mitochondria are responsible for ATP production and regulation of cellular metabolism. Aging is associated with mitochondrial DNA damage, impaired oxidative phosphorylation, and increased ROS generation.

Mitochondrial dysfunction is considered a central hallmark of aging.

Functional Impact

- Reduced ATP production
- Fatigue and reduced endurance

- Increased oxidative stress
- Organ dysfunction
- **Function:** Produces ATP (cellular energy)
- **Decline reason:** DNA damage, oxidative stress
- **Impact:** Fatigue, reduced organ function

Autophagy (Cell Cleanup Process)

Autophagy is a cellular recycling mechanism responsible for removing damaged proteins and organelles.

Causes of Decline

- Dysregulated mTOR signaling
- Reduced AMPK activation
- Oxidative stress

Functional Impact

- Accumulation of dysfunctional proteins
- Increased cellular damage
- Enhanced aging-related degeneration
- **Function:** Removes damaged cellular components
- **Decline reason:** Reduced signaling (e.g., mTOR imbalance)
- **Impact:** Accumulation of waste → aging and disease

3. Genetic and Cellular Aging Markers

Telomere Length

Telomeres protect chromosomal integrity during cell division. Progressive telomere shortening occurs with repeated replication and stress exposure.

Functional Impact

- Cellular senescence
- Reduced regenerative capacity
- Genomic instability
- **Function:** Protects chromosomes
- **Decline reason:** Repeated cell division, stress
- **Impact:** Cellular aging and senescence

Cellular Senescence

Cellular senescence refers to a state of irreversible cell-cycle arrest triggered by stressors such as DNA damage, oxidative stress, and telomere shortening.

Senescent cells accumulate with age and secrete inflammatory mediators collectively known as the senescence-associated secretory phenotype (SASP).

Functional Impact

- Chronic inflammation
- Tissue dysfunction
- Altered intercellular communication
- **Function:** Stops damaged cells from dividing
- **Problem:** Accumulation of senescent cells
- **Impact:** Inflammation and tissue dysfunction

Stem Cells

Stem cells are essential for tissue repair and regeneration. Aging reduces stem cell number and function.

Functional Impact

- Delayed tissue repair
- Reduced regenerative potential
- Organ functional decline
- **Function:** Tissue repair and regeneration
- **Decline reason:** Aging and environmental stress
- **Impact:** Slower healing and regeneration

Klotho Protein

Klotho is an anti-aging protein involved in phosphate metabolism, oxidative stress reduction, and cellular signaling.

Age-Related Decline

Reduced Klotho expression has been associated with:

- Cognitive decline
- Vascular aging
- Kidney dysfunction

4. Decline in Hormones

Growth Hormone (GH)

Growth hormone levels progressively decline after early adulthood.

Functional Impact

- Reduced muscle mass
- Impaired tissue repair
- Increased fat accumulation
- Declines after early adulthood
- Leads to reduced muscle mass and repair

Melatonin

Melatonin regulates circadian rhythm and exhibits antioxidant properties.

Functional Impact

- Sleep disturbances
- Increased oxidative stress
- Circadian dysregulation
- Regulates sleep and antioxidant activity
- Declines with age → sleep disorders

DHEA (Dehydroepiandrosterone)

DHEA is a precursor steroid hormone involved in metabolic and immune regulation.

Functional Impact

- Reduced energy metabolism
- Altered immune function
- Hormonal imbalance
- Precursor hormone
- Decline affects energy and immunity

Testosterone & Estrogen

- Decline with age
- Affect muscle, bone, and reproductive health

5. Structural and Skin-Related Molecules

Collagen

Collagen provides structural integrity to connective tissues and skin.

Functional Impact

- Reduced skin elasticity
- Wrinkle formation
- Tissue fragility
- Provides skin strength
- Declines → wrinkles, weak tissues

Elastin

- Gives skin elasticity
- Declines → sagging skin

Hyaluronic Acid

- Maintains skin hydration
- Declines → dryness and aging

6. Vitamins and Nutrients

Vitamin D

Vitamin D deficiency becomes increasingly common with age due to reduced synthesis and absorption.

Functional Impact

- Reduced bone mineralization
- Impaired immune regulation
- Declines due to less sunlight exposure and absorption
- Affects bone and immune health

Magnesium

Magnesium functions as a cofactor for numerous enzymatic reactions.

Functional Impact

- Neuromuscular dysfunction
- Metabolic imbalance
- Important for enzyme function
- Declines due to poor diet

Vitamin B12

Reduced gastrointestinal absorption contributes to vitamin B12 deficiency in aging populations.

Functional Impact

- Neurological dysfunction
- Fatigue
- Impaired DNA synthesis
- Absorption decreases with age
- Leads to fatigue and nerve issues

Acetyl-Carnitine/Carnitine

Carnitine facilitates fatty acid transport into mitochondria for energy production.

Functional Impact

- Reduced mitochondrial metabolism
- Fatigue and muscle weakness

- Helps transport fatty acids into mitochondria
- Declines → reduced energy production

7. Decline in Metabolic Signaling

AMPK Sensitivity

AMPK functions as a cellular energy sensor regulating metabolism and mitochondrial homeostasis.

Functional Impact

- Impaired metabolic adaptation
- Reduced fatty acid oxidation
- Decline in cellular energy balance
- **Function:** Energy sensor of the cell
- **Decline reason:** Aging, metabolic dysfunction
- **Impact:** Reduced fat metabolism and energy balance

Sirtuins

Sirtuins are NAD^+-dependent proteins involved in DNA repair, stress resistance, and metabolic regulation.

Functional Impact

- Reduced cellular resilience
- Impaired mitochondrial regulation
- Accelerated aging-related dysfunction

mTOR Dysregulation

mTOR regulates cellular growth, nutrient sensing, and protein synthesis.

Chronic mTOR activation during aging suppresses autophagy and contributes to metabolic dysfunction.

8. Brain and Nervous System Aging

Neurotransmitter Decline

Aging is associated with reduced levels of dopamine, serotonin, and acetylcholine.

Functional Impact

- Cognitive decline
- Reduced memory function
- Mood alterations

Cognitive Aging

Age-related neuronal dysfunction contributes to:

- Reduced processing speed
- Memory impairment
- Neurodegenerative disease risk

9. Immune Aging (Immunosenescence)

The aging immune system demonstrates:

- Reduced adaptive immune response
- Chronic low-grade inflammation ("inflammaging")
- Impaired vaccine responsiveness

Functional Impact

- Increased infection susceptibility
- Delayed tissue repair
- Chronic inflammatory disease risk

Thymic Function and Thymosin

The thymus plays a critical role in T-lymphocyte maturation and adaptive immune regulation. Aging is associated with thymic involution and reduced thymosin activity.

Functional Impact

- Reduced T-cell production
- Impaired adaptive immunity
- Increased susceptibility to infections

10. Proteostasis and Protein Quality Control

Proteostasis refers to the maintenance of protein folding, repair, and degradation.

Age-Related Changes

- Decline in heat shock proteins (HSPs)
- Increased protein misfolding

Functional Impact

- Neurodegenerative disorders
- Cellular dysfunction

Heat Shock Proteins (HSPs)

Heat shock proteins are molecular chaperones that assist in proper protein folding, stabilization, and protection against cellular stress.

Age-Related Changes

Aging is associated with reduced heat shock response and impaired chaperone activity.

Functional Impact

- Increased protein misfolding
- Cellular stress accumulation
- Neurodegenerative disease risk

11. Epigenetic Alterations

Aging is associated with changes in:

- DNA methylation
- Histone modification
- Chromatin organization

Functional Impact

- Altered gene expression
- Loss of cellular identity
- Increased disease susceptibility

12. Microbiome Alterations

The gut microbiome undergoes significant changes with aging.

Functional Impact

- Reduced microbial diversity
- Increased inflammation
- Metabolic dysregulation

13. Cardiovascular and Pulmonary Aging

Cardiovascular Aging

- Reduced vascular elasticity
- Increased arterial stiffness
- Declining cardiac efficiency

Pulmonary Aging

- Reduced lung elasticity
- Decreased oxygen exchange capacity

Clinical Impact

- Reduced endurance
- Increased cardiovascular and respiratory disease risk

14. Bone and Musculoskeletal Aging

Bone Density Decline

Aging reduces bone mineral density and structural integrity.

Functional Impact

- Osteoporosis
- Increased fracture risk

Sarcopenia

Age-related muscle loss contributes to:

- Frailty
- Reduced mobility
- Functional decline

15. Altered Intercellular Communication

Aging impairs cellular signaling and systemic coordination between tissues and organs.

Functional Impact

- Chronic inflammation
- Hormonal imbalance
- Reduced physiological adaptability

Conclusion

Aging is not driven by a single molecular event but rather by the progressive decline of interconnected cellular systems, signaling pathways, and physiological processes. Alterations in mitochondrial function, nutrient sensing, genomic stability, proteostasis, stem cell activity, immune regulation, and intercellular communication collectively contribute to the aging phenotype and increased disease susceptibility.

Understanding these mechanisms provides important insight into the biology of aging and forms the scientific foundation for emerging therapeutic strategies aimed at improving health span and reducing age-related dysfunction.

Summary Table (Quick Revision)

Category	Key Declines	Main Effect
Energy Molecules	NAD+, CoQ10, Glutathione	Reduced cellular energy
Cellular Systems	Mitochondria, Autophagy	Accumulation of damage
Genetic Factors	Telomeres, Senescence	Aging of cells
Hormones	GH, Melatonin, DHEA	Reduced repair and function
Structural	Collagen, Elastin	Skin and tissue aging
Nutrients	Vitamin D, B12, Magnesium	Weak metabolism
Signaling	AMPK	Poor energy regulation

1. Energy Molecules Decline

- ↓ NAD+
- ↓ CoQ10
- ↓ Glutathione
- ↓ Nitric Oxide
- ↓ Spermidine

👉 **Effect:**

Reduced ATP, oxidative stress ↑

2. Cellular Energy Systems

- ↓ Mitochondrial Function
- ↓ ATP production
- ↓ Autophagy

👉 **Effect:**

Accumulation of damaged cells, low energy

3. Genetic & Cellular Aging

- ↓ Telomere Length
- ↑ Cellular Senescence
- ↓ Stem Cells
- ↓ DNA repair

👉 **Effect:**

Reduced regeneration, Aging cells, Mutations

4. Hormonal Decline

- ↓ Growth Hormone
- ↓ Melatonin
- ↓ DHEA
- ↓ Testosterone/Estrogen

👉 **Effect:**

Reduced repair, sleep, metabolism

5. Structural Components

- ↓ Collagen
- ↓ Elastin
- ↓ Hyaluronic Acid

👉 **Effect:**

Skin aging, tissue weakness

6. Nutrients & Signaling

- ↓ Vitamin D
- ↓ Vitamin B12
- ↓ Magnesium
- ↓ Carnitine
- ↓ AMPK sensitivity

👉 **Effect:**

Poor metabolism and energy balance

Brain & Neurotransmitters

- ↓ Dopamine
- ↓ Serotonin
- ↓ Acetylcholine

👉 Effect: Memory loss, cognitive decline

Immune System (Immunosenescence)

- ↓ Immune response
- ↑ Chronic inflammation

👉 Effect: Infections, inflammaging

Proteostasis

- ↓ Protein folding
- ↑ Misfolded proteins

👉 Effect: Neurodegenerative diseases

Epigenetic Changes

Related to Epigenetics

- Altered gene regulation

👉 Effect: Abnormal cell function

Microbiome Changes

Related to Microbiome

- ↓ Diversity
- ↑ Harmful bacteria

👉 Effect: Inflammation, metabolic issues

Protein Synthesis

- ↓ Ribosome function

👉 Effect: Slower repair and growth

Cardiovascular System

- ↓ Vessel elasticity
- ↓ heart efficiency

👉 Effect: Heart disease

Cell Communication

- ↓ Signaling efficiency

👉 Effect: Poor organ coordination

Consequences of Aging Decline

- Fatigue
- Chronic inflammation
- Metabolic disorders
- Neurodegeneration
- Reduced lifespan

Conclusion

Aging is not caused by a single factor but by the gradual decline of multiple molecules and cellular processes. These changes reduce the body's ability to produce energy, repair damage, and maintain balance. Understanding these mechanisms helps students and researchers explore ways to improve health, delay aging, and prevent disease.

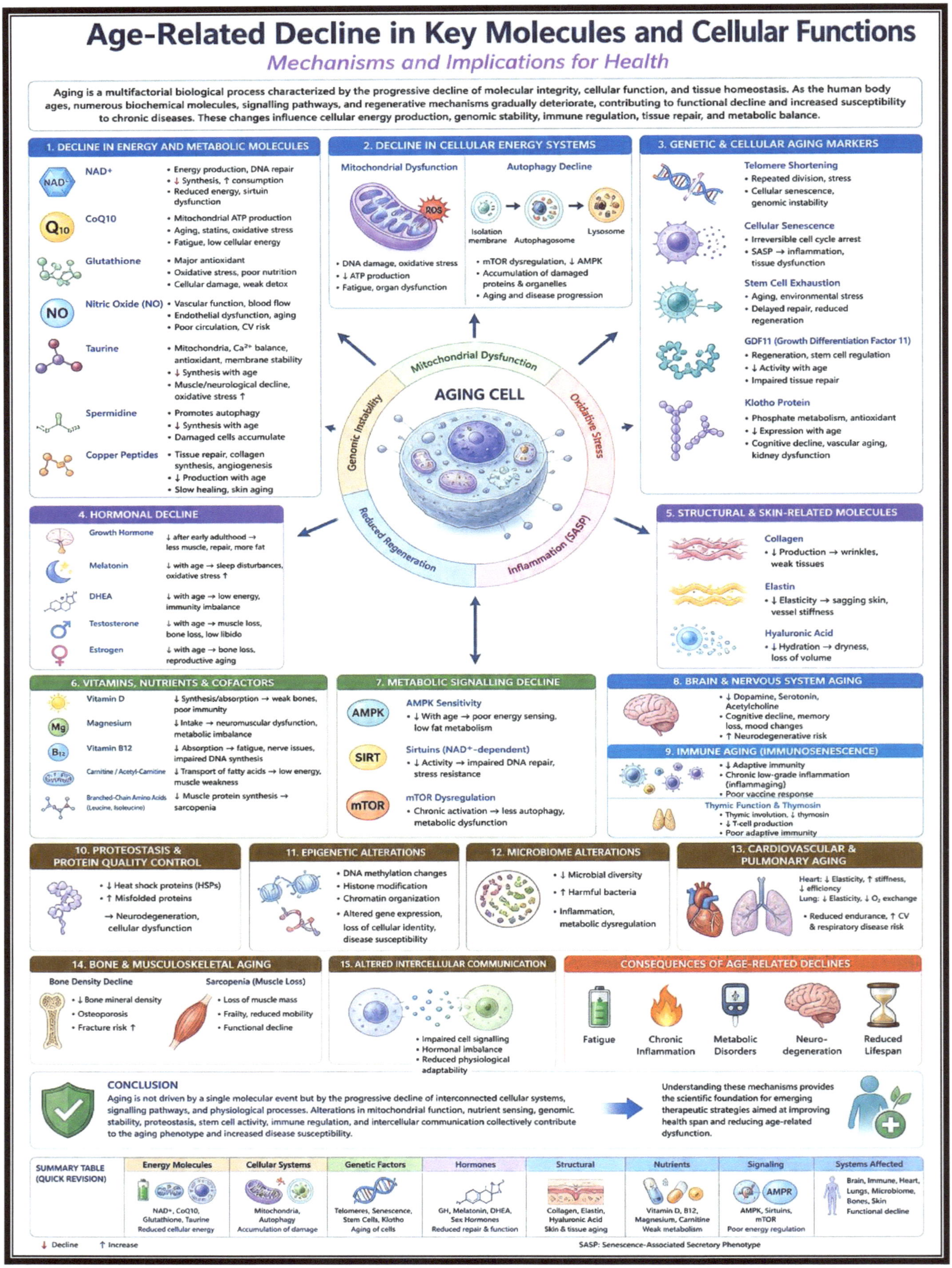
Age-Related Decline in Key Molecules and Cellular Functions
Mechanisms and Implications for Health
Aging is a multifactorial biological process characterized by the progressive decline of molecular integrity, cellular function, and tissue homeostasis. As the human body ages, numerous biochemical molecules, signalling pathways, and regenerative mechanisms gradually deteriorate, contributing to functional decline and increased susceptibility to chronic diseases. These changes influence cellular energy production, genomic stability, immune regulation, tissue repair, and metabolic balance.
1. DECLINE IN ENERGY AND METABOLIC MOLECULES
NAD+
• Energy production, DNA repair
• ↓ Synthesis, ↑ consumption
• Reduced energy, sirtuin dysfunction
CoQ10
• Mitochondrial ATP production
• Aging, statins, oxidative stress
• Fatigue, low cellular energy
Glutathione
• Major antioxidant
• Oxidative stress, poor nutrition
• Cellular damage, weak detox
Nitric Oxide (NO)
• Vascular function, blood flow
• Endothelial dysfunction, aging
• Poor circulation, CV risk
Taurine
• Mitochondria, Ca²⁺ balance, antioxidant, membrane stability
• ↓ Synthesis with age
• Muscle/neurological decline, oxidative stress ↑
Spermidine
• Promotes autophagy
• ↓ Synthesis with age
• Damaged cells accumulate
Copper Peptides
• Tissue repair, collagen synthesis, angiogenesis
• ↓ Production with age
• Slow healing, skin aging
2. DECLINE IN CELLULAR ENERGY SYSTEMS
Mitochondrial Dysfunction
ROS
• DNA damage, oxidative stress
• ↓ ATP production
• Fatigue, organ dysfunction
Autophagy Decline
Isolation membrane
Autophagosome
Lysosome
• mTOR dysregulation, ↓ AMPK
• Accumulation of damaged proteins & organelles
• Aging and disease progression
3. GENETIC & CELLULAR AGING MARKERS
Telomere Shortening
• Repeated division, stress
• Cellular senescence, genomic instability
Cellular Senescence
• Irreversible cell cycle arrest
• SASP → inflammation, tissue dysfunction
Stem Cell Exhaustion
• Aging, environmental stress
• Delayed repair, reduced regeneration
GDF11 (Growth Differentiation Factor 11)
• Regeneration, stem cell regulation
• ↓ Activity with age
• Impaired tissue repair
Klotho Protein
• Phosphate metabolism, antioxidant
• ↓ Expression with age
• Cognitive decline, vascular aging, kidney dysfunction
AGING CELL
Mitochondrial Dysfunction
Oxidative Stress
Inflammation (SASP)
Reduced Regeneration
Genomic Instability
4. HORMONAL DECLINE
Growth Hormone
↓ after early adulthood → less muscle, repair, more fat
Melatonin
↓ with age → sleep disturbances, oxidative stress ↑
DHEA
↓ with age → low energy, immunity imbalance
Testosterone
↓ with age → muscle loss, bone loss, low libido
Estrogen
↓ with age → bone loss, reproductive aging
5. STRUCTURAL & SKIN-RELATED MOLECULES
Collagen
• ↓ Production → wrinkles, weak tissues
Elastin
• ↓ Elasticity → sagging skin, vessel stiffness
Hyaluronic Acid
• ↓ Hydration → dryness, loss of volume
6. VITAMINS, NUTRIENTS & COFACTORS
Vitamin D
↓ Synthesis/absorption → weak bones, poor immunity
Magnesium
↓ Intake → neuromuscular dysfunction, metabolic imbalance
Vitamin B12
↓ Absorption → fatigue, nerve issues, impaired DNA synthesis
Carnitine / Acetyl-Carnitine
↓ Transport of fatty acids → low energy, muscle weakness
Branched-Chain Amino Acids (Leucine, Isoleucine)
↓ Muscle protein synthesis → sarcopenia
7. METABOLIC SIGNALLING DECLINE
AMPK
AMPK Sensitivity
• ↓ With age → poor energy sensing, low fat metabolism
SIRT
Sirtuins (NAD⁺-dependent)
• ↓ Activity → impaired DNA repair, stress resistance
mTOR
mTOR Dysregulation
• Chronic activation → less autophagy, metabolic dysfunction
8. BRAIN & NERVOUS SYSTEM AGING
• ↓ Dopamine, Serotonin, Acetylcholine
• Cognitive decline, memory loss, mood changes
• ↑ Neurodegenerative risk
9. IMMUNE AGING (IMMUNOSENESCENCE)
• ↓ Adaptive immunity
• Chronic low-grade inflammation (inflammaging)
• Poor vaccine response
Thymic Function & Thymosin
• Thymic involution, ↓ thymosin
• ↓ T-cell production
• Poor adaptive immunity
10. PROTEOSTASIS & PROTEIN QUALITY CONTROL
• ↓ Heat shock proteins (HSPs)
• ↑ Misfolded proteins
→ Neurodegeneration, cellular dysfunction
11. EPIGENETIC ALTERATIONS
• DNA methylation changes
• Histone modification
• Chromatin organization
• Altered gene expression, loss of cellular identity, disease susceptibility
12. MICROBIOME ALTERATIONS
• ↓ Microbial diversity
• ↑ Harmful bacteria
• Inflammation, metabolic dysregulation
13. CARDIOVASCULAR & PULMONARY AGING
Heart: ↓ Elasticity, ↑ stiffness, ↓ efficiency
Lung: ↓ Elasticity, ↓ O₂ exchange
• Reduced endurance, ↑ CV & respiratory disease risk
14. BONE & MUSCULOSKELETAL AGING
Bone Density Decline
• ↓ Bone mineral density
• Osteoporosis
• Fracture risk ↑
Sarcopenia (Muscle Loss)
• Loss of muscle mass
• Frailty, reduced mobility
• Functional decline
15. ALTERED INTERCELLULAR COMMUNICATION
• Impaired cell signalling
• Hormonal imbalance
• Reduced physiological adaptability
CONSEQUENCES OF AGE-RELATED DECLINES
Fatigue
Chronic Inflammation
Metabolic Disorders
Neuro-degeneration
Reduced Lifespan
CONCLUSION
Aging is not driven by a single molecular event but by the progressive decline of interconnected cellular systems, signalling pathways, and physiological processes. Alterations in mitochondrial function, nutrient sensing, genomic stability, proteostasis, stem cell activity, immune regulation, and intercellular communication collectively contribute to the aging phenotype and increased disease susceptibility.
Understanding these mechanisms provides the scientific foundation for emerging therapeutic strategies aimed at improving health span and reducing age-related dysfunction.
SUMMARY TABLE (QUICK REVISION)
Energy Molecules
NAD+, CoQ10, Glutathione, Taurine
Reduced cellular energy
Cellular Systems
Mitochondria, Autophagy
Accumulation of damage
Genetic Factors
Telomeres, Senescence, Stem Cells, Klotho
Aging of cells
Hormones
GH, Melatonin, DHEA, Sex Hormones
Reduced repair & function
Structural
Collagen, Elastin, Hyaluronic Acid
Skin & tissue aging
Nutrients
Vitamin D, B12, Magnesium, Carnitine
Weak metabolism
Signaling
AMPK
AMPK, Sirtuins, mTOR
Poor energy regulation
Systems Affected
Brain, Immune, Heart, Lungs, Microbiome, Bones, Skin
Functional decline
↓ Decline
↑ Increase
SASP: Senescence-Associated Secretory Phenotype

There are **several other important molecules, systems, and functions that also decline with age**.

Brain & Nervous System Decline

Neurotransmitters

- Examples: Dopamine, Serotonin, Acetylcholine
- **Function:** Brain signaling, mood, memory
- **Decline effect:**
  - Memory loss
  - Depression
  - Reduced focus

👉 Important for linking aging with neurodegenerative diseases

Immune System Decline (Immunosenescence)

- Reduced immune cell function
- Lower ability to fight infections
- Poor vaccine response

👉 Leads to:

- Increased infections
- Chronic inflammation ("inflammaging")

Proteostasis (Protein Balance)

- Decline in protein folding and repair systems
- Accumulation of misfolded proteins

👉 Leads to:

- Alzheimer's disease
- Parkinson's disease

DNA Repair Capacity

- Reduced efficiency of DNA repair systems
- Increased mutations over time

👉 Leads to:

- Cancer
- Cellular dysfunction

Epigenetic Regulation

Related to Epigenetics

- Changes in DNA methylation patterns
- Loss of gene regulation control

👉 Leads to:

- Abnormal gene expression
- Aging-related diseases

Protein Synthesis & Ribosome Function

- Reduced ability to make new proteins
- Slower cellular repair

👉 Leads to:

- Muscle loss
- Weak tissue repair

Cardiovascular Function

- Reduced elasticity of blood vessels
- Decreased cardiac output

👉 Leads to:

- Hypertension
- Heart disease

Lung Function

- Reduced lung capacity
- Less oxygen exchange

👉 Leads to:

- Fatigue
- Reduced endurance

Bone Density

- Loss of calcium and minerals
- Reduced bone strength

👉 Leads to:

- Osteoporosis
- Fractures

Skin and Barrier Function

- Reduced skin thickness
- Slower wound healing

👉 Leads to:

- Increased infections
- Visible aging

Microbiome Diversity

Related to Microbiome

- Reduced diversity of gut bacteria
- Increase in harmful microbes

👉 Leads to:

- Inflammation
- Metabolic disorders

Cellular Communication

- Cells communicate less efficiently
- Hormone and signaling imbalance

👉 Leads to:

- Poor coordination between organs

Cognitive Function

- Slower processing speed
- Reduced memory

👉 Leads to:

- Cognitive decline

Aging affects not only molecules but also entire systems including the brain, immune system, heart, lungs, and microbiome, leading to reduced function and increased disease risk.

Lysosomal Pathways in Aging: From Dysfunction to Cellular Rejuvenation

Aging is characterized by a progressive decline in cellular homeostasis, resulting in the accumulation of damaged macromolecules and organelles. A central system responsible for intracellular quality control is the lysosomal degradation pathway. Lysosomes serve as the terminal degradative compartment of the cell and play a crucial role in autophagy, endocytosis, and maintenance of proteostasis.

Recent research highlights that activation or restoration of lysosomal function can counteract key aspects of cellular aging by enhancing the clearance of toxic protein aggregates. This positions lysosomal pathways as promising therapeutic targets in aging and age-related diseases.

During aging, lysosomal efficiency declines, leading to:

- Accumulation of misfolded and toxic proteins
- Increased oxidative stress
- Cellular senescence

A key example is progerin, which accumulates when lysosomal degradation is impaired, resulting in DNA damage and premature aging phenotypes.

Enhancing lysosomal activity—through mechanisms such as TFEB activation and mTOR inhibition—leads to:

- Increased autophagic flux
- Improved clearance of toxic proteins
- Reduction in senescence markers
- Restoration of cellular function

Consequently, lysosomal activation supports proteostasis and overall cellular health.

Lysosomal dysfunction is therefore a significant contributor to aging, while its restoration represents a potential therapeutic strategy. It is best understood within the **loss of proteostasis** hallmark of aging and is closely linked to other processes, including:

- Cellular senescence
- Mitochondrial dysfunction
- Deregulated nutrient sensing (mTOR pathway)

Key regulatory pathways that enhance lysosomal function include:

- TFEB activation, which promotes lysosomal biogenesis
- mTOR inhibition, which stimulates autophagy
- AMPK activation, which supports cellular catabolic processes

Scientific References

Core Aging Framework

- https://www.cell.com/S0092-8674(13)00645-4
- https://www.cell.com/S0092-8674(22)01377-0

Energy, Mitochondria, NAD$^+$

- https://www.ncbi.nlm.nih.gov/pmc/articles/PMC3616313
- https://www.ncbi.nlm.nih.gov/pmc/articles/PMC4924200

Oxidative Stress & Antioxidants

- https://www.ncbi.nlm.nih.gov/pmc/articles/PMC4684116

Autophagy & Cellular Cleanup

- https://www.ncbi.nlm.nih.gov/pmc/articles/PMC3898688

🧬 **Telomeres, Senescence, Stem Cells**

- https://www.ncbi.nlm.nih.gov/pmc/articles/PMC3836174
- https://www.ncbi.nlm.nih.gov/pmc/articles/PMC3370421

💉 **Hormonal Aging**

- https://www.ncbi.nlm.nih.gov/pmc/articles/PMC3666679

🧴 **Skin & Structural Aging**

- https://www.ncbi.nlm.nih.gov/pmc/articles/PMC3583892

💊 **Nutrients (Vitamin D, B12)**

- https://ods.od.nih.gov

🔋 **Metabolic Signaling (AMPK)**

- https://www.ncbi.nlm.nih.gov/pmc/articles/PMC2998669

🧠 **Brain & Neuro aging**

- https://www.ncbi.nlm.nih.gov/pmc/articles/PMC6770068

🦠 **Immune Aging**

- https://www.ncbi.nlm.nih.gov/pmc/articles/PMC4031968

🧬 **Epigenetics & Proteostasis**

- https://www.ncbi.nlm.nih.gov/pmc/articles/PMC5372957

🦠 **Microbiome**

- https://www.ncbi.nlm.nih.gov/pmc/articles/PMC3535073

🧡 **Cardiovascular & Bone Aging**

- https://www.ncbi.nlm.nih.gov/pmc/articles/PMC4609308

1. The Crucial Impact of Lysosomes in Aging and Longevity

https://pmc.ncbi.nlm.nih.gov/articles/PMC5081277/

2. Lysosomes as a Therapeutic Target (Nature Reviews Drug Discovery)

https://www.nature.com/articles/s41573-019-0036-1

3. Lysosomes as Coordinators of Cellular Catabolism and Metabolic Signaling

https://www.nature.com/articles/s41580-023-00676-x

4. TFEB and TFE3: Linking Lysosomes to Cellular Adaptation to Stress

https://www.annualreviews.org/doi/10.1146/annurev-cellbio-111315-125407

5. Lysosome Biogenesis in Health and Disease

https://pmc.ncbi.nlm.nih.gov/articles/PMC6368902/

6. Lysosomal Activation and Progerin Clearance (Your Core Paper)

https://link.springer.com/article/10.1007/s11427-025-2983-2

Cell Turnover, Regeneration, and the Hallmarks of Aging: A Dynamic View of Biological Renewal

🧠 1. Core Concept

The human body is not static. It is a dynamic system in which billions of cells are continuously formed, renewed, and removed. The rate at which different cells regenerate reflects both biological function and biological aging.

👉 "Your biological age is not only determined by your genes, but by how efficiently your cells renew, repair, and maintain themselves."

🔄 2. Cell Turnover Timeline

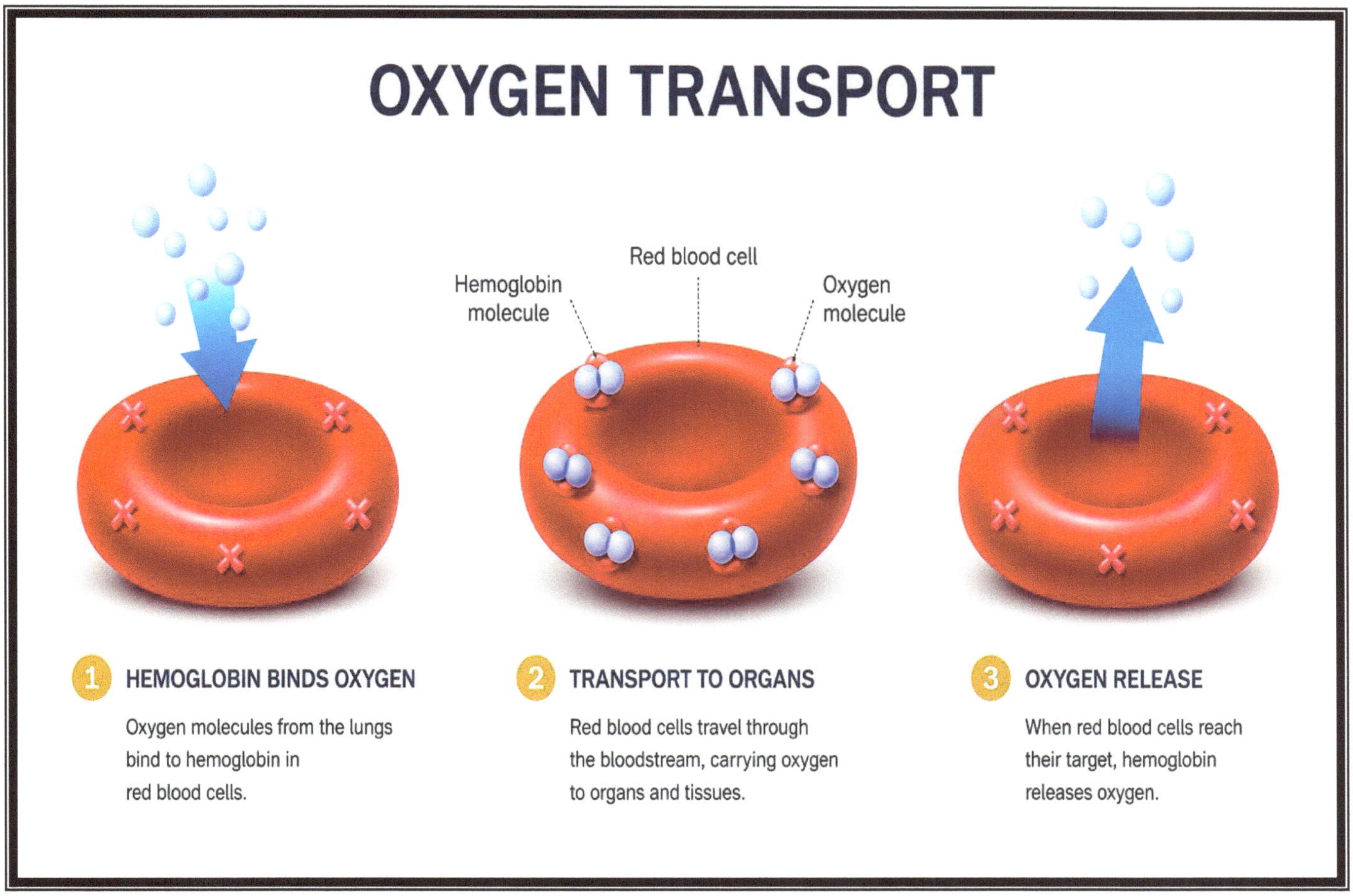

- Formation: ~**7 days (erythropoiesis)**
- Lifespan: ~**120 days**
- Production rate: ~**2–3 million cells/second**

👉 Key function: Oxygen transport

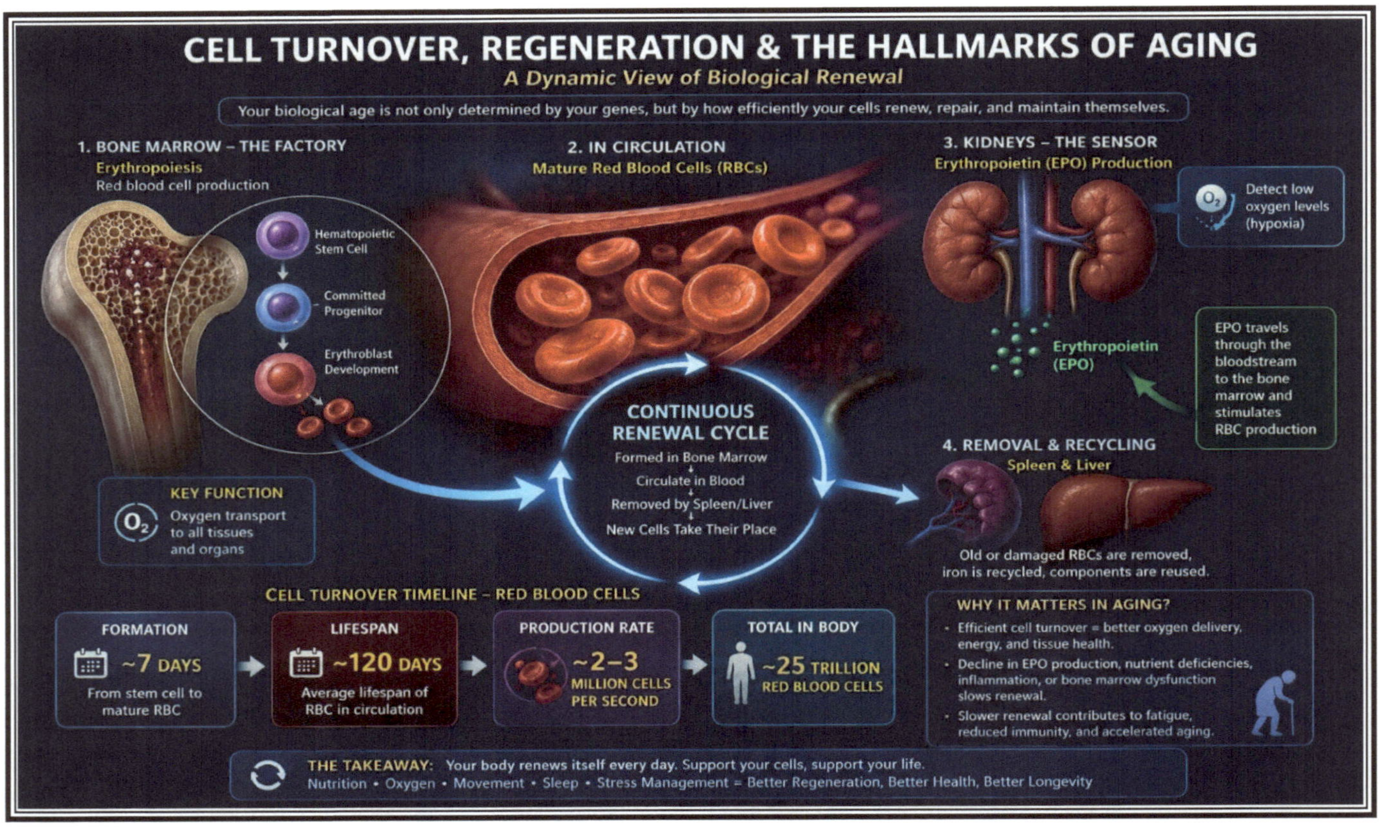

Skin Cells (Epidermis)

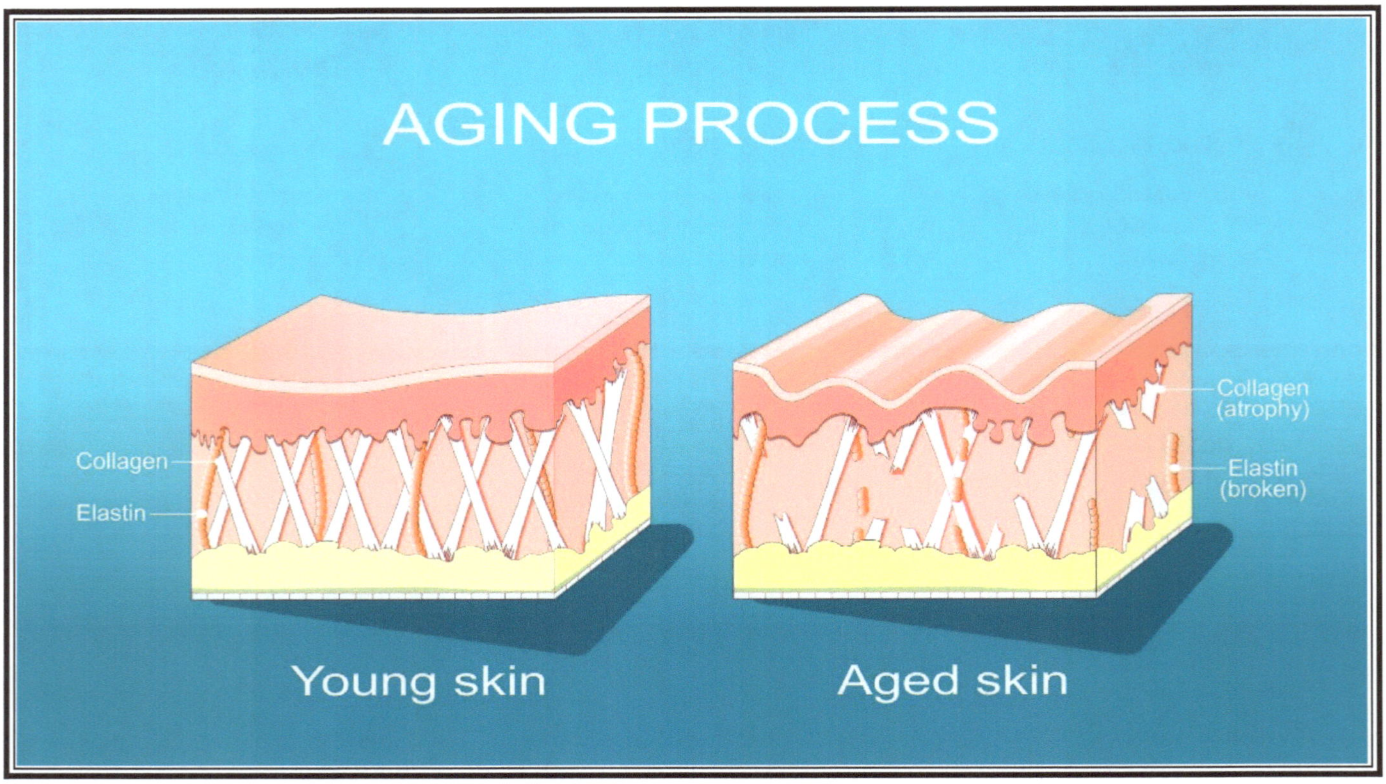

- Turnover: **28–40 days (young adults)**
- With aging: **up to 60–80 days**

👉 Key function: Barrier + protection

⚡ **Other Rapidly Renewing Cells**

Cell Type	Turnover Time
Gut lining cells	3–5 days
White blood cells	Hours to days
Liver cells	~300–500 days
Fat cells	~8–10 years
Muscle cells	Very slow (~10–15 years)

Some cells such as neurons and cardiac muscle cells have very limited regenerative capacity, but they are not completely non-renewable. Low-level regeneration may occur under specific conditions.

🔗 **3. Why Cell Turnover Matters in Aging**

👉 Transition:

Efficient cell turnover reflects a healthy balance between damage and repair. Aging disrupts this balance.

🧬 **4. Connection to Hallmarks of Aging (CORE SECTION)**

🔬 **1. Stem Cell Exhaustion**

- RBCs depend on bone marrow stem cells
- Aging → ↓ stem cell function

👉 Result:

- Poor RBC quality
- Reduced oxygen delivery

🧬 **2. Telomere Attrition**

- Fast-dividing cells (skin, gut) → faster telomere shortening

👉 Result:

- Slower regeneration
- Thinner skin, delayed healing

🔥 **3. Inflammaging (Chronic Inflammation)**

- Old RBCs → rigid → poor circulation
- Damaged cells → immune activation

👉 Result:

- Chronic low-grade inflammation

⚙️ **4. Loss of Proteostasis**

- Skin cells accumulate damaged proteins

👉 Result:

- Wrinkles
- Loss of elasticity

🔋 **5. Mitochondrial Dysfunction**

- ↓ energy production

👉 Result:

- Slower cell turnover
- Poor repair

🧠 **6. Altered Intercellular Communication**

- Hormones & cytokines become dysregulated

👉 Result:

- Poor signaling for regeneration

🎯 Integrating with Epigenome Concept

Cell renewal is not automatic in isolation—it is regulated by epigenetic mechanisms that respond to internal and external signals such as nutrition, hormones, and stress.

👉 Gene expression controlling cell regeneration is not simply ON or OFF, but operates like a volume knob.

🔑 **Key Insight:**

- DNA = blueprint
- Epigenome = regulator
- Cell turnover = output

Example:

- Low expression → slow skin repair
- Optimal expression → healthy renewal
- Dysregulated expression → aging + disease

🧠 Aging can be understood as a progressive decline in the body's ability to renew its cells efficiently, driven by interconnected hallmarks such as stem cell exhaustion, epigenetic alterations, mitochondrial dysfunction, and chronic inflammation.

⚠️ **8. Scientific Boundaries**

While cell turnover can be influenced by lifestyle, nutrition, and metabolic health, it cannot be fully controlled or reversed, and varies significantly between individuals.

📌 **9. Key Takeaways (Student-Friendly)**

- Body is constantly renewing itself
- Different cells have different lifespans
- Aging slows regeneration
- Hallmarks of aging disrupt cell turnover
- Epigenetics regulates how efficiently cells renew

📊 **1. Master Flow: Cell Renewal & Aging**

DNA (Genetic Blueprint)

↓

Epigenetic Regulation (Control Layer)

↓

Gene Expression (Volume Control 🎚️)

↓

Protein Synthesis

↓

Cell Function

↓

Cell Turnover (RBC, Skin, Gut, etc.)
↓
Tissue Health
↓
Aging Process
↓
Disease Risk

🧬 2. Cell Turnover Timeline Diagram

FAST RENEWAL
↓
Gut Cells → 3–5 days
WBCs → Hours to days
↓
MODERATE RENEWAL
↓
RBC Formation → ~7 days
RBC Lifespan → ~120 days
Skin Cells → 28–40 days (↑ with age)
↓
SLOW RENEWAL
↓
Liver Cells → 300–500 days
Fat Cells → ~10 years
Muscle Cells → ~10–15 years
↓
VERY LIMITED RENEWAL
↓
Neurons/Cardiac Cells

🎚 3. Gene Expression

Gene Expression Level

LOW	MEDIUM	HIGH
Poor Repair	Normal Function	High Activity
Slow Renewal	Healthy Cells	Rapid Growth

Epigenetic Control = 🎚 Volume Knob (Not ON/OFF switch)

🔬 4. Hallmarks of Aging → Cell Turnover Impact

Hallmarks of Aging
↓

Stem Cell Exhaustion → ↓ RBC & tissue regeneration
Telomere Attrition → ↓ cell division capacity
Mitochondrial Dysfunction → ↓ energy for renewal
Loss of Proteostasis → damaged proteins accumulate
Inflammaging → chronic inflammation damages cells
Altered Communication → poor repair signaling

↓
Reduced Cell Turnover Efficiency
↓
Aging & Disease

🔗 **5. Integrated System (VERY IMPORTANT DIAGRAM)**

Food/Nutrition
↓
Metabolism → Cofactors → Enzymes
↓
Epigenetic Modifications
↓
Gene Expression (↕ regulation)
↓
Cell Renewal Rate
↓
Organ Function
↓
Aging Outcome

🧠 **6. RBC Formation Flow**

Bone Marrow Stem Cell
↓
Erythropoiesis (~7 days)
↓
Mature RBC
↓
Circulation (~120 days)
↓
Removal (Spleen)
↓
New RBC Formation

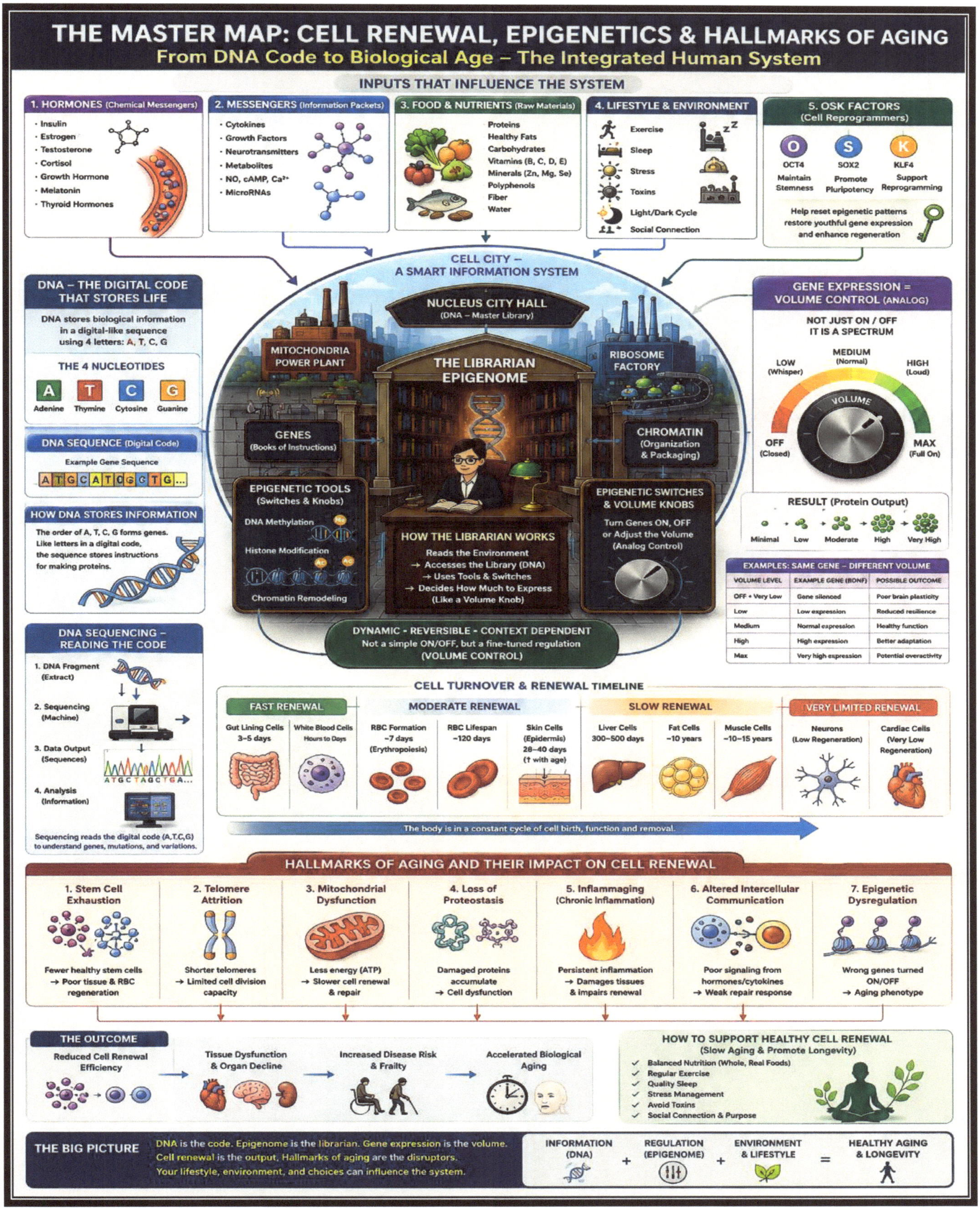

THE MASTER MAP: CELL RENEWAL, EPIGENETICS & HALLMARKS OF AGING
From DNA Code to Biological Age – The Integrated Human System
INPUTS THAT INFLUENCE THE SYSTEM
1. HORMONES (Chemical Messengers)
• Insulin
• Estrogen
• Testosterone
• Cortisol
• Growth Hormone
• Melatonin
• Thyroid Hormones
2. MESSENGERS (Information Packets)
• Cytokines
• Growth Factors
• Neurotransmitters
• Metabolites
• NO, cAMP, Ca²⁺
• MicroRNAs
3. FOOD & NUTRIENTS (Raw Materials)
Proteins
Healthy Fats
Carbohydrates
Vitamins (B, C, D, E)
Minerals (Zn, Mg, Se)
Polyphenols
Fiber
Water
4. LIFESTYLE & ENVIRONMENT
Exercise
Sleep
Stress
Toxins
Light/Dark Cycle
Social Connection
5. OSK FACTORS (Cell Reprogrammers)
O S K
OCT4 Maintain Stemness
SOX2 Promote Pluripotency
KLF4 Support Reprogramming
Help reset epigenetic patterns restore youthful gene expression and enhance regeneration
CELL CITY – A SMART INFORMATION SYSTEM
DNA – THE DIGITAL CODE THAT STORES LIFE
DNA stores biological information in a digital-like sequence using 4 letters: A, T, C, G
THE 4 NUCLEOTIDES
A Adenine
T Thymine
C Cytosine
G Guanine
DNA SEQUENCE (Digital Code)
Example Gene Sequence
ATGCATGGCTG...
HOW DNA STORES INFORMATION
The order of A, T, C, G forms genes. Like letters in a digital code, the sequence stores instructions for making proteins.
DNA SEQUENCING – READING THE CODE
1. DNA Fragment (Extract)
2. Sequencing (Machine)
3. Data Output (Sequences)
ATGCTAGCTGA...
4. Analysis (Information)
Sequencing reads the digital code (A,T,C,G) to understand genes, mutations, and variations.
NUCLEUS CITY HALL (DNA – Master Library)
MITOCHONDRIA POWER PLANT
RIBOSOME FACTORY
THE LIBRARIAN EPIGENOME
GENES (Books of Instructions)
CHROMATIN (Organization & Packaging)
EPIGENETIC TOOLS (Switches & Knobs)
DNA Methylation
Me
Histone Modification
Ac
Chromatin Remodeling
HOW THE LIBRARIAN WORKS
Reads the Environment
→ Accesses the Library (DNA)
→ Uses Tools & Switches
→ Decides How Much to Express (Like a Volume Knob)
EPIGENETIC SWITCHES & VOLUME KNOBS
Turn Genes ON, OFF or Adjust the Volume (Analog Control)
DYNAMIC • REVERSIBLE • CONTEXT DEPENDENT
Not a simple ON/OFF, but a fine-tuned regulation (VOLUME CONTROL)
GENE EXPRESSION = VOLUME CONTROL (ANALOG)
NOT JUST ON / OFF IT IS A SPECTRUM
LOW (Whisper)
MEDIUM (Normal)
HIGH (Loud)
VOLUME
OFF (Closed)
MAX (Full On)
RESULT (Protein Output)
Minimal Low Moderate High Very High
EXAMPLES: SAME GENE – DIFFERENT VOLUME
VOLUME LEVEL | EXAMPLE GENE (BDNF) | POSSIBLE OUTCOME
OFF • Very Low | Gene silenced | Poor brain plasticity
Low | Low expression | Reduced resilience
Medium | Normal expression | Healthy function
High | High expression | Better adaptation
Max | Very high expression | Potential overactivity
CELL TURNOVER & RENEWAL TIMELINE
FAST RENEWAL
Gut Lining Cells 3–5 days
White Blood Cells Hours to Days
MODERATE RENEWAL
RBC Formation ~7 days (Erythropoiesis)
RBC Lifespan ~120 days
Skin Cells (Epidermis) 28–40 days (↑ with age)
SLOW RENEWAL
Liver Cells 300–500 days
Fat Cells ~10 years
Muscle Cells ~10–15 years
VERY LIMITED RENEWAL
Neurons (Low Regeneration)
Cardiac Cells (Very Low Regeneration)
The body is in a constant cycle of cell birth, function and removal.
HALLMARKS OF AGING AND THEIR IMPACT ON CELL RENEWAL
1. Stem Cell Exhaustion
Fewer healthy stem cells → Poor tissue & RBC regeneration
2. Telomere Attrition
Shorter telomeres → Limited cell division capacity
3. Mitochondrial Dysfunction
Less energy (ATP) → Slower cell renewal & repair
4. Loss of Proteostasis
Damaged proteins accumulate → Cell dysfunction
5. Inflammaging (Chronic Inflammation)
Persistent inflammation → Damages tissues & impairs renewal
6. Altered Intercellular Communication
Poor signaling from hormones/cytokines → Weak repair response
7. Epigenetic Dysregulation
Wrong genes turned ON/OFF → Aging phenotype
THE OUTCOME
Reduced Cell Renewal Efficiency
Tissue Dysfunction & Organ Decline
Increased Disease Risk & Frailty
Accelerated Biological Aging
HOW TO SUPPORT HEALTHY CELL RENEWAL (Slow Aging & Promote Longevity)
✓ Balanced Nutrition (Whole, Real Foods)
✓ Regular Exercise
✓ Quality Sleep
✓ Stress Management
✓ Avoid Toxins
✓ Social Connection & Purpose
THE BIG PICTURE
DNA is the code. Epigenome is the librarian. Gene expression is the volume. Cell renewal is the output. Hallmarks of aging are the disruptors. Your lifestyle, environment, and choices can influence the system.
INFORMATION (DNA) + REGULATION (EPIGENOME) + ENVIRONMENT & LIFESTYLE = HEALTHY AGING & LONGEVITY

🧴 7. Skin Renewal Flow

Basal Layer (Stem Cells)
↓
Cell Division
↓
Keratinocyte Migration Upwards
↓
Differentiation
↓
Dead Skin Layer (Shedding)
↓
Cycle Repeats (28–40 days → slower with age)

⚡ 8. Aging Effect on Cell Renewal (Simple Visual)

YOUNG STATE
Fast Renewal → Efficient Repair → Healthy Tissue

↓ Aging ↓

AGED STATE
Slow Renewal → Accumulated Damage → Disease Risk

🎯 9. One-Line Master Diagram

DNA → Epigenome → Gene Expression → Cell Renewal → Aging

🔗 Step-by-Step Biological Connection

1 Age-Related Decline in Molecules (Root Cause)

Decline in key molecules → leads to poor cellular function → which slows cell turnover → which accelerates aging (hallmarks).

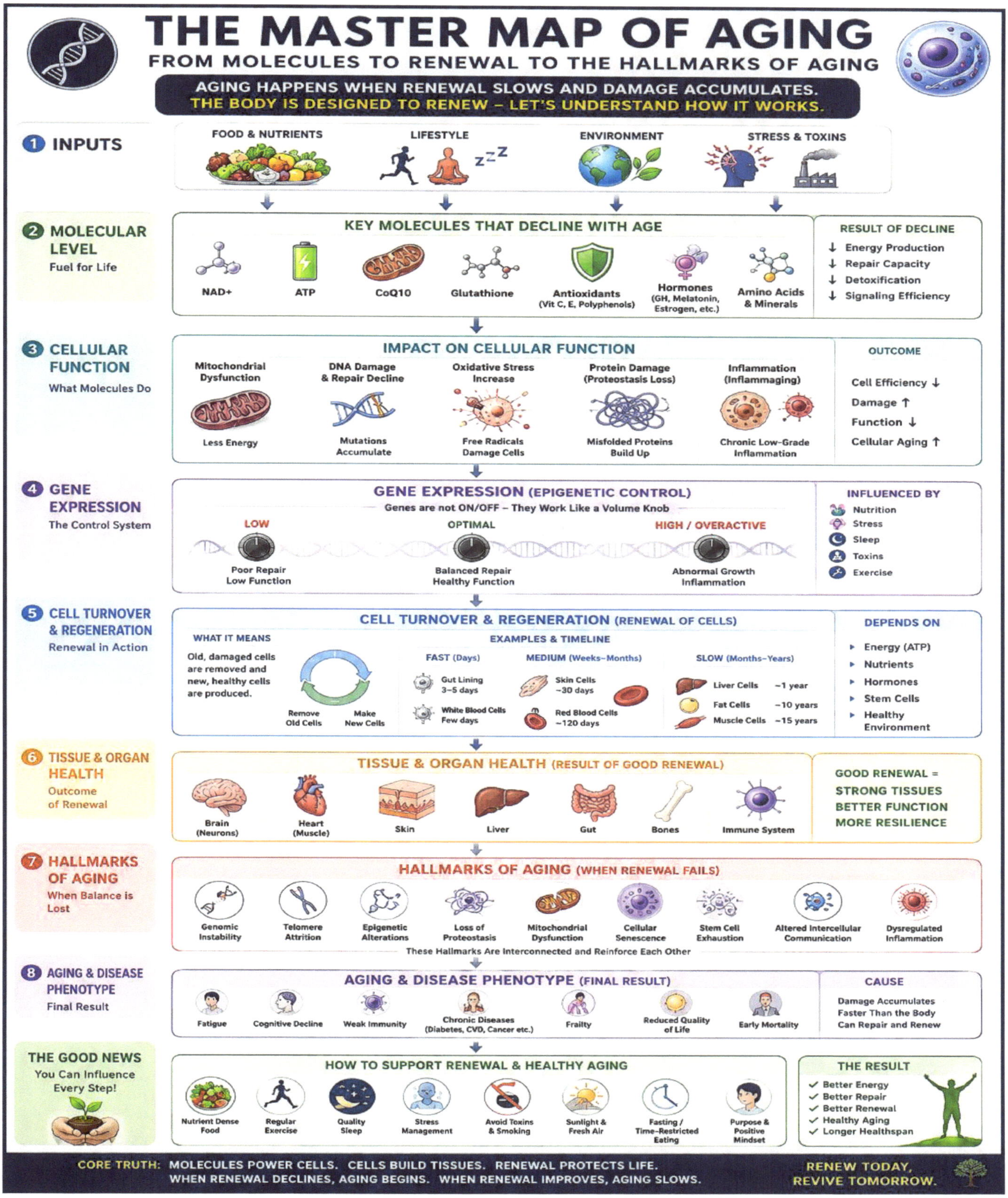

With aging, important molecules decrease:

- NAD^+ ↓
- ATP ↓
- Glutathione ↓
- CoQ10 ↓
- Hormonal signals ↓

👉 These molecules are essential for:

- Energy
- Repair
- Detox
- Gene regulation

2️⃣ Impact on Cellular Function

When these molecules decline:

- Mitochondria produce less energy ⚡
- DNA repair becomes inefficient 🧬
- Oxidative stress increases 🔥
- Protein damage accumulates ⚙️

👉 Cells become:

- Slower
- Less efficient
- More damaged

3️⃣ Effect on Cell Turnover & Regeneration

Now how these process or functions connect with each other:

👉 Cell renewal depends on:

- Energy (ATP)
- Stem cell function
- Gene expression (epigenetics)

When molecules decline:

- RBC production quality ↓
- Skin renewal slows
- Gut repair weakens
- Stem cells become exhausted

🔁 Flow Connection

Molecular Decline
↓
Cellular Dysfunction
↓
Reduced Cell Turnover
↓
Tissue Aging
↓
Hallmarks of Aging Activated

🧬 4 Direct Link to Hallmarks of Aging

🔬 Mitochondrial Dysfunction

- Caused by ↓ NAD^+, ↓ CoQ10
- Leads to ↓ energy → slower regeneration

🧬 Stem Cell Exhaustion

- Molecule decline → stem cells lose efficiency
- → Poor RBC & tissue renewal

⚙️ Loss of Proteostasis

- ↓ glutathione → ↑ damaged proteins

🔥 Inflammaging

- Damaged cells → chronic inflammation

🧠 Epigenetic Alterations

- Nutrients & molecules regulate gene expression
- Decline → improper gene control

🎯 5 Simple Analogy

Think of the body like a city:

- Molecules = fuel + electricity
- Cells = workers
- Cell turnover = maintenance system

👉 If fuel supply drops:

- Workers slow down
- Maintenance stops
- City starts deteriorating

🧠 6 Integration

Age-related molecular decline forms the biochemical foundation of impaired cellular function, which directly disrupts cell turnover and regeneration, ultimately manifesting as the hallmarks of aging.

📊 7 Master Combined Flow

Food/Environment
↓
Key Molecules (NAD+, ATP, Antioxidants)
↓
Cellular Function (Energy, Repair, Signaling)
↓
Cell Turnover (RBC, Skin, Gut)
↓
Tissue Health
↓
Hallmarks of Aging
↓
Disease & Aging Phenotype

Important Scientific Note

While decline in molecules contributes to aging, it is part of a complex, multi-factorial system and cannot fully explain aging independently.

⚡ One-Line Memory Trick

"Less Energy → Less Repair → Less Renewal → More Aging"

📚 Scientific References

1. López-Otín C, Blasco MA, Partridge L, Serrano M, Kroemer G. The hallmarks of aging. *Cell*. 2013;153(6):1194–1217.
2. Hattangadi SM, Wong P, Zhang L, Flygare J, Lodish HF. From stem cell to red cell: regulation of erythropoiesis. *Genes Dev*. 2011;25(7):656–669.
3. Rittié L, Fisher GJ. Natural and sun-induced aging of human skin. *Cold Spring Harb Perspect Med*. 2015;5(1):a015370.
4. van der Flier LG, Clevers H. Stem cells in the intestinal epithelium. *Annu Rev Physiol*. 2009;71:241–260.
5. Blackburn EH, Epel ES, Lin J. Telomere biology and aging. *Science*. 2015;350(6265):1193–1198.
6. Franceschi C, Campisi J. Inflammaging and age-related diseases. *J Gerontol A Biol Sci Med Sci*. 2014;69 Suppl 1:S4–S9.
7. Sun N, Youle RJ, Finkel T. The mitochondrial basis of aging. *Mol Cell*. 2016;61(5):654–666.
8. Sen P, Shah PP, Nativio R, Berger SL. Epigenetic mechanisms of aging. *Cell*. 2016;166(4):822–839.

Chapter-2

The NAD+ – CD38 – Sirtuin Pathway Linking Mitochondrial Dysfunction to Aging

Mitochondria are producing a low level of free radicals all of the time. Since mitochondrial DNA is stored within the mitochondria, it is particularly exposed to this source of damage, and is thought to mutate roughly 10 times faster than nuclear DNA.

Cellular levels of antioxidants and free radical-scavengers that protect against this damage also decline with age. Consequently, an increasing proportion of the mitochondria within our cells become dysfunctional as we age, meaning that they do not produce ATP as efficiently as they should.

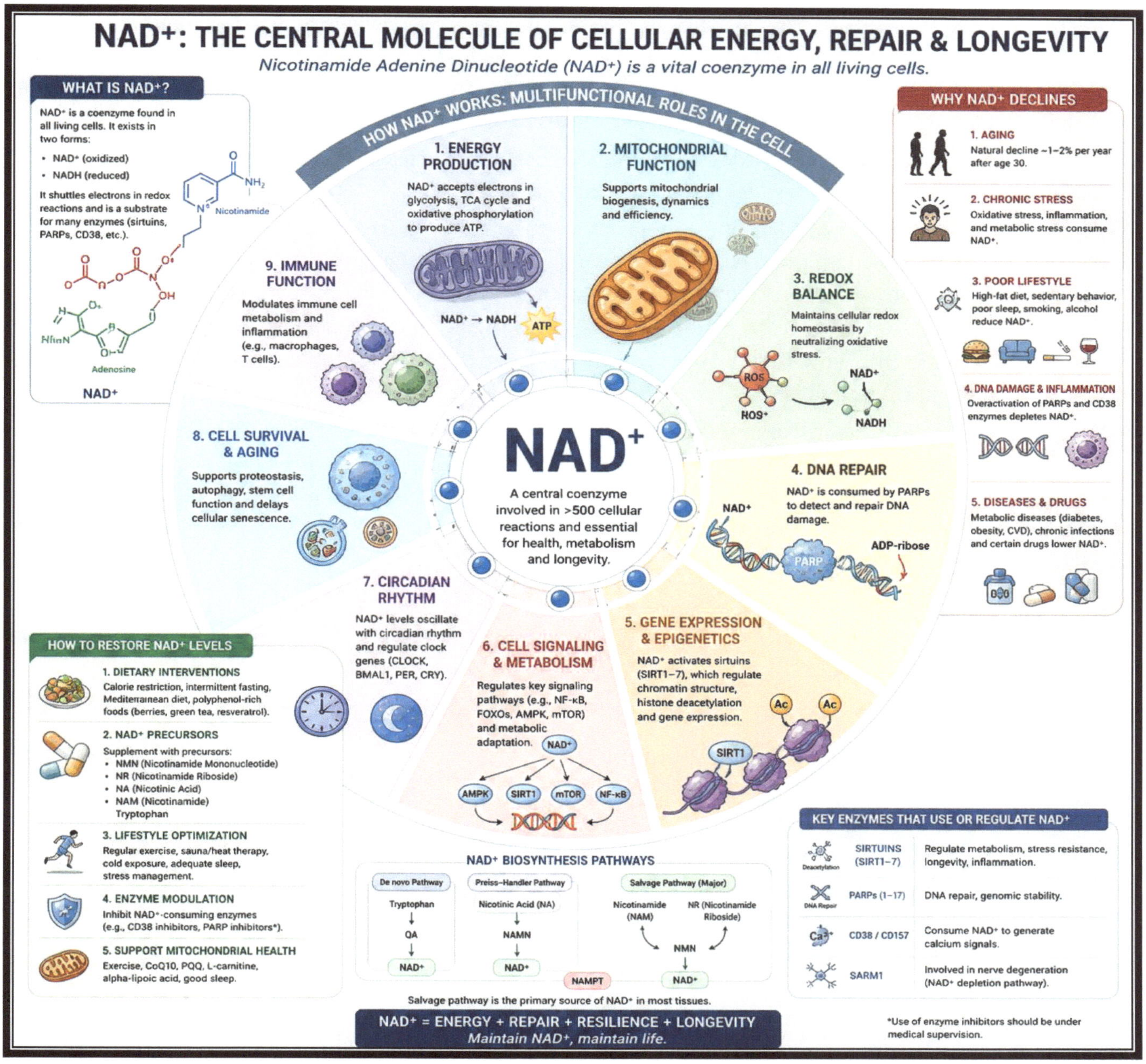

These dysfunctional mitochondria are supposed to be destroyed by the cell in a recycling process called autophagy (also called mitophagy where mitochondria specifically are concerned).

However, this process becomes disrupted with age (loss of proteostasis - causing misfolded proteins to accumulate and create toxic aggregates). Consequently, entire cells can eventually be 'taken over' by dysfunctional mitochondria.

One way in which mitochondrial dysfunction may contribute to ageing and its diseases is through inefficient ATP production. ATP is an essential fuel for cells of all types. It provides the energy necessary for muscles to contract, for neurons to send electrical impulses, and for cells to control the concentration of ions inside their membranes.

It is suggested that a deficit of energy may be responsible for some aspects of ageing, particularly in tissues that demand a lot of energy-like muscle. ATP is also required for processes that remove toxic proteins such as amyloid, thought to play a role in many age-associated diseases including Alzheimer's.

Mitochondria are important to the cell in more ways than merely producing energy. Products of mitochondrial metabolism act as signaling molecules that influence a wide range of cellular processes, including apoptosis (cell suicide), autophagy (the disposal of damaged cell components), inflammation, and glucose metabolism.

These processes may all be disrupted by mitochondrial dysfunction. The accumulation of dysfunctional mitochondria also depletes an essential molecule called nicotinamide adenine dinucleotide (NAD). NAD is necessary for the production of ATP, but is also used in many processes that are vital to the cell such as the repair of damaged DNA, the recycling of damaged cell components, and the growth and division of existing mitochondria.

NAD, or nicotinamide adenine dinucleotide, is a molecule or coenzyme found in every cell in your body. The part of the NAD coenzyme that performs essential functions is known as NAD+.

NAD+ has two important roles—helping proteins regulate the functions in your cells and turning nutrients into energy. The process of converting food to energy is what helps you stay alive. NAD+ supports all the crucial functions of your cells, affecting your sleeping and waking cycles, your neurological health, and the health of your vital organs.

As people grow older, their levels of NAD+ naturally decrease. Stress on the body and mind may cause NAD+ levels to decline even further. Low NAD+ levels increase your risk for many health conditions, like heart disease, Alzheimer's disease, and Type 2 diabetes.

NAD+ and Nicotinamide mononucleotide (NMN) are in the same cellular pathway; NMN is the precursor of NAD+, and the body turns naturally into NAD+. NMN is more stable than NAD+. Boosting NMN levels can increase NAD+ biosynthesis and has been shown to mitigate aging-related dysfunctions. A recent Japanese double-blind, randomized trial on healthy humans shows that NMN is safe and well-tolerated and can replenish cellular NAD+ levels to mitigate aging-related NAD+ biosynthesis.

CD38 and NAD^+ Decline in Aging — Mechanisms and Therapeutic Implications

CD38 is a **cell-surface enzyme (ectoenzyme)** that primarily functions as an **NAD^+ hydrolase**, meaning it **breaks down NAD^+** into smaller molecules.

It sits at a very important intersection of **NAD^+ metabolism, inflammation, and cellular senescence**—all core aging biology themes.

Key Functions

- Degrades NAD^+ → reduces cellular energy capacity
- Produces signaling molecules (like cyclic ADP-ribose)
- Regulates calcium signaling
- Highly expressed in immune cells

Location:

- Immune cells (macrophages, lymphocytes)
- Endothelial cells
- Various tissues including brain

Aging is associated with a progressive decline in cellular energy, increased inflammation, and reduced repair capacity. A central molecular change underlying these processes is the depletion of **NAD+**, a critical coenzyme in metabolism and cellular maintenance.

One of the key drivers of this decline is **CD38**, an enzyme whose expression increases with age and inflammation.

🧠 **Why is CD38 important in Aging?**

The central issue is this:

👉 **CD38 ↑ with age → NAD^+ ↓ → cellular dysfunction**

🔬 **Mechanism (Core Concept)**

Stepwise process:

1. Aging → chronic inflammation ("inflammaging")
2. Immune cells (especially macrophages) ↑ CD38 expression
3. CD38 consumes NAD^+ excessively
4. NAD^+ levels decline
5. Key longevity pathways fail

⚠️ **What problems does CD38 cause in aging?**

1. NAD^+ depletion

NAD^+ is essential for:

- Energy production (ATP)
- DNA repair
- Sirtuin activation

👉 CD38 directly reduces NAD^+ availability

2. Mitochondrial dysfunction

- Reduced NAD^+ → impaired oxidative phosphorylation
- Leads to fatigue and organ decline

3. Reduced Sirtuin Activity

- Sirtuins (SIRT1, SIRT3) depend on NAD^+
- Reduced activity → accelerated aging

4. Increased Inflammation

- CD38 is highly expressed in inflammatory immune cells
- Creates a **feedback loop of aging + inflammation**

5. Stem Cell Decline

- NAD^+ depletion reduces regenerative capacity

🔗 **Relation to Hallmarks of Aging**

Hallmark	CD38 Connection
Deregulated nutrient sensing	NAD^+–Sirtuin axis disrupted
Mitochondrial dysfunction	Energy failure
Cellular senescence	Promotes inflammatory environment
Genomic instability	Reduced DNA repair
Altered intercellular communication	Inflammation ↑

👉 CD38 is a "central metabolic regulator" linking multiple hallmarks

CD38 connects to multiple hallmarks:

Hallmark	Connection
Deregulated nutrient sensing	NAD^+ decline affects AMPK/sirtuins
Mitochondrial dysfunction	Reduced energy production
Cellular senescence	Senescent cells increase CD38
Altered intercellular communication	Inflammation-driven CD38
Genomic instability	Impaired DNA repair

🔷 CD38 in Aging: What Goes Wrong?

Key Observation:

👉 CD38 expression **increases with age**

Why does it increase?

- Chronic inflammation (**inflammaging**)
- Accumulation of senescent cells
- Immune system activation

🔻 Consequences:

1. NAD^+ Decline

- Reduced cellular energy
- Impaired metabolism

2. Reduced Sirtuin Activity

- Sirtuins depend on NAD^+
- Leads to:
  - Poor DNA repair
  - Mitochondrial dysfunction

Mitochondrial Dysfunction

- Less ATP production
- Increased ROS

Increased Aging Phenotypes

- Fatigue
- Metabolic disorders
- Neurodegeneration

Flow:

Aging → Inflammation ↑ → CD38 ↑

→ NAD^+ breakdown ↑

→ NAD^+ ↓

→ Sirtuins ↓

→ Mitochondrial dysfunction → Aging

Lifestyle Interventions

✔ **Fasting**

- Reduces CD38 expression
- Increases NAD$^+$

✔ **Exercise**

- Enhances mitochondrial function
- Improves NAD$^+$ metabolism

✔ **Caloric restriction**

- One of the strongest natural modulators - reduces CD38 activity

Senolytics

- Remove senescent cells
- Reduce CD38-inducing inflammation

📊 **Therapeutic Strategies**

CD38 ↑ → NAD$^+$ ↓

Intervention:

├── CD38 inhibitors

├── NAD$^+$ boosters

├── Fasting/Exercise

└── Senolytics

→ NAD$^+$ restoration → Healthy aging

◆ **Summary**

- CD38 is a major NAD$^+$-consuming enzyme
- Its levels increase with aging and inflammation
- Leads to metabolic decline and cellular dysfunction
- Targeting CD38 may improve healthspan

◆ **Conclusion**

CD38 plays a pivotal role in aging by driving NAD$^+$ depletion and disrupting cellular homeostasis. Its interaction with inflammation, senescence, and metabolism makes it a **key molecular target** in aging research. Therapeutic strategies aimed at modulating CD38 activity and restoring NAD$^+$ levels hold promise for delaying aging and preventing age-related diseases.

◆ **Diagram**

AGING/INFLAMMATION (Inflammaging)

↓

↑ CD38

(NAD+ consuming enzyme)

↓

NAD+ DEPLETION

↓

↓ ↓ ↓

↓ SIRTUINS ↓ PARPs ↓ DNA Repair

(SIRT1,3) ↓

↓ ↓

Mitochondrial Genomic Instability

Dysfunction ↓

↓ ↓

↓ ATP Production Cellular Damage

↓ ↓

↓

CELLULAR AGING

↓

Organ Dysfunction

Scientific References

1. Camacho-Pereira J et al. CD38 dictates age-related NAD decline (*Cell Metabolism*)
2. Covarrubias AJ et al. NAD^+ metabolism and aging (*Nature Reviews*)
3. Chini CCS et al. CD38 inhibitors in aging (*Trends in Endocrinology*)
4. Verdin E. NAD^+ and longevity (*Science*)

NMN, NAMPT, PNC1 and the NAD$^+$ Salvage Pathway: Central Regulators of Cellular Metabolism and Aging

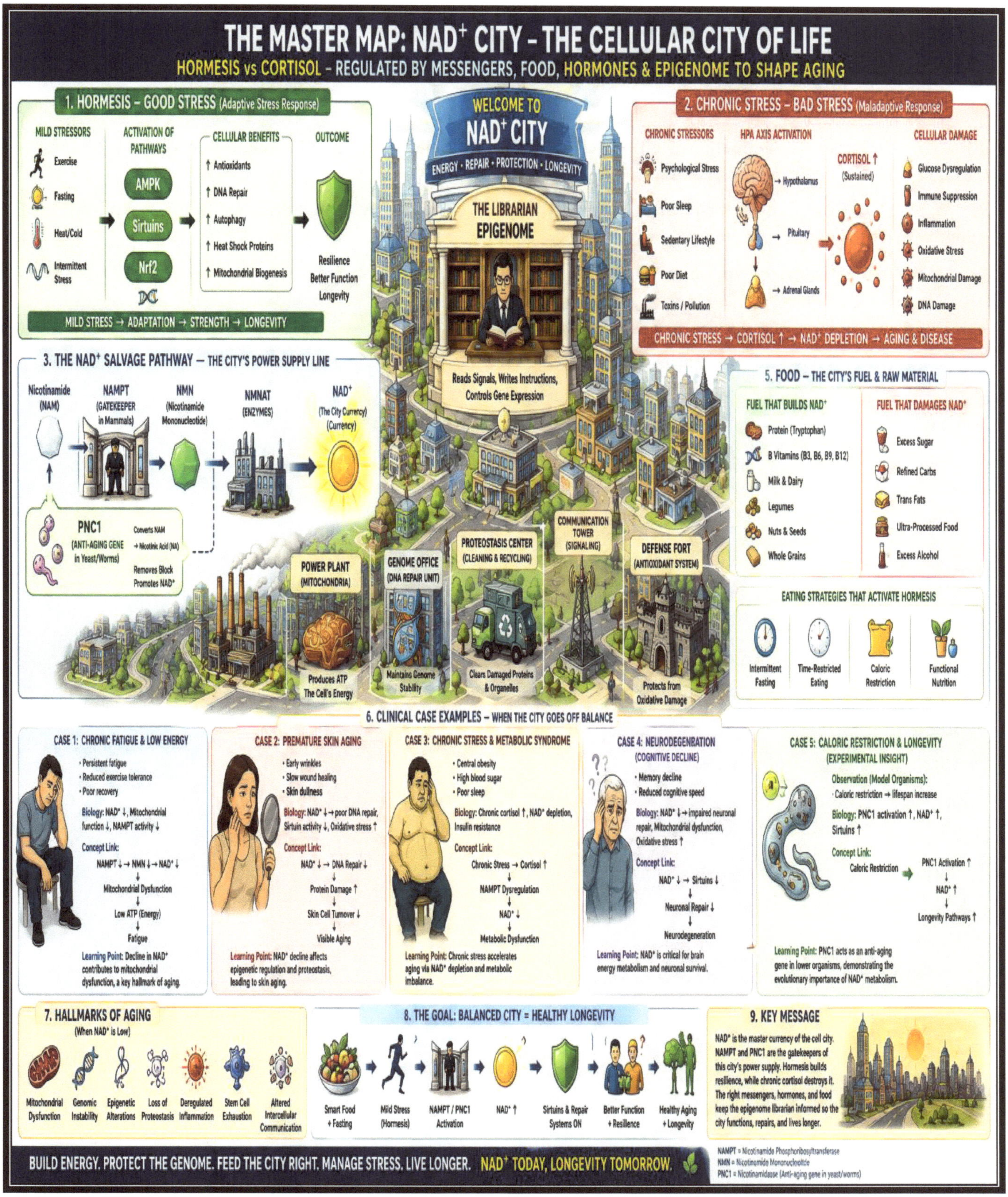

🧠 1. Introduction

Nicotinamide adenine dinucleotide (NAD^+) is a **fundamental coenzyme in cellular metabolism**, playing a critical role in:

- Redox reactions (energy metabolism)
- DNA repair
- Epigenetic regulation
- Cellular signaling

With aging, **NAD^+ levels decline**, contributing to multiple **hallmarks of aging**, including mitochondrial dysfunction, genomic instability, and impaired cellular repair.

The **NAD^+ salvage pathway** is the primary mechanism by which cells recycle nicotinamide (NAM) into NAD^+. Key components of this pathway include:

- **NMN (Nicotinamide Mononucleotide)**
- **NAMPT (rate-limiting enzyme in mammals)**
- **PNC1 (functional analog in lower organisms)**

🔁 2. What is the NAD^+ Salvage Pathway?

The body does not waste important molecules.
It **recycles nicotinamide (NAM)** back into NAD^+.

Nicotinamide (NAM)
↓
NMN
↓
NAD^+
↓
Energy + Repair + Survival

👉 This recycling system is called the **NAD^+ salvage pathway**.

🧬 3. NMN (Nicotinamide Mononucleotide)

📌 Simple Role

NMN is a **middle step molecule** that becomes NAD^+.

🧠 Easy Understanding

Think of NMN as:

"The raw material that becomes cellular energy"

🧬 4. NAMPT – The Key Controller (Mammals)

📌 Definition

NAMPT is the **most important enzyme** in this pathway.

⚙️ What it does

It converts:

Nicotinamide (NAM) → NMN → NAD^+

🧠 Simple Meaning

NAMPT controls how much NAD^+ your body can make

🔑 **Important Points**

- It is the **rate-limiting step** (slowest and most important step)
- Activated by:
  - Exercise
  - Fasting
  - Caloric restriction

👉 This is why lifestyle affects aging

🧬 5. PNC1 – The Anti-Aging Gene (Lower Organisms)

📌 **Definition**

PNC1 is a gene found in:

- Yeast
- Worms
- Lower organisms

⚙️ **What it does**

Nicotinamide (NAM)
↓
Nicotinic Acid (NA)
↓
NAD^+

🔥 **Why PNC1 is Called an Anti-Aging Gene**

Scientific studies show:

- PNC1 is activated during:
  - Stress
  - Caloric restriction
- It **removes excess nicotinamide**, which otherwise:
  - Blocks longevity enzymes (sirtuins)

👉 Result:

- NAD^+ levels increase
- Sirtuins become active
- Lifespan increases (in yeast models)

🧠 **Simple Explanation**

PNC1 helps the cell remove "bad accumulation" and supports "good energy production," which is why it is considered an anti-aging gene.

🔗 6. Functional Relationship: NMN, NAMPT, and PNC1

Component	Organism	Function	Role in Aging
NMN	All	NAD^+ precursor	Supports repair & energy
NAMPT	Mammals	Converts NAM → NMN	Controls NAD^+ levels
PNC1	Yeast	Converts NAM → NA	Enhances longevity pathways

🩺 Clinical Case Examples

🧠 Case 1: Chronic Fatigue & Low Energy

📌 Presentation

A 52-year-old male presents with:

- Persistent fatigue
- Reduced exercise tolerance
- Poor recovery after exertion

🔬 Underlying Biology

- NAD^+ levels ↓ with age
- Mitochondrial function ↓
- NAMPT activity ↓

🔗 Concept Link

NAMPT ↓ → NMN ↓ → NAD^+ ↓
↓
Mitochondrial Dysfunction
↓
Low ATP (Energy)
↓
Fatigue

🎯 Learning Point

Decline in NAD^+ contributes to **mitochondrial dysfunction**, a key hallmark of aging.

🧴 Case 2: Premature Skin Aging

📌 Presentation

A 45-year-old female with:

- Early wrinkles
- Slow wound healing
- Skin dullness

🔬 Underlying Biology

- Reduced NAD^+ → poor DNA repair
- Reduced sirtuin activity
- Increased oxidative stress

🔗 Concept Link

NAD^+ ↓ → DNA Repair ↓
↓
Protein Damage ↑
↓
Skin Cell Turnover ↓
↓
Visible Aging

🎯 Learning Point

NAD^+ decline affects **epigenetic regulation and proteostasis**, leading to skin aging.

🧠 Case 3: Chronic Stress & Metabolic Syndrome

📌 **Presentation**

A 48-year-old executive with:

- Central obesity
- High blood sugar
- Poor sleep

🔬 **Underlying Biology**

- Chronic cortisol ↑
- NAD^+ depletion
- Insulin resistance

🔗 **Concept Link**

Chronic Stress → Cortisol ↑
↓
NAMPT Dysregulation
↓
NAD^+ ↓
↓
Metabolic Dysfunction

🎯 **Learning Point**

Chronic stress accelerates aging via **NAD^+ depletion and metabolic imbalance**.

🧠 **Case 4: Neurodegeneration (Cognitive Decline)**

📌 **Presentation**

A 65-year-old patient with:

- Memory decline
- Reduced cognitive speed

🔬 **Underlying Biology**

- NAD^+ ↓ → impaired neuronal repair
- Mitochondrial dysfunction
- Increased oxidative stress

🔗 **Concept Link**

NAD^+ ↓ → Sirtuins ↓
↓
Neuronal Repair ↓
↓
Neurodegeneration

🎯 **Learning Point**

NAD^+ is critical for **brain energy metabolism and neuronal survival**.

🧪 **Case 5: Caloric Restriction & Longevity (Experimental Insight)**

📌 **Observation (Model Organisms)**

- Caloric restriction → lifespan increase

🔬 **Underlying Biology**

- PNC1 activation ↑
- NAD^+ ↑
- Sirtuins ↑

🔗 **Concept Link**

Caloric Restriction
↓
PNC1 Activation ↑
↓
NAD^+ ↑
↓
Longevity Pathways ↑

🎯 **Learning Point**

PNC1 acts as an **anti-aging gene in lower organisms**, demonstrating the evolutionary importance of NAD^+ metabolism.

📚 **Scientific References**

1. Revollo JR, Grimm AA, Imai S. The NAD biosynthesis pathway mediated by NAMPT. *Circ Res*. 2007.
   👉 http://pubmed.ncbi.nlm.nih.gov/17673663/
2. Yoshino J, Mills KF, Yoon MJ, Imai S. Nicotinamide mononucleotide increases NAD^+. *Cell Metab*. 2011.
   👉 http://pubmed.ncbi.nlm.nih.gov/21803291/
3. Anderson RM, Bitterman KJ, Wood JG, et al. Nicotinamide and PNC1 regulate lifespan. *Nature*. 2003.
   👉 http://pubmed.ncbi.nlm.nih.gov/12646908/
4. López-Otín C et al. The hallmarks of aging. *Cell*. 2013.
   👉 http://pubmed.ncbi.nlm.nih.gov/23746838/

Assessing and Modulating Mitochondrial Dysfunction in Aging Biology

Mitochondrial dysfunction represents one of the central biological processes underlying aging and is closely interconnected with multiple hallmarks of aging, including **deregulated nutrient sensing, genomic instability, loss of proteostasis, and cellular senescence**. As cellular energy systems decline, the ability of cells to maintain repair, regeneration, and metabolic balance becomes progressively impaired.

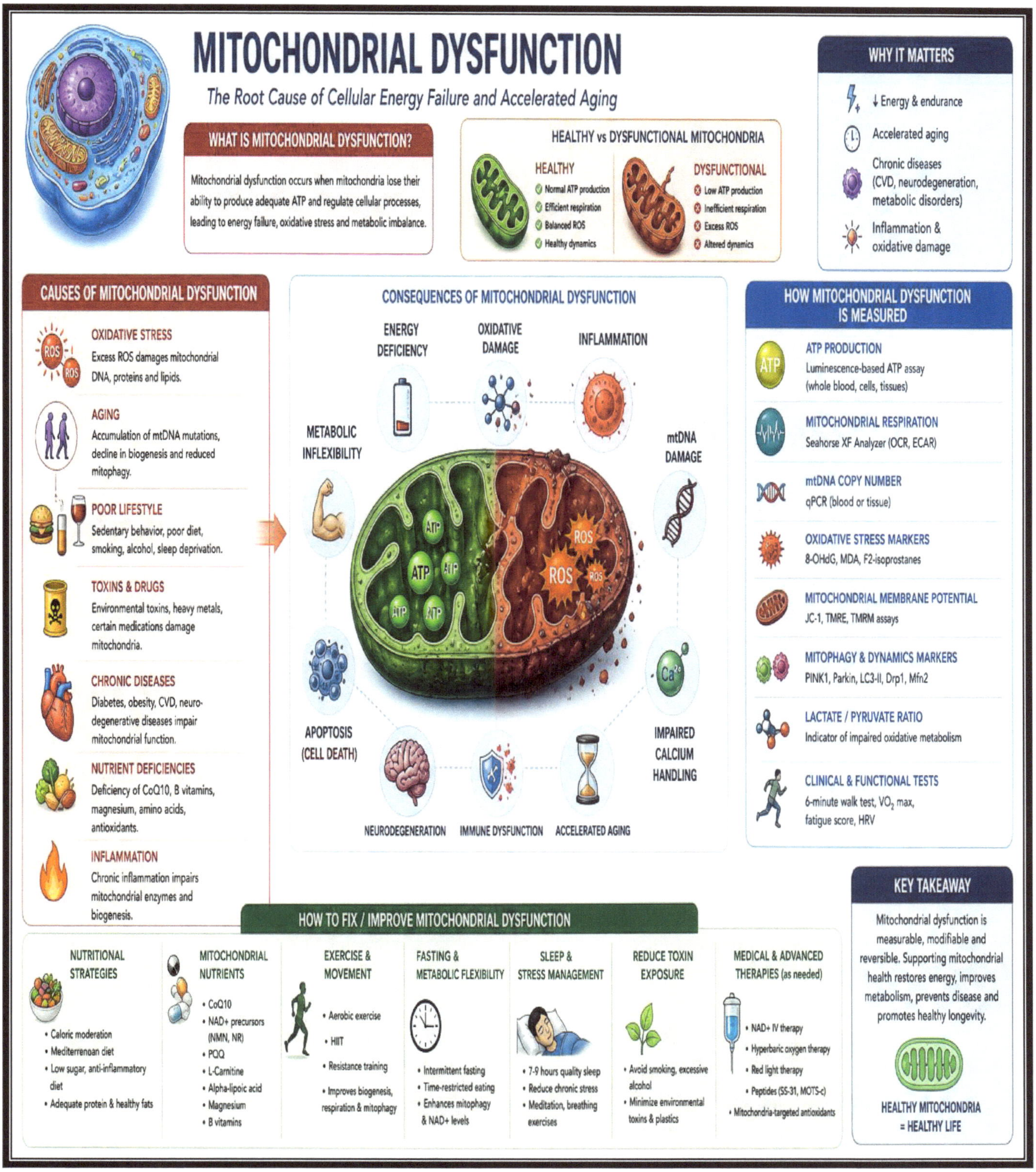

How Mitochondrial Dysfunction Is Measured

Mitochondrial function can be evaluated at structural, genetic, and functional levels. At a structural level, microscopy techniques allow visualization of mitochondrial morphology. Changes in size, number, or shape—such as fragmentation or swelling—often indicate impaired mitochondrial dynamics, reflecting disruptions in fusion, fission, or mitophagy processes. These alterations are strongly associated with aging-related loss of cellular quality control mechanisms.

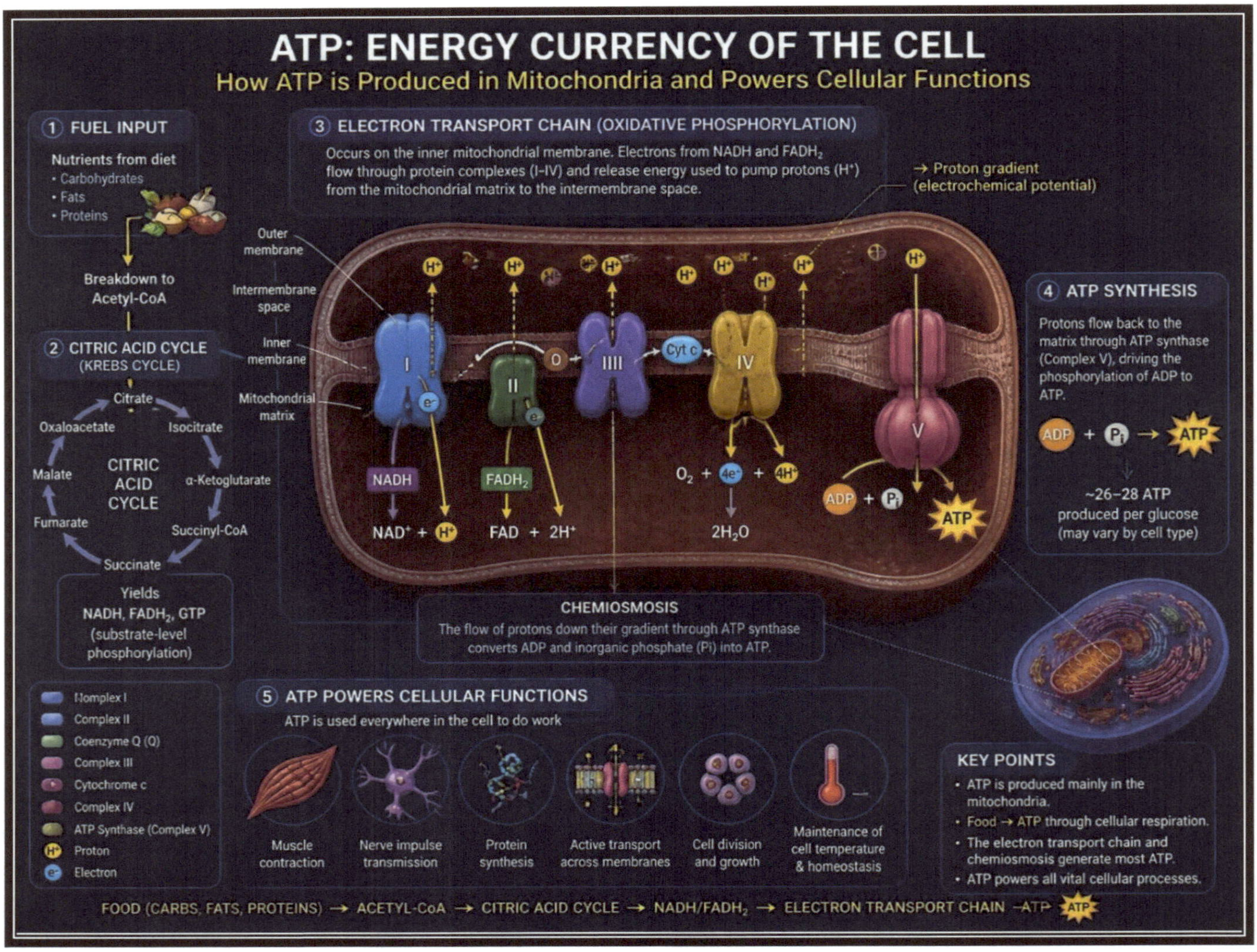

At a molecular level, researchers assess the expression of genes involved in mitochondrial biogenesis, including regulators such as PGC-1α, as well as pathways linked to stress responses and repair. Disruptions in these regulatory networks suggest impaired mitochondrial renewal and are frequently linked to declining cellular resilience with age.

Functionally, one of the most important indicators is ATP production. Mitochondria generate ATP through oxidative phosphorylation, a process dependent on the mitochondrial membrane potential. A reduction in this electrochemical gradient reflects diminished energy production capacity and is a hallmark of mitochondrial decline.

Another key parameter is oxidative stress. Mitochondria are the primary source of reactive oxygen species (ROS), and excessive ROS production leads to damage of DNA, proteins, and lipids. This contributes directly to several hallmarks of aging, including genomic instability and altered intercellular communication.

Because mitochondria consume the majority of cellular oxygen, oxygen consumption rate (OCR) is widely used as a proxy for mitochondrial activity. Additionally, physiological measures such as exercise tolerance and recovery can indirectly reflect mitochondrial efficiency, particularly in high-energy tissues like muscle.

However, mitochondrial function is influenced not only by oxygen availability but also by nutrient supply, including glucose and fatty acids. This highlights the close relationship between mitochondrial health and nutrient-sensing pathways—another key hallmark of aging.

Importantly, many experimental measurements are conducted in cell culture systems, which may not fully replicate the complexity of living organisms. In vivo assessments provide more physiologically relevant insights but are technically more challenging.

⚡ NAD^+, CD38, and the Energy Decline of Aging

A critical molecular link connecting mitochondrial dysfunction to aging is the decline of **nicotinamide adenine dinucleotide (NAD^+)**, an essential coenzyme required for energy metabolism, DNA repair, and cellular signaling.

With aging, NAD^+ levels progressively decrease. One of the primary drivers of this decline is **CD38**, an enzyme whose expression increases in response to chronic inflammation (inflammaging). CD38 acts as a major NAD^+-consuming enzyme, accelerating its depletion.

This creates a cascade of dysfunction:

- ↓ NAD^+ → ↓ Sirtuin activity (SIRT1, SIRT3)
- ↓ Sirtuins → impaired mitochondrial biogenesis and DNA repair
- ↓ Mitochondrial function → reduced ATP and increased ROS
- ↑ ROS + ↓ repair → cellular damage and aging phenotypes

Thus, the **CD38–NAD^+ axis** serves as a central regulatory pathway linking multiple hallmarks of aging, including mitochondrial dysfunction, cellular senescence, and altered metabolic signaling.

🔄 Can Mitochondrial Dysfunction Be Improved?

Although mitochondrial DNA mutations accumulate with age and are difficult to reverse, mitochondrial dysfunction is not entirely irreversible. Several strategies aim to restore mitochondrial health and improve cellular resilience.

💊 1. Antioxidant and Mitochondrial Support

Compounds such as coenzyme Q10 play a role in the electron transport chain and may help improve ATP production while reducing oxidative damage. These interventions target oxidative stress, one of the key drivers of mitochondrial decline.

🔋 2. NAD^+ Restoration Strategies

Given the central role of NAD^+ depletion in aging, considerable attention has been directed toward NAD^+-boosting approaches:

- NAD^+ precursors (e.g., nicotinamide riboside, NMN)
- Sirtuin activators (e.g., resveratrol)

These interventions aim to restore metabolic balance, enhance mitochondrial function, and improve cellular repair mechanisms. However, while promising in experimental models, clinical evidence in humans is still evolving.

🧬 3. Targeting CD38 and Inflammation

Reducing CD38 activity represents a novel therapeutic strategy. By limiting NAD^+ degradation, it may be possible to restore cellular energy metabolism and counteract age-related decline. This also highlights the importance of controlling chronic inflammation, which drives CD38 expression.

🔁 4. Enhancing Mitophagy and Biogenesis

Promoting the removal of damaged mitochondria (mitophagy) and stimulating the formation of new mitochondria are essential for maintaining cellular energy balance. Lifestyle interventions such as exercise and caloric restriction have been shown to support these processes.

🧠 5. Advanced Genetic Approaches

Emerging strategies, such as transferring mitochondrial genes into the nuclear genome, aim to protect genetic material from damage. Although still experimental, such approaches represent a future direction in longevity science.

🔷 Conclusion

Mitochondrial dysfunction is not an isolated event but a central node in the network of aging biology. Its interaction with NAD⁺ depletion, CD38 activation, oxidative stress, and impaired cellular repair forms a self-amplifying cycle that drives aging and age-related diseases.

Understanding this interconnected system provides a strong foundation for exploring the **hallmarks of aging**, where mitochondrial dysfunction emerges not only as a hallmark itself but also as a key driver influencing multiple biological pathways.

📚 Scientific Reference

🔬 Core Aging Biology & Hallmarks

1. López-Otín C, et al. *The Hallmarks of Aging.* Cell, 2013.
   - https://pubmed.ncbi.nlm.nih.gov/23746838/
2. Barzilai N, et al. *The Critical Role of Metabolic Pathways in Aging.* Diabetes, 2012.
   - https://pubmed.ncbi.nlm.nih.gov/22618766/

⚡ NAD⁺ Biology & Aging Mechanisms

3. Covarrubias AJ, et al. *NAD⁺ metabolism and its roles in cellular processes during ageing.* Nature Reviews Molecular Cell Biology, 2021.
   - https://www.nature.com/articles/s41580-020-00313-x
4. Verdin E. *NAD⁺ in aging, metabolism, and neurodegeneration.*
   - https://pubmed.ncbi.nlm.nih.gov/24786309/
5. Imai S, Guarente L. *NAD⁺ and the aging process.*
   - https://pubmed.ncbi.nlm.nih.gov/27825999/
6. Yoshino J, et al. *NAD⁺ Intermediates: The Biology and Therapeutic Potential.*
   - https://pubmed.ncbi.nlm.nih.gov/28899755/
7. Strømland Ø, et al. *NAD⁺ metabolism and balance in ageing.*
   - https://pubmed.ncbi.nlm.nih.gov/34509469/

🔁 Mitochondrial Function & Dysfunction

8. Petersen KF, et al. *Mitochondrial dysfunction in aging and insulin resistance.* Science, 2003.
   - https://pubmed.ncbi.nlm.nih.gov/12750520/
9. Morino K, et al. *Molecular mechanisms of insulin resistance and mitochondrial dysfunction.* Diabetes, 2006.
   - https://pubmed.ncbi.nlm.nih.gov/17130651/

🔗 Additional Supporting Reviews

10. ScienceDirect Review on NAD⁺ Biology
    - https://www.sciencedirect.com/science/article/pii/S1550413116302443
11. NIH/PMC Full-text Review on NAD⁺ and Aging
    - https://pmc.ncbi.nlm.nih.gov/articles/PMC8917930/

Sirtuins, NAD$^+$, and the Mitochondrial Axis in Aging

1. Introduction: Sirtuins as Longevity Regulators

Sirtuins (SIRT1–SIRT7) are a family of NAD$^+$-dependent enzymes that play a central role in maintaining cellular health, metabolic balance, and genomic stability. Although often referred to as "anti-aging genes," they are more accurately described as metabolic sensors that link cellular energy status to gene regulation and survival pathways.

A defining feature of sirtuins is their dependence on nicotinamide adenine dinucleotide (NAD$^+$). As NAD$^+$ levels decline with age, the activity of sirtuins decreases, contributing to many of the biological changes associated with aging.

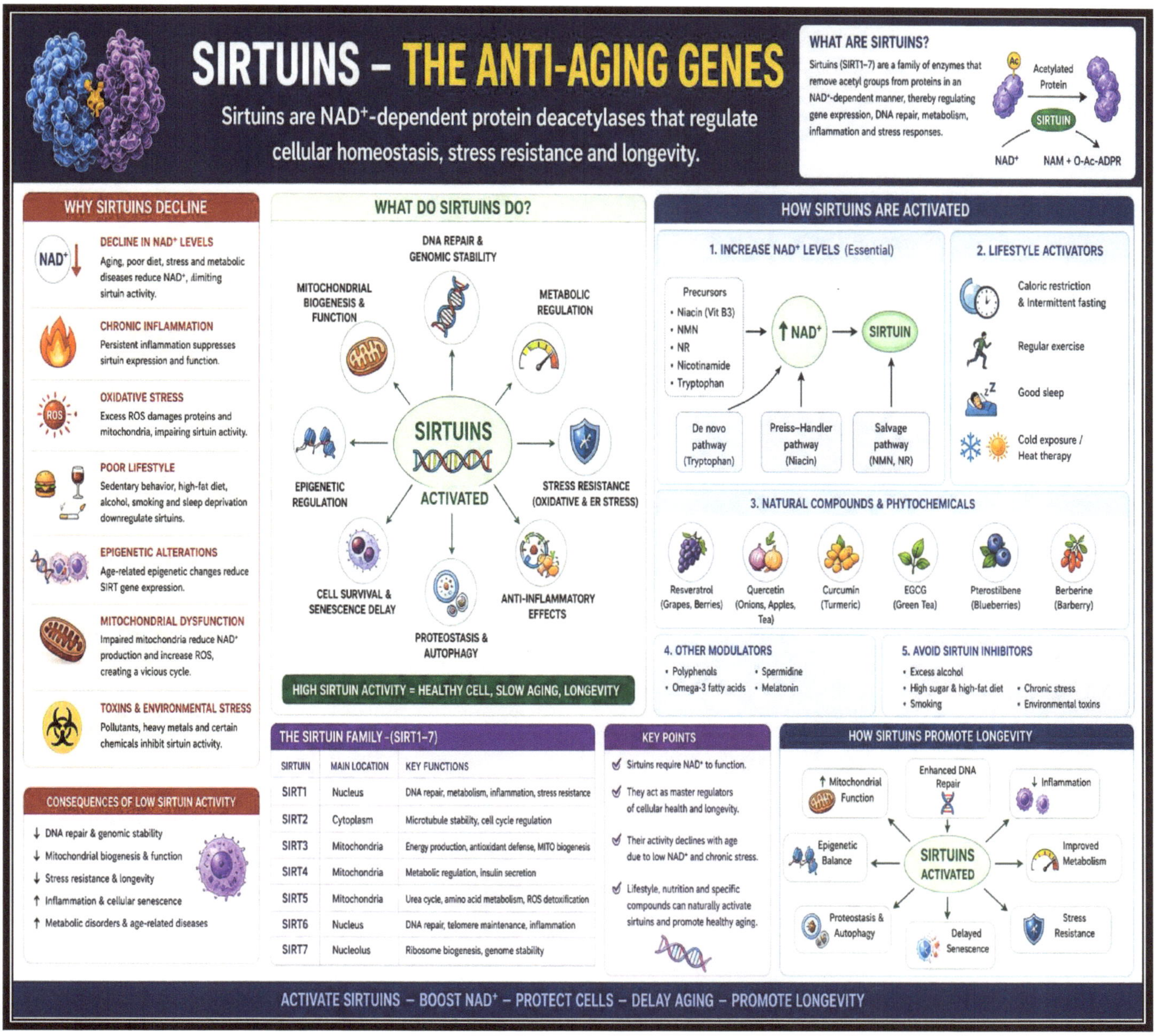

2. The NAD$^+$– CD38 – Sirtuin Connection

Aging is characterized by a progressive decline in NAD$^+$ levels. One of the major drivers of this decline is **CD38**, an enzyme that degrades NAD$^+$.

Key Mechanism

- Aging and chronic inflammation ("inflammaging") increase CD38 expression
- CD38 consumes NAD$^+$ → reduces its availability

- Reduced NAD^+ → decreased sirtuin activity
- Impaired sirtuins → mitochondrial dysfunction, DNA damage, and metabolic decline

👉 This creates a cascade:

CD38 ↑ → NAD^+ ↓ → Sirtuins ↓ → Mitochondrial dysfunction → Reduced ATP → Cellular aging

3. Sirtuins and Mitochondrial Function

Sirtuins play a critical role in maintaining mitochondrial health—the central hub of cellular energy production.

Key Functions

- Enhance mitochondrial biogenesis (via PGC-1α activation)
- Improve oxidative phosphorylation and ATP production
- Reduce oxidative stress (ROS generation)
- Promote mitophagy (removal of damaged mitochondria)

When sirtuin activity declines:

- ATP production decreases
- Reactive oxygen species (ROS) increase
- Damaged mitochondria accumulate
- Cellular energy crisis accelerates aging

4. Role of Sirtuins in ATP and Energy Metabolism

ATP is the primary energy currency of the cell, and its production depends heavily on mitochondrial efficiency.

Sirtuins regulate:

- Glucose and lipid metabolism
- Insulin sensitivity
- Cellular adaptation to stress

Low NAD^+ → reduced sirtuin activity → impaired ATP generation → fatigue, organ dysfunction, and metabolic disease.

5. Biological Functions of Sirtuins

Sirtuins influence multiple hallmarks of aging:

a. DNA Repair and Genomic Stability

- Maintain DNA integrity
- Reduce mutations and genomic instability

b. Inflammation Control

- Suppress chronic inflammation (inflammaging)
- Regulate immune signaling pathways

c. Metabolic Regulation

- Control glucose and lipid metabolism
- Adapt to caloric restriction and energy stress

d. Cellular Survival

- Enhance stress resistance
- Promote autophagy and cell repair mechanisms

6. The Seven Sirtuins (SIRT1–SIRT7): Roles and Localization

SIRT1 (Nucleus/Cytoplasm)

- Master regulator of metabolism and stress response
- Activates longevity pathways (e.g., **FOXO**, PGC-1α)

SIRT2 (Cytoplasm)

- Regulates cell cycle and cytoskeletal organization
- Involved in oxidative stress response

SIRT3 (Mitochondria)

- Enhances mitochondrial respiration
- Reduces oxidative stress
- Key regulator of ATP production

SIRT4 (Mitochondria)

- Controls amino acid metabolism
- Modulates insulin secretion

SIRT5 (Mitochondria)

- Regulates metabolic enzymes
- Detoxifies ammonia and reactive intermediates

SIRT6 (Nucleus)

- Critical for DNA repair and metabolic regulation
- Strongly linked to longevity (detailed below)

SIRT7 (Nucleolus)

- Regulates ribosome production
- Supports cellular growth and cardiac health

7. SIRT6: A Central Guardian of Aging

SIRT6 is one of the most important sirtuins in aging biology due to its powerful effects on **DNA repair, metabolism, and inflammation**.

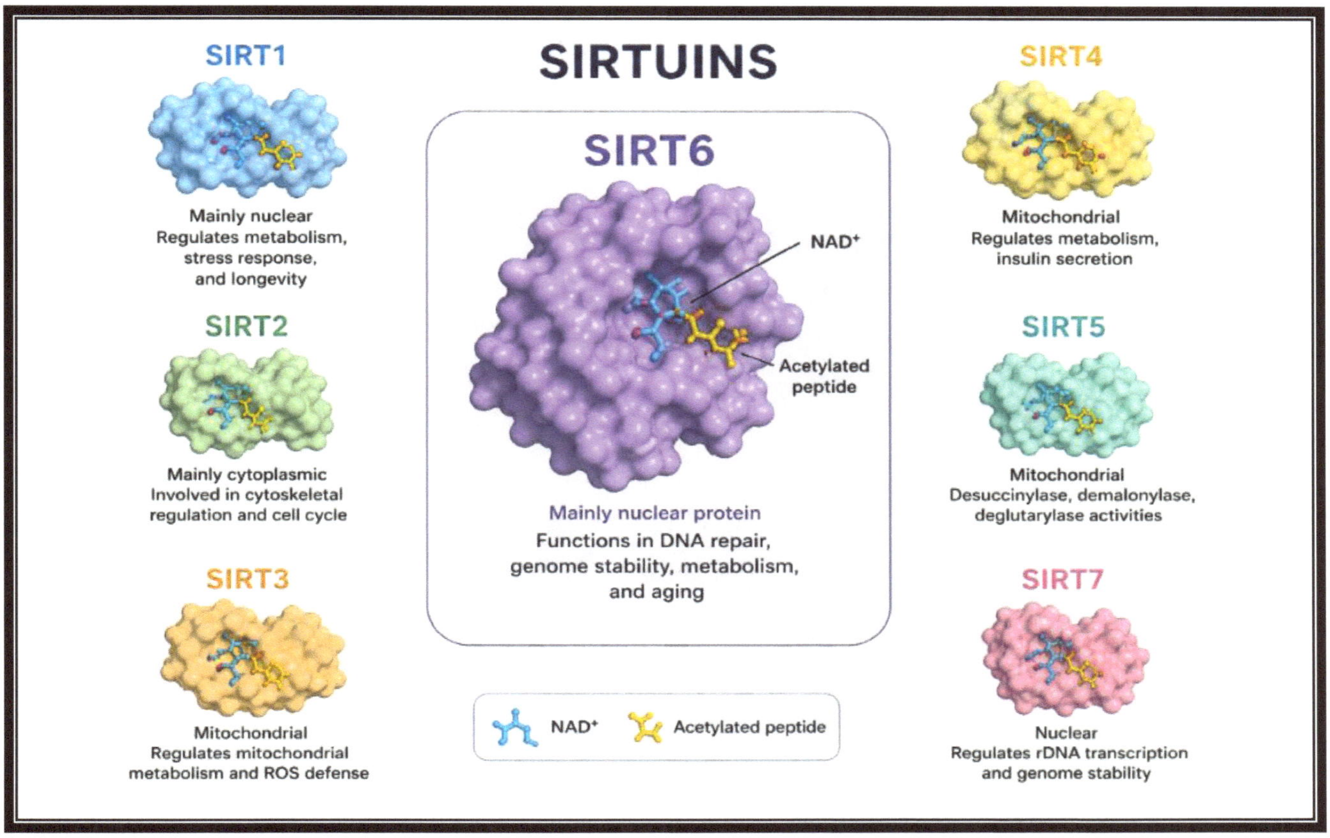

7.1 DNA Repair and Genomic Stability

- Repairs DNA double-strand breaks
- Maintains telomere integrity
- Prevents genomic instability

👉 Directly linked to the hallmark: **Genomic Instability**

7.2 Metabolic Regulation

- Controls glucose metabolism
- Maintains energy homeostasis
- Supports NAD^+ balance

👉 Linked to: **Deregulated Nutrient Sensing**

7.3 Inflammation and Immune Control

- Suppresses pro-inflammatory cytokines
- Regulates immune cell Behavior
- Reduces chronic inflammation

👉 Linked to: **Altered Intercellular Communication (Inflammaging)**

7.4 Cellular Senescence and SASP Control

- Reduces senescence-associated secretory phenotype (SASP)
- Limits tissue damage from aging cells

7.5 Evidence from Animal Studies

- SIRT6 deficiency leads to:
  - Severe metabolic disorders
  - Loss of fat tissue
  - Growth defects
  - Early death

👉 Demonstrates that SIRT6 is essential for survival and healthy aging.

8. Integrated Aging Pathway

The interaction between CD38, NAD^+, sirtuins, and mitochondria forms a central axis of aging:

Aging → Inflammation ↑ → CD38 ↑ → NAD^+ ↓

→ Sirtuins ↓ → Mitochondrial dysfunction

→ ATP ↓ + ROS ↑ → Cellular damage → Aging phenotypes

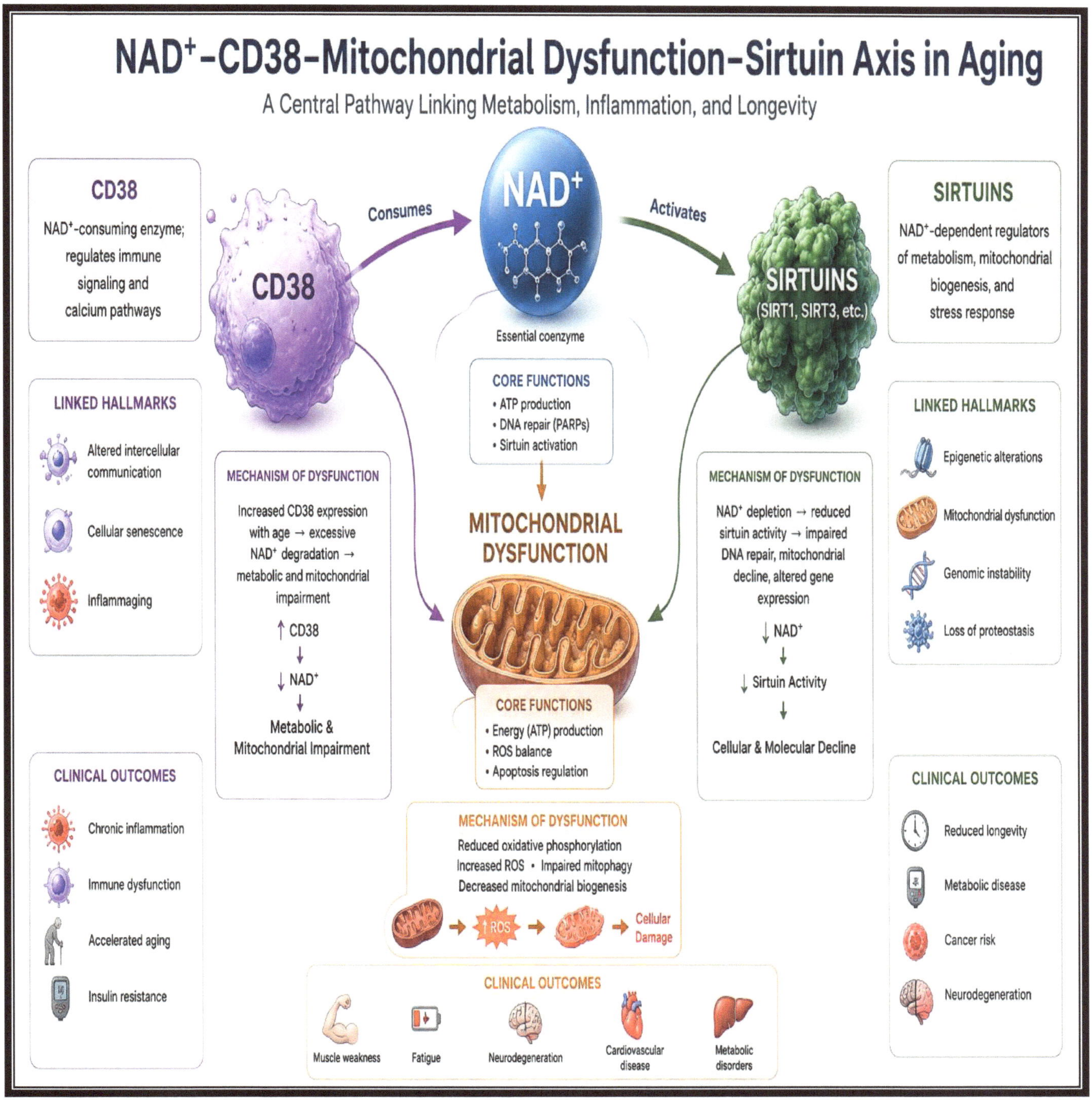

9. Summary

Sirtuins act as a critical bridge between metabolism, energy production, and longevity. Their dependence on NAD^+ places them at the center of aging biology, while CD38-driven NAD^+ depletion represents a key mechanism of age-related decline.

Among all sirtuins, **SIRT6 stands out as a central regulator**, protecting DNA, controlling metabolism, and suppressing inflammation. Together, the **NAD^+–CD38–Sirtuin–Mitochondrial axis** represents one of the most important interconnected pathways driving aging and age-related diseases.

🔷 NAD⁺–CD38–Mitochondrial Dysfunction–Sirtuin Axis in Aging

Component	Core Function	Linked Hallmark(s) of Aging	Mechanism of Dysfunction	Clinical Outcomes
NAD^+ (Nicotinamide Adenine Dinucleotide)	Essential coenzyme for ATP production, DNA repair (PARPs), and sirtuin activation	Deregulated nutrient sensing, mitochondrial dysfunction, genomic instability, cellular senescence	Age-related NAD^+ decline reduces energy metabolism, impairs DNA repair, and decreases sirtuin activity	Fatigue, metabolic syndrome, neurodegeneration (Alzheimer's), type 2 diabetes, cardiovascular disease
CD38	NAD^+-consuming enzyme; regulates immune signaling and calcium pathways	Altered intercellular communication, cellular senescence, inflammaging	Increased CD38 expression with age → excessive NAD^+ degradation → metabolic and mitochondrial impairment	Chronic inflammation, immune dysfunction, accelerated aging, insulin resistance
Mitochondrial Dysfunction	Energy (ATP) production, ROS balance, apoptosis regulation	Mitochondrial dysfunction (hallmark), genomic instability, loss of proteostasis	Reduced oxidative phosphorylation, increased ROS, impaired mitophagy, decreased mitochondrial biogenesis	Muscle weakness, fatigue, neurodegeneration, cardiovascular disease, metabolic disorders
Sirtuins (SIRT1, SIRT3, etc.)	NAD^+-dependent regulators of metabolism, mitochondrial biogenesis, and stress response	Epigenetic alterations, mitochondrial dysfunction, genomic instability, loss of proteostasis	NAD^+ depletion → reduced sirtuin activity → impaired DNA repair, mitochondrial decline, altered gene expression	Reduced longevity, metabolic disease, cancer risk, neurodegen

📚 Scientific References

🔬 Core Aging Biology (Hallmarks of Aging)

1. **López-Otín C, et al. (2013)**
2. *The Hallmarks of Aging. Cell*
3. 🔗 https://pubmed.ncbi.nlm.nih.gov/23746838/
4. *(Foundational paper defining key biological drivers of aging)*

⚡ NAD^+ Biology & Aging Mechanisms

1. **Verdin E. (2015)**
2. *NAD^+ in Aging, Metabolism, and Neurodegeneration*
3. 🔗 https://pubmed.ncbi.nlm.nih.gov/24786309/
4. **Imai S & Guarente L. (2016)**
5. *NAD^+ and the Aging Process*
6. 🔗 https://pubmed.ncbi.nlm.nih.gov/27825999/
7. **Fang EF, et al. (2017)**
8. *NAD^+ in Aging: Molecular Mechanisms and Implications*
9. 🔗 https://pubmed.ncbi.nlm.nih.gov/28899755/
10. **Strømland Ø, et al. (2021)**
11. *NAD^+ Metabolism and Aging*
12. 🔗 https://pubmed.ncbi.nlm.nih.gov/34509469/

Sirtuins, NAD+ & Cellular Regulation

1. **Imai S, Guarente L. (2014)**
2. *NAD+ and Sirtuins in Aging and Disease*
3. https://pubmed.ncbi.nlm.nih.gov/24786309/
4. **Petersen MC, Shulman GI. (2018)**
5. *Mechanisms of Insulin Action and Resistance*
6. https://pubmed.ncbi.nlm.nih.gov/30067154/

Mitochondrial Dysfunction & Metabolic Aging

1. **Morino K, Petersen KF, Shulman GI. (2006)**
2. *Mitochondrial Dysfunction and Insulin Resistance*
3. https://pubmed.ncbi.nlm.nih.gov/17130651/

Comprehensive Reviews & Open Access Sources

1. **Nature Reviews Molecular Cell Biology (2021)**
2. *NAD+ Metabolism in Ageing*
3. https://www.nature.com/articles/s41580-020-00313-x
4. **NIH/PMC Review Article**
5. *NAD+ and Aging (Full Text)*
6. https://pmc.ncbi.nlm.nih.gov/articles/PMC8917930/

Metabolic Syndrome

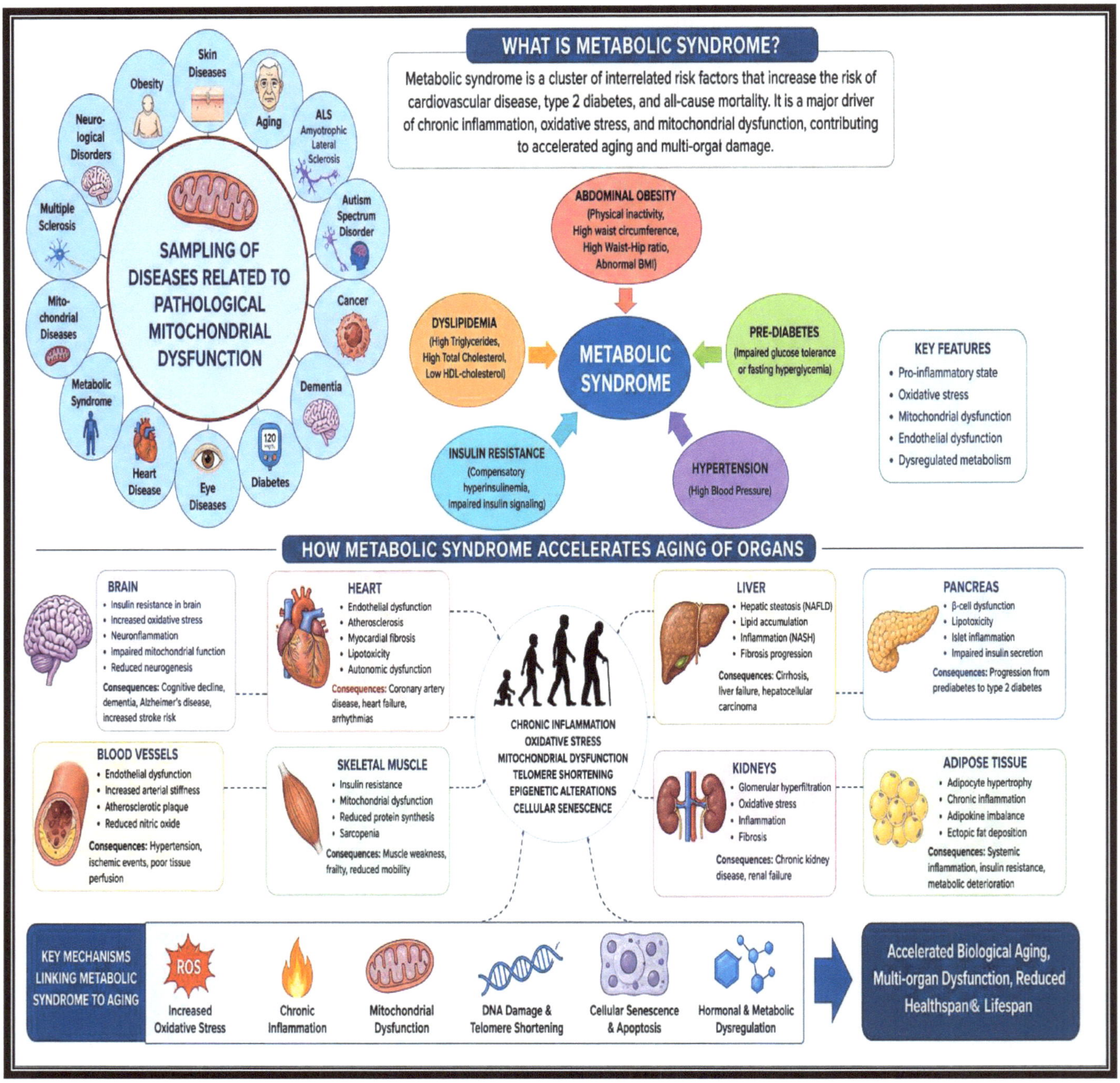

Metabolic Syndrome and Its Connection to the Hallmarks of Aging

Metabolic syndrome is not a single disease but a cluster of interrelated metabolic abnormalities that occur together, significantly increasing the risk of cardiovascular disease, stroke, and type 2 diabetes. It is characterized by:

- Central (abdominal) obesity
- Elevated blood pressure

- High fasting blood glucose (insulin resistance)
- Elevated triglycerides
- Reduced HDL ("good") cholesterol

Rather than being a primary cause of aging, metabolic syndrome is best understood as both a consequence and an accelerator of underlying biological aging processes.

Insulin, Glucose, and Metabolic Balance

The pancreas plays a central role in metabolic regulation by producing insulin, a hormone that enables glucose to enter cells and be used for energy. Under normal conditions, this system maintains blood sugar balance.

However, in insulin resistance, cells fail to respond effectively to insulin. As a result:

- Glucose remains in the bloodstream
- Blood sugar levels rise
- The pancreas compensates by producing more insulin

Over time, this leads to metabolic imbalance and may progress to type 2 diabetes. Insulin resistance is therefore a core feature of metabolic syndrome and a major contributor to age-related metabolic disorders.

Metabolic Syndrome and Cellular Dysfunction

At the cellular level, metabolic syndrome is closely associated with disturbances in energy metabolism, particularly involving mitochondria—the energy-producing structures of the cell.

1. Mitochondrial Dysfunction

Impaired mitochondrial function leads to:

- Reduced ATP (energy) production
- Increased generation of reactive oxygen species (ROS)
- Altered cellular metabolism

This dysfunction is central to many metabolic diseases, including obesity, diabetes, and cardiovascular disorders.

2. Oxidative Stress

Oxidative stress occurs when the production of reactive oxygen species exceeds the body's antioxidant defences.

👉 Effects include:

- Damage to DNA, proteins, and lipids
- Structural and functional changes in mitochondria
- Acceleration of cellular aging processes

3. Lipid Accumulation and Impaired Signaling

Disruption of insulin signaling leads to the accumulation of lipids and free fatty acids (FFA) in tissues. This contributes to:

- Insulin resistance
- Chronic inflammation
- Further metabolic imbalance

Role of Aging in Metabolic Syndrome

Several age-related changes contribute to the development of metabolic syndrome:

- Reduced mitochondrial efficiency
- Decline in antioxidant defences
- Altered metabolic regulation
- Increased inflammation

Lifestyle factors such as physical inactivity, poor diet, and chronic stress further amplify these effects.

A Vicious Cycle: Aging and Metabolic Syndrome

Metabolic syndrome and aging are linked in a bidirectional relationship:

- Aging processes promote metabolic dysfunction
- Metabolic syndrome accelerates biological aging

This creates a self-reinforcing cycle, where each condition worsens the other over time.

Connection with the Hallmarks of Aging

Although metabolic syndrome is not classified as a primary hallmark, it is strongly associated with several key hallmarks:

Primary Hallmarks

- Genomic instability (DNA damage)
- Telomere attrition
- Epigenetic alterations
- Loss of proteostasis
- Impaired autophagy

Antagonistic Hallmarks

- Mitochondrial dysfunction
- Deregulated nutrient sensing

Mechanisms Linking Metabolic Syndrome to Aging

1. Insulin Resistance

- Leads to elevated insulin and growth signaling
- Promotes abnormal cell proliferation
- Increases risk of DNA damage and metabolic disease

2. Oxidative Stress

- Excess ROS damages cellular components
- Contributes to mitochondrial dysfunction
- Accelerates aging at the molecular level

3. Chronic Inflammation

Often referred to as low-grade "inflammaging," chronic inflammation:

- Releases cytokines and inflammatory mediators
- Damages DNA and cellular structures
- Amplifies oxidative stress

Clinical Implications

Metabolic syndrome significantly increases the risk of:

- Type 2 diabetes
- Cardiovascular disease
- Fatty liver disease
- Certain cancers

These conditions are not only diseases but also manifestations of accelerated biological aging.

Key Perspective

Metabolic syndrome should not be viewed as an isolated condition, but rather as a visible clinical expression of deeper cellular dysfunctions. It reflects disturbances in energy balance, nutrient sensing, and mitochondrial health—core processes that underlie aging itself.

Simple Takeaway

- Metabolic syndrome is not a direct cause of aging, but it accelerates aging processes
- It is closely linked to insulin resistance, oxidative stress, and inflammation
- It forms a vicious cycle with aging, where both reinforce each other

Metabolic Syndrome, Hallmarks of Aging, and Clinical Outcomes

Metabolic Component	Underlying Biological Mechanism	Associated Hallmark(s) of Aging	Clinical Outcomes/ Diseases
Insulin Resistance/ Hyperglycaemia	Impaired insulin signaling, elevated glucose, increased ROS production	Deregulated nutrient sensing, Mitochondrial dysfunction, Genomic instability	Type 2 diabetes, cardiovascular disease, neuropathy
Central Obesity (Visceral Fat)	Excess fat accumulation, adipokine imbalance, chronic inflammation	Altered intercellular communication, Chronic inflammation ("inflammaging")	Metabolic syndrome progression, heart disease, fatty liver
Dyslipidaemia (High triglycerides, Low HDL)	Lipid imbalance, increased free fatty acids, oxidative stress	Loss of proteostasis, Mitochondrial dysfunction	Atherosclerosis, coronary artery disease, stroke
Hypertension	Endothelial dysfunction, oxidative stress, vascular stiffness	Genomic instability, Cellular senescence	Stroke, heart failure, kidney disease
Chronic Inflammation	Persistent cytokine release, immune dysregulation	Altered intercellular communication, Cellular senescence	Cancer, autoimmune disorders, age-related diseases
Oxidative Stress (↑ ROS)	Imbalance between ROS and antioxidants leading to cellular damage	Genomic instability, Mitochondrial dysfunction	Neurodegeneration, cancer, accelerated aging
Mitochondrial Dysfunction	Reduced ATP production, increased ROS, impaired energy metabolism	Mitochondrial dysfunction (core hallmark), Deregulated nutrient sensing	Diabetes, muscle weakness, neurodegenerative diseases
Impaired Autophagy	Reduced cellular "cleanup" and accumulation of damaged proteins	Disabled macro autophagy, Loss of proteostasis	Aging-related degeneration, metabolic diseases
Hormonal Imbalance (e.g., insulin, leptin)	Disrupted signaling pathways affecting metabolism	Deregulated nutrient sensing, Epigenetic alterations	Obesity, diabetes, endocrine disorders

⚠️ **Important Note for Scientific Accuracy**

Metabolic syndrome is not a primary hallmark of aging but represents a clinical manifestation of underlying processes such as mitochondrial dysfunction, oxidative stress, and deregulated nutrient sensing.

📚 **Scientific References**

1. Metabolic Syndrome – Definition & Risk Factors

- https://www.mdpi.com/1422-0067/24/9/7898
- 👉 **Explains metabolic syndrome as a cluster of conditions (obesity, hypertension, dyslipidaemia, insulin resistance) and its link to chronic diseases**

2. Oxidative Stress in Metabolic Syndrome

- https://www.mdpi.com/1422-0067/24/9/7898
- 👉 **Highlights that oxidative stress and inflammation are central drivers of metabolic syndrome and its complications**

3. Mitochondrial Dysfunction and Metabolic Disorders

- https://www.sciencedirect.com/science/article/pii/S0925443916302927
- 👉 **Shows that mitochondrial dysfunction and oxidative stress are strongly involved in metabolic syndrome, aging, and related diseases**

4. Mitochondria, ROS, and Cellular Damage

- https://pmc.ncbi.nlm.nih.gov/articles/PMID/27836629/
- 👉 **Describes how excess ROS damages DNA, proteins, and lipids, linking mitochondrial dysfunction to aging and metabolic diseases**

5. Oxidative Stress & Mitochondrial Damage Mechanism

- https://www.mdpi.com/2077-0383/6/7/71
- 👉 **Explains oxidative stress as an imbalance between ROS and antioxidants leading to cellular damage**

6. Mitochondrial Dysfunction in Metabolic Syndrome (Cardiac Link)

- https://link.springer.com/article/10.1007/s10741-021-10109-6
- 👉 **Shows how oxidative stress damages mitochondrial DNA and contributes to metabolic syndrome complications**

7. Mitochondrial Oxidative Stress & Metabolic Syndrome

- https://pubmed.ncbi.nlm.nih.gov/22831852/
- 👉 **Describes how mitochondrial oxidative stress contributes to insulin resistance and metabolic syndrome development**

The association between metabolic syndrome, oxidative stress, and mitochondrial dysfunction is well established in scientific literature, highlighting their collective role in accelerating cellular damage and contributing to age-related diseases.

Insulin Resistance

Insulin Resistance: A Central Driver of Metabolic Aging

Insulin resistance (IR) is a fundamental metabolic disturbance in which the body's cells—particularly in the liver, skeletal muscle, and adipose tissue—fail to respond effectively to insulin. As a result, glucose uptake is impaired, leading to elevated blood glucose levels (hyperglycaemia) and compensatory overproduction of insulin (hyperinsulinemia).

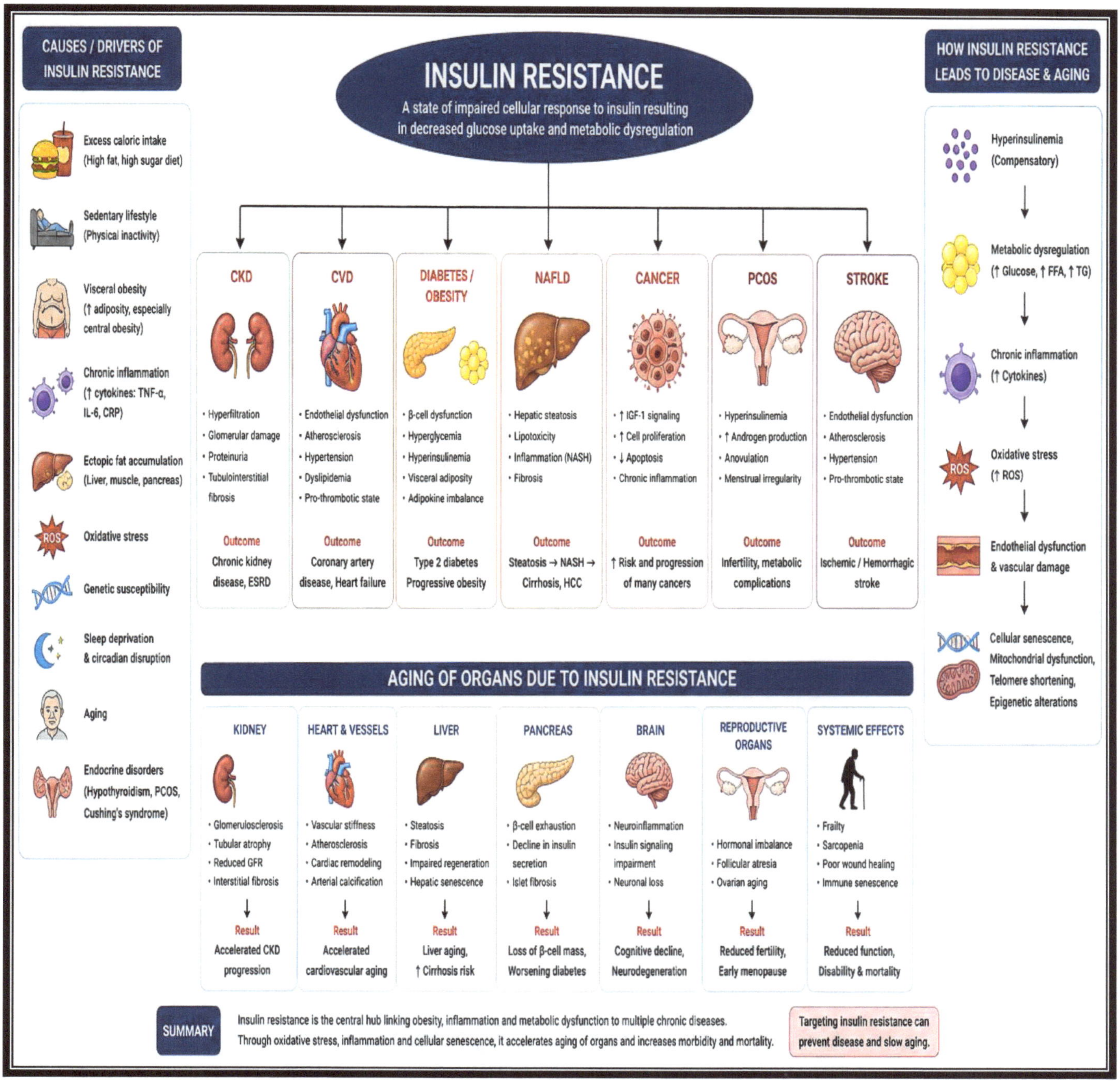

While insulin resistance is a clinical condition, it also represents a **key biological interface between metabolism and aging**, closely linked to several hallmarks of aging—especially **deregulated nutrient sensing, mitochondrial dysfunction, chronic inflammation, and genomic instability**.

Physiological Basis of Insulin Resistance

Under normal conditions, insulin facilitates the uptake of glucose into cells for energy production. However, in insulin resistance:

- Cells become less responsive to insulin signaling
- Glucose remains in the bloodstream
- The pancreas compensates by producing more insulin
- Over time, pancreatic β-cells become dysfunctional

This progressive dysfunction can culminate in **prediabetes and type 2 diabetes mellitus (T2DM).**

Insulin Resistance and the Hallmarks of Aging

Insulin resistance is not itself a primary hallmark but acts as a **driver and amplifier of multiple aging mechanisms**:

1. Deregulated Nutrient Sensing

Insulin resistance disrupts key metabolic signaling pathways, including insulin/IGF-1 signaling, leading to impaired energy homeostasis and metabolic imbalance.

2. Mitochondrial Dysfunction

Reduced mitochondrial efficiency leads to:

- Decreased ATP production
- Increased generation of reactive oxygen species (ROS)
- Impaired metabolic flexibility

3. Oxidative Stress

Chronic hyperglycemia increases ROS production, which damages:

- DNA
- Proteins
- Lipids

This contributes directly to cellular aging.

4. Chronic Inflammation (Inflammaging)

Adipose tissue in insulin-resistant states releases pro-inflammatory cytokines, promoting systemic low-grade inflammation.

5. Genomic Instability

Oxidative stress and inflammation increase DNA damage, elevating the risk of mutations and age-related diseases, including cancer.

Systemic Consequences of Insulin Resistance

Insulin resistance is a **multi-organ disorder**, affecting nearly every physiological system:

Metabolic Disorders

- Prediabetes and Type 2 Diabetes
- Dyslipidaemia (high triglycerides, low HDL)
- Obesity (especially visceral fat accumulation)

Cardiovascular System

- Endothelial dysfunction
- Atherosclerosis
- Coronary artery disease (CAD)
- Stroke

Reduced nitric oxide availability and increased vascular inflammation impair blood flow and increase cardiovascular risk.

Liver

- Non-Alcoholic Fatty Liver Disease (NAFLD)
- Non-Alcoholic Steatohepatitis (NASH)

Excess insulin promotes lipid accumulation in hepatocytes, impairing liver function.

Kidneys

- Chronic Kidney Disease (CKD)
- Glomerular damage due to hyperglycaemia

Reproductive System

In Females:

- Polycystic Ovary Syndrome (PCOS)
- Hormonal imbalance (increased androgens)
- Anovulation and infertility

In Males:

- Reduced testosterone
- Impaired sperm quality and motility

Endocrine System

- Thyroid dysfunction
- Hormonal imbalance due to disrupted metabolic signaling

Nervous System

- Diabetic neuropathy
- Cognitive decline linked to metabolic dysfunction

Immune System

- Increased susceptibility to infections
- Higher risk of autoimmune disorders

Skin and Connective Tissue

- Skin tags
- Psoriasis and inflammatory skin conditions

Insulin Resistance and Cancer Risk

Chronic hyperinsulinemia and inflammation create a pro-growth environment that may promote tumor development. Mechanisms include:

- Increased insulin and IGF-1 signaling
- Enhanced cellular proliferation
- Reduced apoptosis
- DNA damage due to oxidative stress

This is associated with increased risk of cancers such as:

- Liver cancer
- Breast cancer
- Colorectal cancer
- Pancreatic cancer

The Vicious Cycle: Aging and Insulin Resistance

Aging and insulin resistance are interconnected in a **self-reinforcing cycle**:

- Aging promotes mitochondrial dysfunction, inflammation, and hormonal imbalance
- These changes lead to insulin resistance
- Insulin resistance further accelerates cellular damage and aging

Key Contributing Factors

Major risk factors for insulin resistance include:

- Aging
- Physical inactivity
- Visceral obesity
- Chronic stress (cortisol dysregulation)
- Poor diet (high refined carbohydrates and fats)
- Genetic predisposition

Conceptual Summary

Insulin resistance is not merely a metabolic disorder—it is a **central node in the biology of aging**. It reflects a breakdown in the body's ability to efficiently manage energy, maintain cellular integrity, and regulate inflammation.

Although it is not classified as a primary hallmark of aging, insulin resistance acts as a **powerful accelerator of aging processes**, bridging molecular damage with systemic disease.

Key Takeaways

- Insulin resistance impairs glucose metabolism and leads to hyperinsulinemia
- It is strongly linked to multiple hallmarks of aging
- It contributes to major chronic diseases across organ systems
- It forms a vicious cycle with aging, accelerating biological decline
- Targeting insulin resistance is crucial for promoting healthy aging and longevity

Insulin Resistance, Hallmarks of Aging, and Scientific Evidence

Insulin Resistance Mechanism	Associated Hallmark(s) of Aging	Scientific Evidence (with Links)
Impaired insulin/IGF-1 signaling and chronic hyperinsulinemia	Deregulated nutrient sensing	Insulin resistance disrupts nutrient-sensing pathways (IIS, mTOR), contributing to metabolic diseases and aging
Reduced mitochondrial oxidative capacity and ATP production	Mitochondrial dysfunction	Age-related insulin resistance is linked to ~40% reduction in mitochondrial activity in muscle tissue
Increased reactive oxygen species (ROS) due to hyperglycaemia	Genomic instability, Oxidative stress	Oxidative stress associated with insulin resistance damages DNA, proteins, and lipids
Chronic low-grade inflammation (inflammaging) driven by adipose tissue dysfunction	Altered intercellular communication, Chronic inflammation	Insulin resistance promotes cytokine release and systemic inflammation, reinforcing aging pathways

Insulin Resistance Mechanism	Associated Hallmark(s) of Aging	Scientific Evidence (with Links)
Lipid accumulation and free fatty acid toxicity	Loss of proteostasis, Mitochondrial dysfunction	Fat accumulation in liver and muscle contributes to mitochondrial impairment and metabolic decline
Adipose tissue dysfunction and senescent cell accumulation	Cellular senescence, Stem cell exhaustion	Aging adipose tissue promotes insulin resistance via inflammatory cytokines and senescence-associated secretory phenotype (SASP)
Persistent inflammation and ROS interaction	Crosstalk of multiple hallmarks (network effect)	Chronic inflammation interacts with mitochondrial dysfunction, nutrient sensing, and DNA damage in a feedback loop accelerating aging
Altered energy metabolism and imbalance between energy intake and utilization	Deregulated nutrient sensing, Mitochondrial dysfunction	Aging and insulin resistance both alter energy expenditure and metabolic efficiency

Key Insight

Insulin resistance acts as a biological bridge between metabolic dysfunction and the hallmarks of aging, linking altered nutrient sensing, mitochondrial decline, inflammation, and genomic damage into a unified aging network.

The relationship between insulin resistance and aging is not linear but network-driven, where a single metabolic defect influences multiple hallmarks simultaneously, accelerating systemic aging.

Scientific References

1. López-Otín C, et al. *The Hallmarks of Aging.* Cell. 2013.
    - https://pubmed.ncbi.nlm.nih.gov/23746838/
2. Petersen KF, et al. *Mitochondrial dysfunction and insulin resistance.* Science. 2003.
    - https://pubmed.ncbi.nlm.nih.gov/12750520/
3. Shulman GI. *Cellular mechanisms of insulin resistance.* J Clin Invest. 2000.
    - https://pubmed.ncbi.nlm.nih.gov/10903330/
4. DeFronzo RA, et al. *Type 2 diabetes mellitus.* Nat Rev Dis Primers. 2015.
    - https://pubmed.ncbi.nlm.nih.gov/27189025/
5. Houstis N, et al. *Reactive oxygen species and insulin resistance.* Nature. 2006.
    - https://pubmed.ncbi.nlm.nih.gov/16612386/
6. Hotamisligil GS. *Inflammation and metabolic disorders.* Nature. 2006.
    - https://pubmed.ncbi.nlm.nih.gov/17167474/
7. Franceschi C, et al. *Inflammaging and age-related diseases.* Nat Rev Endocrinol. 2018.
    - https://pubmed.ncbi.nlm.nih.gov/30046148/
8. Petersen MC, Shulman GI. *Mechanisms of insulin action and resistance.* Physiol Rev. 2018.
    - https://pubmed.ncbi.nlm.nih.gov/30067154/

Chapter-4

Genomic instability – Hallmark of aging

1. Definition

Genomic instability refers to the **progressive accumulation of DNA damage, mutations, and chromosomal alterations over time**, resulting in **loss of genome integrity and fidelity of genetic information**.

In the context of aging, it represents a **primary initiating hallmark** that drives downstream cellular dysfunction and systemic decline.

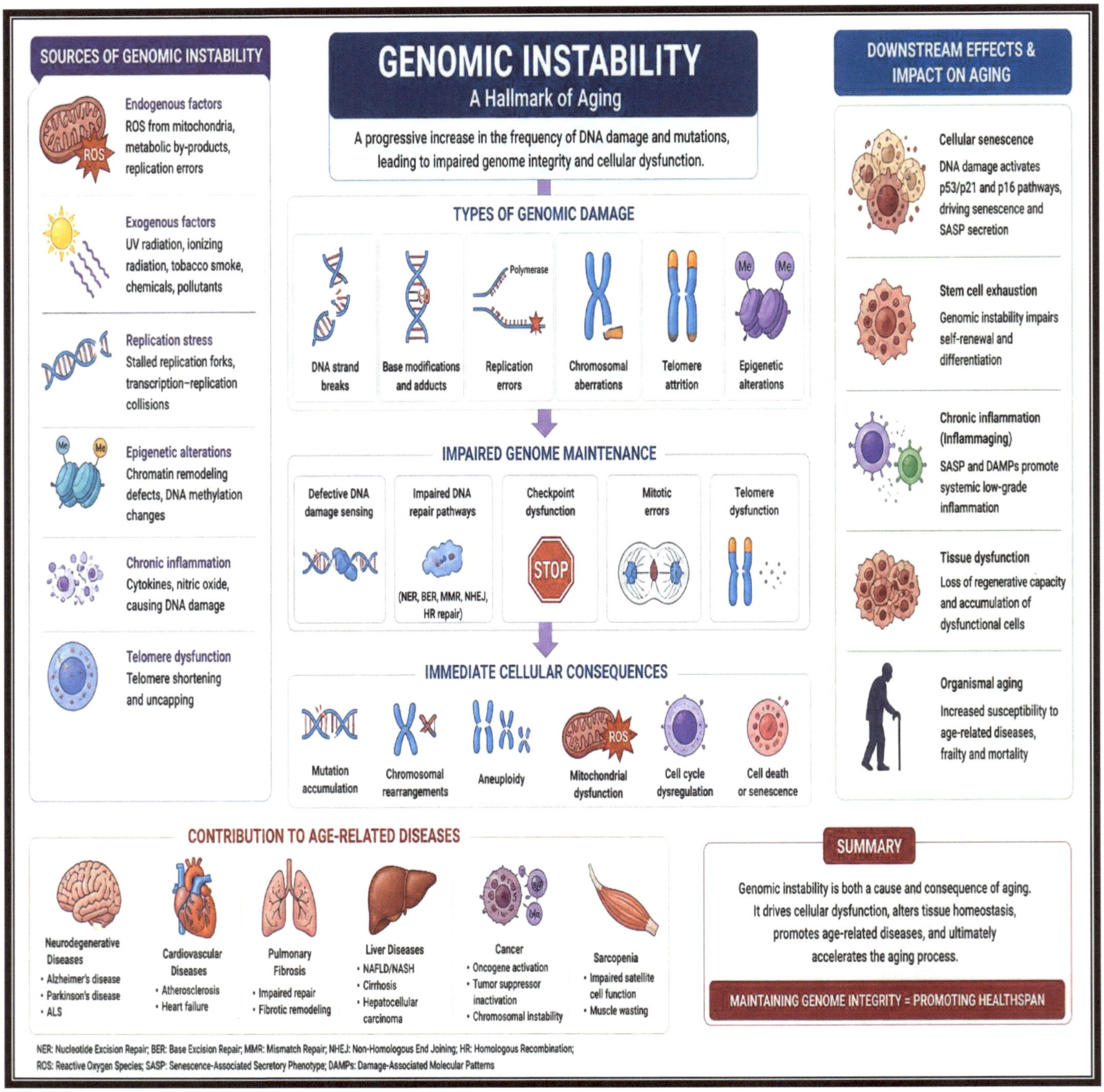

2. Conceptual Understanding (Narrative Explanation)

Think of the genome as the **instruction manual of the cell**. In youth, this manual is continuously **proofread, repaired, and maintained**. However, with aging:

- DNA damage **occurs more frequently**
- Repair systems become **less efficient**
- Errors begin to **accumulate and propagate**

Over time, this leads to a situation where:

Cells are functioning with **faulty instructions**, resulting in impaired function, stress responses, and eventual failure.

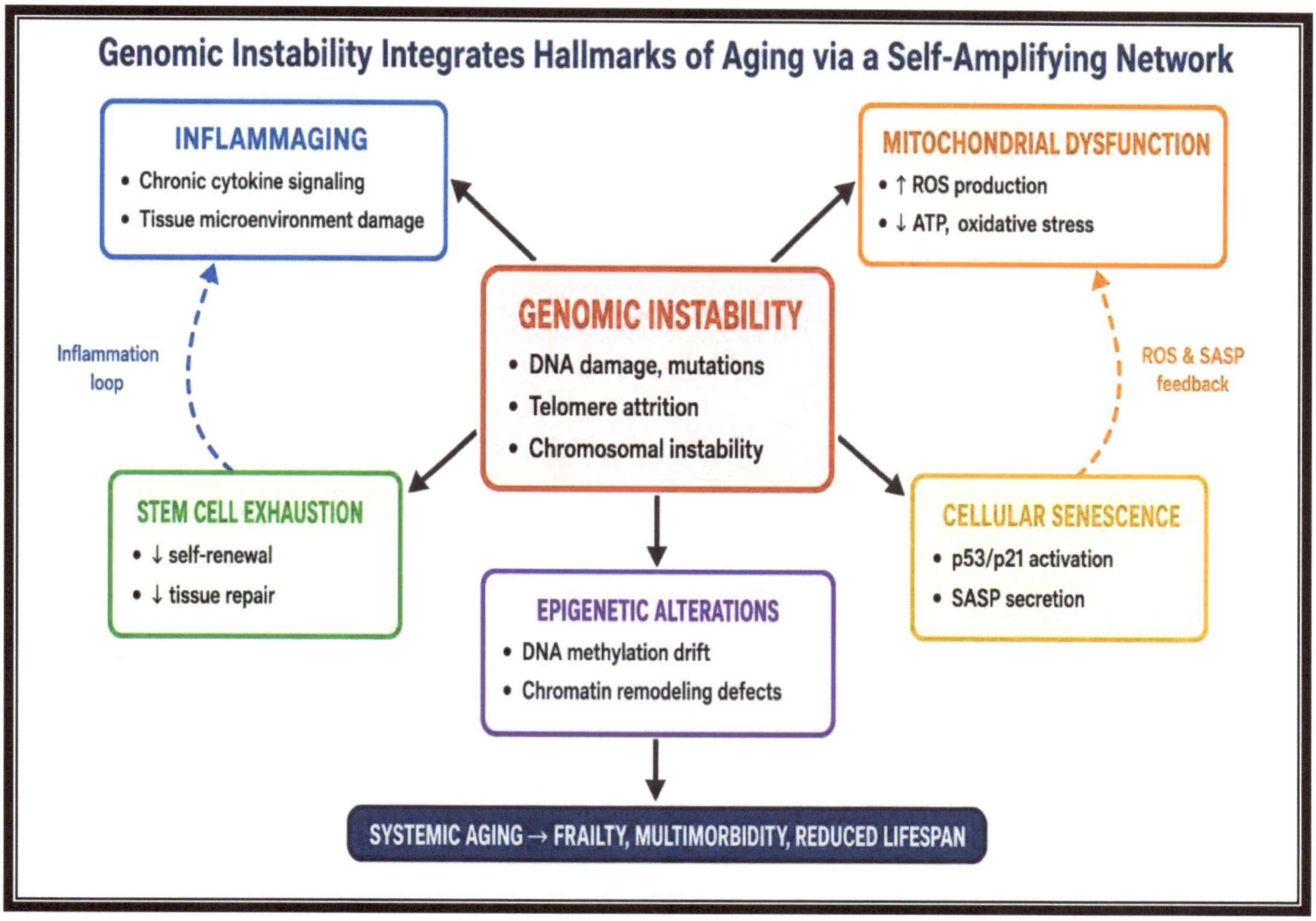

3. Causes of Genomic Instability

A. Endogenous (Internal) Causes

- **Reactive Oxygen Species (ROS):** Byproducts of mitochondrial metabolism damaging DNA
- **Replication errors:** DNA polymerase mistakes during cell division
- **Spontaneous base modifications:** e.g., deamination, oxidation
- **Telomere shortening:** Loss of chromosomal protection with each division

B. Exogenous (External) Causes

- **Ultraviolet (UV) radiation:** Causes thymine dimers
- **Ionizing radiation:** Double-strand breaks
- **Environmental toxins:** Smoking, pollutants, chemicals
- **Dietary factors:** Advanced glycation end products, oxidative stress

C. Age-related Decline in Repair Systems

- Reduced efficiency of:
    - **NER (Nucleotide Excision Repair)**
    - **BER (Base Excision Repair)**
    - **MMR (Mismatch Repair)**
    - **HR/NHEJ (Double-strand break repair)**

4. Types of Genomic Damage

- **DNA strand breaks** (single and double strand)
- **Point mutations**
- **Chromosomal rearrangements** (translocations, deletions)
- **Aneuploidy**
- **Telomere attrition**

5. Chain Reaction (Pathophysiological Cascade)

Step 1: DNA Damage Accumulation

↓

Step 2: Impaired DNA Repair Mechanisms

↓

Step 3: Mutation Accumulation & Genomic Errors

↓

Step 4: Cellular Responses

- Cell cycle arrest (p53 pathway)
- Apoptosis
- Cellular senescence

↓

Step 5: Secondary Effects

- **Mitochondrial dysfunction → ↑ ROS**
- **Epigenetic alterations**
- **Loss of proteostasis**

↓

Step 6: Tissue-Level Changes

- Stem cell exhaustion
- Chronic inflammation (inflammaging)
- Reduced regeneration

↓

Step 7: Organ Dysfunction

- Brain → Neurodegeneration
- Heart → Atherosclerosis
- Liver → Fibrosis
- Kidney → Chronic disease

↓

Step 8: Systemic Aging

- Frailty
- Multimorbidity
- Reduced lifespan

6. Real-Life Examples (Clinical Correlation)

1. Xeroderma Pigmentosum (XP)

- Defect in **NER pathway**
- Extreme sensitivity to UV
- Early onset skin cancers
- 👉 Demonstrates how **failure of DNA repair accelerates aging-like damage**

2. Werner Syndrome (Adult Progeria)

- Mutation in DNA helicase (WRN gene)
- Features:
  - Premature graying
  - Cataracts
  - Diabetes
  - 👉 Classic example of **accelerated aging due to genomic instability**

3. Cancer Development

- Accumulation of mutations:
  - Activation of oncogenes
  - Loss of tumor suppressor genes
  - 👉 Cancer is essentially a **disease of genomic instability**

4. Neurodegenerative Disorders

- Example: Alzheimer's disease
- DNA damage + defective repair in neurons
- 👉 Leads to **progressive neuronal loss**

7. Integrative Insight (High-Yield Concept)

Genomic instability is not just a **cause** but also a **self-amplifying process**:

- DNA damage → mitochondrial dysfunction → ↑ ROS
- ROS → further DNA damage
- Senescence → inflammation → more genomic stress

👉 This creates a **vicious cycle** driving aging.

8. Key Takeaway (Summary)

- **Primary hallmark** initiating aging
- Caused by **DNA damage + impaired repair**
- Leads to **mutations, senescence, and organ dysfunction**
- Acts via **feedback loops (ROS, inflammation)**
- Central to **aging, cancer, and degenerative diseases**

📚 Scientific References

These are **high-impact, widely accepted sources** used globally in textbooks and reviews:

Core Hallmarks of Aging Papers

1. **The Hallmarks of Aging**
   - López-Otín C, et al. *Cell*. 2013;153(6):1194–1217
   - DOI: 10.1016/j.cell.2013.05.039
   - 👉 Foundational paper defining genomic instability as a hallmark

2. **Hallmarks of Aging: An Expanding Universe**
    - López-Otín C, et al. *Cell.* 2023;186(2):243–278
    - DOI: 10.1016/j.cell.2022.11.001
    - 👉 Updated model with 12 hallmarks

Genomic Instability & DNA Damage

3. **DNA Damage and Aging**
    - *Annual Review of Physiology*
    - 👉 Strong mechanistic explanation of DNA damage accumulation
4. **Genomic Instability and Aging**
    - *Nature Reviews Molecular Cell Biology*
    - 👉 Classic review linking DNA repair defects to aging

Oxidative Stress & Mitochondrial Link

5. **Free Radicals and Aging**
    - Harman D. (1956)
    - 👉 Foundational oxidative stress theory
6. **Mitochondrial Dysfunction in Aging**
    - *Nature Reviews Molecular Cell Biology*

Clinical/Genetic Disorders (Real-life examples)

7. **Werner Syndrome**
8. **Xeroderma Pigmentosum**

(Reference from the textbooks like *Robbins Pathologic Basis of Disease* for these.)

📖 **Standard Textbooks**

- *Robbins & Cotran Pathologic Basis of Disease*
- *Harper's Illustrated Biochemistry*
- *Molecular Biology of the Cell* (Alberts et al.)

What is p53?

The p53 protein, encoded by the TP53 gene, is one of the most extensively studied molecules in molecular biology and oncology. Often referred to as the "guardian of the genome," p53 plays a critical role in maintaining genomic stability and preventing malignant transformation. Since its discovery in 1979, p53 has been recognized as a central regulator of cellular stress responses, integrating signals from DNA damage, oncogene activation, hypoxia, and metabolic imbalance.

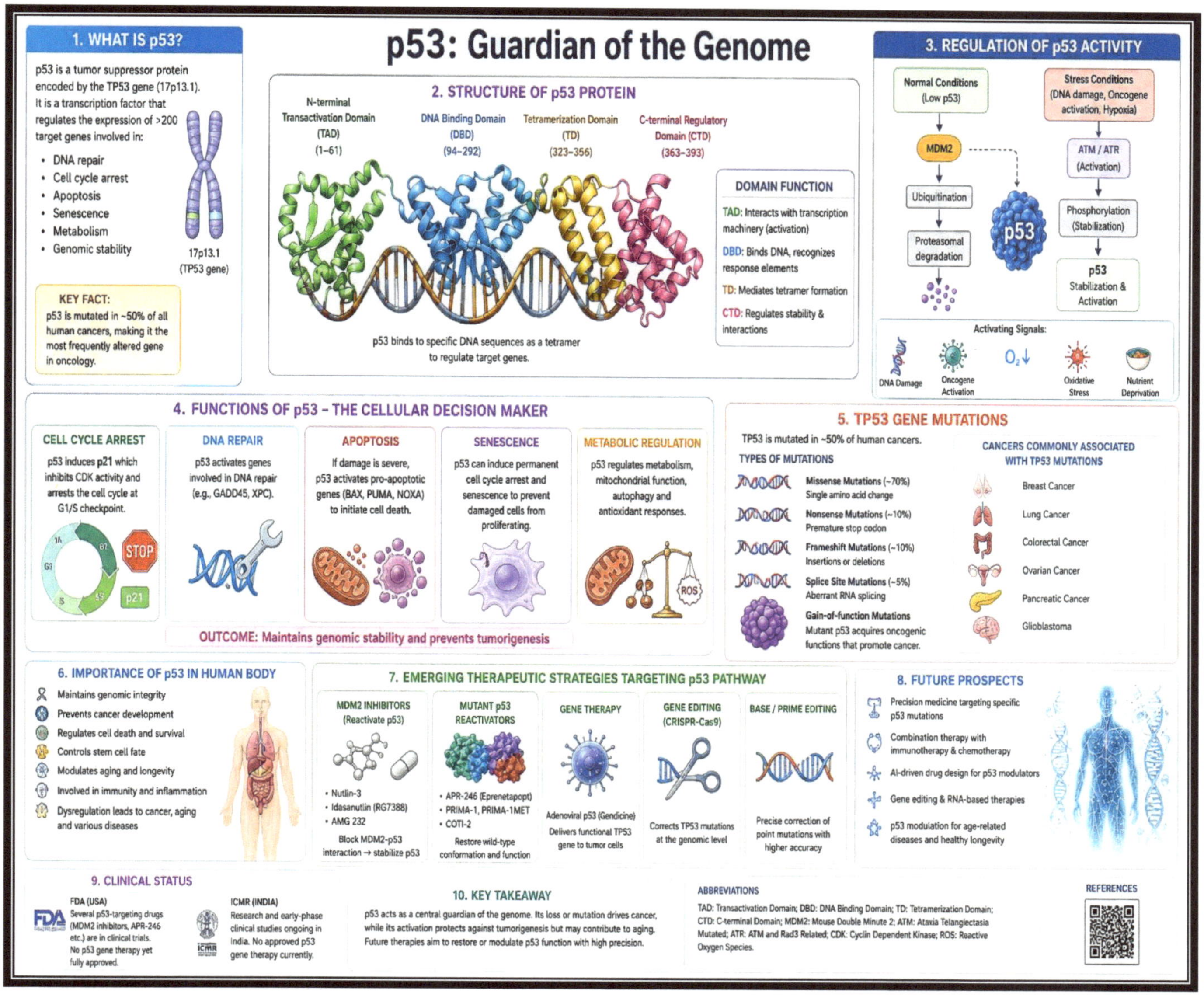

Mutations in TP53 are found in approximately 50% of all human cancers, making it the most frequently altered gene in malignancies. Beyond cancer, p53 is also deeply involved in aging and age-related diseases due to its role in cellular senescence and stem cell regulation.

Is it a gene or protein?

- **p53 is both:**
  - A **gene**: **TP53 gene**
  - A **protein**: p53 protein (transcription factor)

👉 The **TP53 gene encodes the p53 protein**, which regulates many downstream genes.

- It is called the **"guardian of the genome"** because it protects DNA integrity.

🧬 2. What does p53 do? (Core functions)

p53 is a **stress-response transcription factor** activated by DNA damage, oncogene activation, hypoxia, etc.

Major functions:

1. **Cell cycle arrest**
   - Stops cell cycle at **G1/S checkpoint**
   - Allows DNA repair

2. **DNA repair activation**
    - Activates repair genes (NER, BER, MMR pathways)
3. **Apoptosis (programmed cell death)**
    - If damage is irreparable → eliminates cell
4. **Cellular senescence**
    - Permanent growth arrest (anti-cancer mechanism)
5. **Metabolic regulation & stress response**

👉 These effects occur because p53 **binds DNA and regulates transcription of target genes**.

⚙️ **3. How p53 works (Mechanism)**

Under normal conditions:

- p53 is kept **low by MDM2 (ubiquitin-mediated degradation)**

Under stress (DNA damage):

1. p53 is **stabilized (phosphorylation, acetylation)**
2. Accumulates in nucleus
3. Binds DNA
4. Activates genes such as:
    - **p21 → cell cycle arrest**
    - **BAX → apoptosis**
    - DNA repair genes

👉 Outcome depends on severity:

- Mild damage → repair
- Severe damage → apoptosis/senescence

🧪 **4. Is p53 a tumor suppressor?**

✔️ Yes — **the most important tumor suppressor gene**

- Mutated in **~50% of human cancers**

Mechanisms of Tumor Suppression

p53 exerts its tumor suppressive effects through multiple pathways:

Cell Cycle Arrest

p53 induces expression of p21, a cyclin-dependent kinase inhibitor, leading to arrest at the G1/S checkpoint. This allows time for DNA repair.

DNA Repair

p53 regulates genes involved in nucleotide excision repair (NER), base excision repair (BER), and mismatch repair (MMR).

Apoptosis

p53 promotes apoptosis via:

- Intrinsic pathway (BAX, PUMA activation)
- Mitochondrial membrane permeabilization

Cellular Senescence

p53 can induce permanent growth arrest, preventing proliferation of damaged cells.

Metabolic Regulation

p53 modulates glycolysis, oxidative phosphorylation, and antioxidant responses.

Why loss of p53 causes cancer:

- No cell cycle checkpoint
- Damaged DNA propagates
- Cells evade apoptosis

Types of cancers:

p53 mutation is seen in **almost all major cancers**, including:

- Breast cancer
- Lung cancer
- Colorectal cancer
- Ovarian cancer
- Pancreatic cancer
- Brain tumor

👉 So: **not specific — it is a universal tumor suppressor**

🧠 **5. Role of p53 beyond cancer**

p53 is also involved in:

1. Aging

- Regulates **cellular senescence**
- Balances tumor suppression vs aging

👉 Increased p53:

- ↓ cancer risk
- ↑ aging (due to stem cell depletion)

👉 Reduced p53:

- ↑ cancer risk
- ↓ aging control

2. Other diseases

- Neurodegeneration
- Fibrosis
- Inflammation
- Metabolic disorders

👴 **6. P53 in Hallmarks of Aging**

It fits under multiple hallmarks:

✅ **Primary placement:**

1. Genomic Instability

- p53 maintains DNA integrity

✅ **Strong association:**

2. Cellular Senescence

- p53 induces senescence

✅ **Also linked:**

- **Stem cell exhaustion**
- **Altered intercellular communication (via SASP indirectly)**

💊 **7. Senolytics Vs p53?**

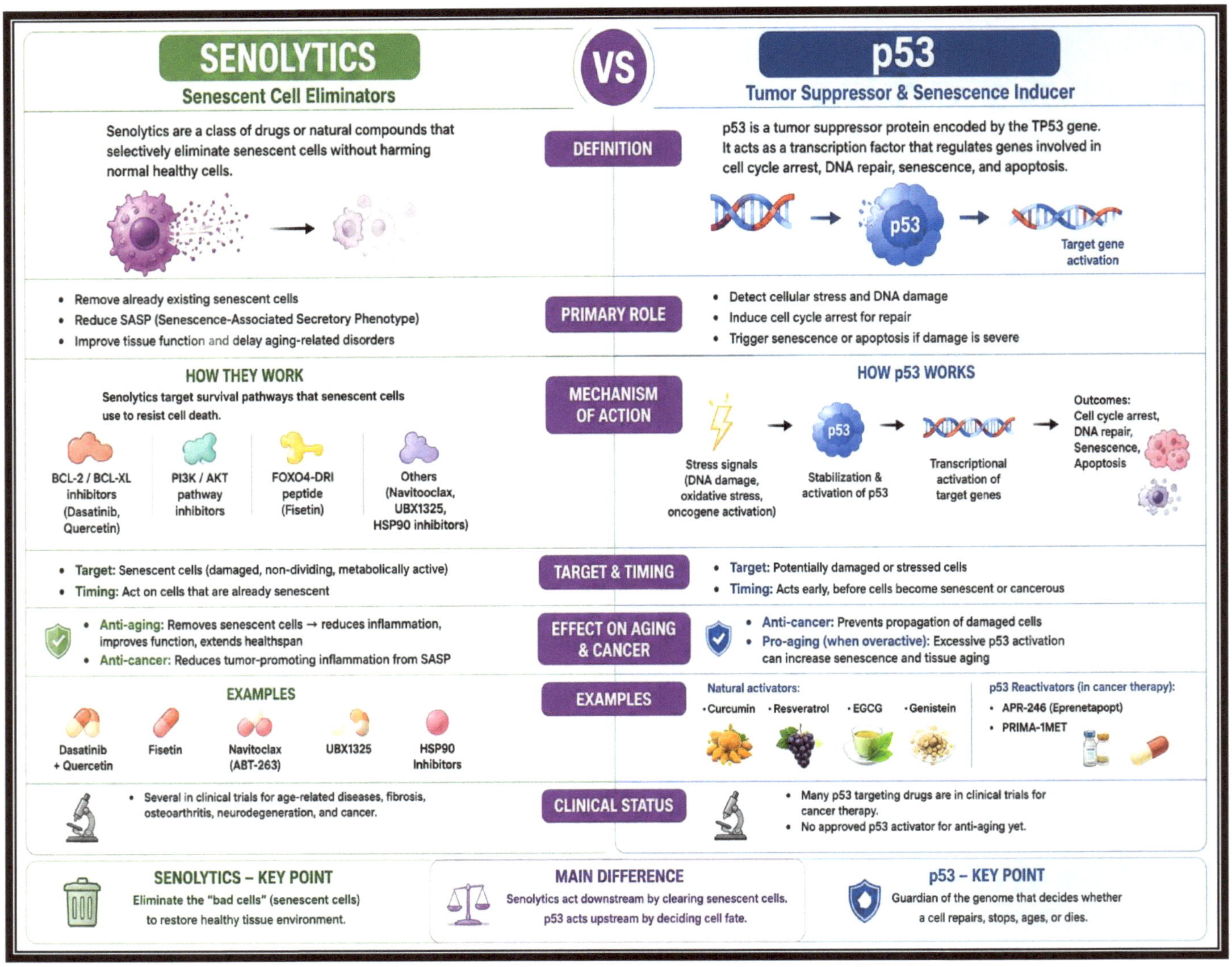

⚠️ **Important clarification:**

- **Senolytics ≠ p53 activators**
- Senolytics remove senescent cells
- p53 activation often **creates senescence**

Senolytics selectively eliminate senescent cells

- Senescent cells = old/damaged cells that have stopped dividing but are still alive
- They often secrete inflammatory factors (SASP), contributing to aging and disease

👉 **Senolytics are drugs that:**

- specifically kill these senescent cells
- Do not target normal healthy cells (ideally)

✔️ **So:**

Senolytics = *"clean-up drugs" that remove already aged/dysfunctional cells*

p53 contributes to senescence induction

This is a completely different step in the timeline.

- p53 does NOT remove cells
- Instead, it forces damaged cells to stop dividing

👉 **When DNA damage occurs:**

- p53 gets activated
- It can:
    - Pause the cell cycle (repair)
    - Trigger apoptosis (cell death)
    - OR induce senescence

✔ **So:**

p53 = *"decision-maker" that can push a cell into senescence*

🧠 **Simple analogy**

- p53 = police officer → stops a dangerous cell from dividing
- Senescent cell = retired but problematic citizen
- Senolytics = cleanup crew → removes that retired problematic cell

⚠ **Key takeaway**

- p53 → induces senescence (anti-cancer mechanism)
- Senolytics → remove senescent cells (anti-aging strategy)
- They act at different stages

🔬 **Why these matters?**

- Too much p53 activity → ↑ senescence → ↑ aging
- Too little p53 → ↓ senescence → ↑ cancer

👉 That's why:

p53 is a double-edged sword in cancer vs aging biology

💊 **Drugs targeting p53 pathway**

1. MDM2 inhibitors (activate p53)

Examples:

- Nutlin-3 (research)
- Idasanutlin
- RG7112

👉 Mechanism:

- Block MDM2 → stabilize p53

2. Mutant p53 reactivators

Examples:

- APR-246 (Eprenetapopt)
- PRIMA-1

👉 Restore wild-type function

FDA approval status

- Some drugs targeting p53 pathway are in **clinical trials**
- Limited approvals in specific contexts

👉 There are **FDA-approved drugs targeting p53 pathways**, but:

- Mostly indirect targeting
- Many still experimental

ICMR/India status

- No specific **ICMR-approved p53 activator drug**
- Mostly used in:
    - Clinical trials
    - Oncology research settings

⚠️ **Important point**

- **Direct "p53 activator therapy" is still evolving**
- No widely used standard clinical drug purely for aging or senolysis via p53

🔮 8. Future prospects

p53 is one of the **most promising therapeutic targets**:

Emerging areas:

1. **Precision oncology**
    - Targeting mutant p53 cancers
2. **Gene therapy**
    - Restoring TP53 function
3. **Synthetic lethality approaches**
4. **Aging interventions**
    - Fine-tuning p53 (not overactivation)

👉 Challenge:

- Too much p53 → aging
- Too little p53 → cancer

👉 Goal:

"Balanced p53 modulation"

📚 9. Future Perspectives

Precision Medicine

Targeting specific TP53 mutations in personalized cancer therapy.

Aging Interventions

Modulating p53 to balance cancer prevention and longevity.

CRISPR-Based Approaches

Gene editing to correct TP53 mutations.

Combination Therapies

Integrating p53 targeting with chemotherapy, radiotherapy, and immunotherapy.

Conclusion

p53 remains a cornerstone in understanding both cancer biology and aging. Its role as a tumor suppressor is well established, but its involvement in senescence and aging highlights the complexity of its function. Future research aims to harness p53 in a way that maximizes its protective effects while minimizing adverse outcomes related to aging.

Scientific References

1. p53 overview
    - https://en.wikipedia.org/wiki/P53
2. p53 in cancer therapy
    - https://www.mdpi.com/2072-6694/15/2/429
3. p53 and aging
    - https://www.nature.com/articles/onc2012640
4. p53 in senescence and aging diseases
    - https://pmc.ncbi.nlm.nih.gov/articles/PMC7422622/
5. Clinical translation of p53 therapies
    - https://www.nature.com/articles/s41568-023-00658-3

Chapter-5

Mitochondria and Their Functional Role in Health and Disease

Mitochondria: Structure and Functional Overview

Mitochondria are semi-autonomous, double membrane–bound organelles located in the cytoplasm of eukaryotic cells. They play a central role in cellular homeostasis and are increasingly recognized as key regulators of health, disease, and aging.

Beyond their classical role in ATP production, mitochondria are critical regulators of intracellular signaling pathways. They are major sources and modulators of Reactive Oxygen Species (ROS), which function not only as damaging agents but also as signaling molecules in redox-sensitive pathways. Through retrograde signaling, mitochondria communicate with the nucleus and cytosol, influencing gene expression and cellular adaptation to metabolic stress.

Mitochondria are deeply integrated into cellular metabolic networks, driving both catabolic and anabolic processes. They generate key metabolites required for biosynthesis and epigenetic regulation, thereby linking metabolism with gene expression. Additionally, mitochondria maintain bidirectional communication with the nucleus, coordinating cellular responses through dynamic regulation of gene expression.

Another critical function of mitochondria is the regulation of cell fate. They play a central role in apoptosis and necrosis through mechanisms involving calcium (Ca^{2+}) overload and the opening of the mitochondrial permeability transition pore (mPTP), which ultimately leads to cell death.

Mitochondria and Vascular Function

In vascular cells, particularly endothelial cells, mitochondria are major contributors to redox homeostasis. Although enzymes such as NADPH oxidase, cyclooxygenases, and xanthine oxidase also produce ROS, mitochondrial oxidative phosphorylation remains the predominant source of intracellular ROS.

At physiological levels, ROS act as signaling molecules regulating vascular tone, endothelial function, and cellular adaptation. However, excessive mitochondrial ROS production disrupts redox balance, leading to oxidative stress and endothelial dysfunction—key events in the development of cardiovascular diseases.

Mitochondria and Type 2 Diabetes Mellitus (T2DM)

Type 2 diabetes mellitus (T2DM) is a chronic metabolic disorder characterized by persistent hyperglycaemia and insulin resistance. Mitochondrial dysfunction plays a crucial role in both the development and progression of T2DM.

Mitochondria regulate multiple cellular pathways involved in glucose and lipid metabolism. Impairment in mitochondrial function leads to reduced oxidative capacity, increased lipid accumulation, and altered insulin signaling, thereby contributing to insulin resistance.

Emerging evidence highlights the role of mitochondrial epigenetics, such as mitochondrial DNA (mtDNA) methylation, in modulating mitochondrial function. These epigenetic modifications can be influenced by environmental and lifestyle factors, making them important targets for therapeutic intervention in T2DM.

Mitochondrial ROS and Oxidative Damage

Mitochondrial oxidative phosphorylation is a major source of intracellular ROS. While a controlled level of ROS is necessary for normal cellular signaling, excessive ROS production leads to oxidative damage of critical cellular components.

Mitochondrial ROS can induce:

- Lipid peroxidation of polyunsaturated fatty acids (PUFAs) in cell membranes
- DNA damage, including single- and double-strand breaks
- Protein oxidation, affecting structure and function

Damage to mitochondrial DNA (mtDNA) is particularly significant, as it impairs the expression and function of electron transport chain (ETC) components. This results in further ROS generation, creating a **self-perpetuating vicious cycle of oxidative damage**.

Clinical Implications

Mitochondrial dysfunction is implicated in a wide range of diseases, including:

- Type 2 diabetes mellitus
- Obesity and dyslipidaemia
- Hypertension
- Atherosclerosis
- Cardiac arrhythmias
- Sudden cardiac death

Experimental studies have shown that mtDNA damage correlates with the severity of atherosclerosis in both animal models and human tissues, highlighting its clinical significance.

Summary

Mitochondria are central regulators of cellular metabolism, redox balance, and cell survival. Their dysfunction leads to excessive ROS production, oxidative damage, and impaired cellular signaling, contributing to the development of metabolic and cardiovascular diseases. Understanding mitochondrial biology and its regulatory mechanisms is essential for developing targeted therapeutic strategies in chronic diseases such as T2DM.

Mitochondrial Dysfunction – Hallmark of Aging

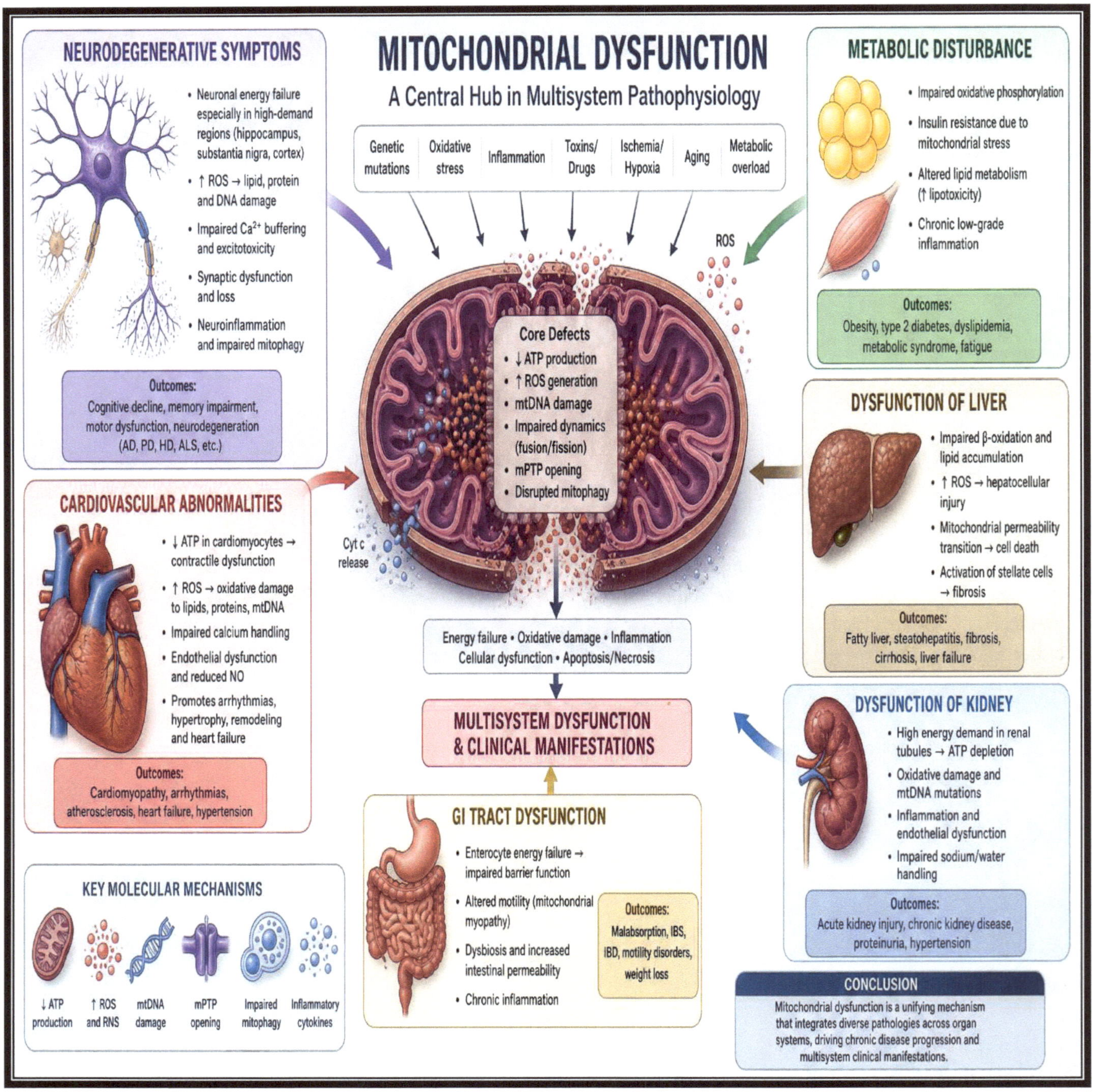

Mitochondrial diseases, also referred to as mitochondrial disorders, comprise a heterogeneous group of conditions characterized by impaired structure or function of mitochondria—specialized intracellular organelles responsible for cellular energy production. Mitochondria generate energy primarily in the form of adenosine triphosphate (ATP), which is essential for sustaining cellular and organ function.

Organs with high energy demands, such as the heart, skeletal muscles, and brain, contain a large number of mitochondria. Consequently, any disruption in mitochondrial number, integrity, or function leads to reduced ATP production and subsequent organ dysfunction.

Clinical Manifestations

The clinical presentation of mitochondrial disorders is highly variable and depends on the tissues affected. Common manifestations include:

- Fatigue and muscle weakness
- Neurological symptoms (seizures, cognitive impairment, developmental delay)
- Cardiovascular abnormalities (cardiomyopathy, arrhythmias)
- Metabolic disturbances (e.g., diabetes mellitus)
- Sensory impairments (hearing and vision loss)
- Dysfunction of liver, kidney, and gastrointestinal systems

These symptoms may manifest at any stage of life, from infancy to late adulthood, reflecting the systemic nature of mitochondrial dysfunction.

Mitochondrial Dysfunction in Cardiovascular Disease

Mitochondrial dysfunction is a key feature in the pathophysiology of cardiovascular diseases, particularly heart failure. It is associated with a progressive decline in cellular bioenergetic capacity. One hallmark metabolic alteration in failing hearts is a shift from mitochondrial fatty acid oxidation to less efficient glycolytic pathways, leading to reduced ATP generation.

Excessive production of Reactive Oxygen Species (ROS) during impaired oxidative phosphorylation further exacerbates mitochondrial damage, promotes cellular apoptosis, and contributes to disease progression.

Structure and Functional Characteristics of Mitochondria

Mitochondria are semi-autonomous organelles located in the cytoplasm. Unlike most other organelles, they possess their own genome (mitochondrial DNA, mtDNA), which is circular and double-stranded. Mitochondria are enclosed by a double membrane consisting of an outer mitochondrial membrane (OMM) and an inner mitochondrial membrane (IMM), the latter housing the components of the electron transport chain (ETC).

In addition to ATP production, mitochondria play critical roles in:

- Regulation of metabolic pathways
- Calcium homeostasis
- Apoptosis and cell survival

Mitochondria in Cardiac Bioenergetics

The heart is one of the most energy-demanding organs in the human body. To meet this continuous demand, mitochondria constitute approximately **20–40% of the total volume of cardiomyocytes**, reflecting their central role in cardiac function. These organelles generate large amounts of **adenosine triphosphate (ATP)** required to sustain constant myocardial contraction and overall cardiac performance.

In adult cardiomyocytes, **fatty acid oxidation** serves as the predominant source of energy. This metabolic process is closely linked to **mitochondrial oxidative phosphorylation**, through which reducing equivalents are utilized to drive ATP synthesis efficiently.

🔬 Clinical Correlation: Heart Failure and Mitochondrial Dysfunction

Mitochondrial dysfunction is a central feature in the pathophysiology of **heart failure**.

⚙ Key Mechanisms:

- **Reduced ATP production** → impaired contractile function of the myocardium
- **Metabolic shift** → decreased fatty acid oxidation and increased reliance on less efficient glycolysis
- **Excess reactive oxygen species (ROS)** → oxidative damage to mitochondrial DNA, proteins, and lipids
- **Impaired oxidative phosphorylation** → reduced energy efficiency
- **Defective mitochondrial dynamics** (fusion/fission imbalance) and reduced mitophagy

🧠 **Pathophysiological Consequences:**

- Energy starvation of cardiomyocytes
- Increased apoptosis and cell death
- Progressive myocardial remodelling
- Decline in cardiac output

📌 **Clinical Insight:**

In failing hearts, the inability of mitochondria to meet energy demands contributes directly to **contractile dysfunction and disease progression**. Targeting mitochondrial pathways—such as improving oxidative phosphorylation, reducing oxidative stress, and enhancing mitophagy—is an emerging therapeutic strategy in cardiovascular medicine.

🎯 **High-Yield Summary**

👉 *Heart failure can be viewed as a state of "bioenergetic failure," where mitochondrial dysfunction leads to reduced ATP production, increased oxidative stress, and progressive cardiac dysfunction.*

Mechanism of ATP Production (Oxidative Phosphorylation)

ATP generation in cardiac mitochondria involves a series of tightly regulated biochemical steps:

1. **Activation of Fatty Acids**
2. Fatty acids are converted into fatty acyl-CoA by acyl-CoA synthetase.
3. **Transport into Mitochondria**
4. Fatty acyl-CoA is converted into acylcarnitine by carnitine palmitoyltransferase 1 (CPT1), allowing its transport across the mitochondrial membranes.
5. **β-Oxidation**
6. Inside the mitochondria, fatty acyl-CoA undergoes β-oxidation, producing acetyl-CoA.
7. **Krebs Cycle (TCA Cycle)**
8. Acetyl-CoA enters the Krebs cycle, generating reducing equivalents:
    - NADH (reduced nicotinamide adenine dinucleotide)
    - $FADH_2$ (reduced flavin adenine dinucleotide)
9. **Electron Transport Chain (ETC)**
10. NADH and $FADH_2$ donate electrons to the ETC located in the inner mitochondrial membrane. Electron flow through complexes I–IV drives proton pumping across the membrane.
11. **ATP Synthesis**
12. The resulting proton gradient powers ATP synthase (Complex V), leading to the production of ATP.

Pathophysiological Insight

Under pathological conditions, such as mitochondrial dysfunction:

- Electron leakage from the ETC increases ROS production
- ATP synthesis becomes inefficient
- Cellular energy deficit develops
- Apoptosis and tissue damage are triggered

These processes are central to the development of cardiovascular diseases and other age-related disorders.

Biological or cellular aging is related to a continuous decline in mitochondrial respiratory activity, i.e., mitochondrial dysfunction, which is responsible for reduced ATP production (responsible for tissue homeostasis and stress response) and elevation in oxidative stress that could damage proteins, lipids, and DNA.

Mitochondrial dysfunction is one of the Hallmarks of Aging. As they age, mitochondria lose their ability to provide chemical ATP energy and release reactive oxygen species that harm Mitochondrial DNA (DNA Mutation) in cells.

One way to understand mitochondrial dysfunction is through inefficient ATP production, an essential fuel for cells of all types.

Aging is associated with the functional decline of diverse body organs, which can alter their capacity to cope with stress induced by metabolism, pathogens, and infections from an external toxic environment. This can damage the cellular macromolecules, posing a risk of several health issues that stimulate aging from cells to tissues to organs and give rise to cancer, cardiovascular disease, autoimmune disease, etc.

Aging is a degenerative process caused by accumulated oxidative stress that leads to cellular dysfunction by producing free radicals (natural byproducts of energy production) in mitochondria.

Mitochondrial ROS production increases with age because of a decline in mitochondrial function. When a mitochondrion is damaged, its ability to power the cell is impaired. This is caused by Free radicals, which are highly reactive and may damage proteins and DNA.

As this damage accumulates, the mitochondria become less effective at producing energy (ATP), leading to mitochondrial dysfunction.

Age-related changes in mitochondria are associated with a decline in mitochondrial function due to oxidative damage induced by reactive oxygen species (ROS).

As aging progresses, NAD+ levels in human cells decrease. Increased ROS, DNA mutations, and oxidized proteins cause mitochondrial dysfunction in aging.

Mitochondrial dysfunction with increased oxidative damage contributes to biological aging. Antioxidants on Cellular levels and free radical scavengers that protect against this damage also decline with age. Subsequently, mitochondria within our cells become dysfunctional over the years, and they do not produce ATP as efficiently as they should. The accumulation of dysfunctional mitochondria also depletes an essential molecule called nicotinamide adenine dinucleotide (NAD).

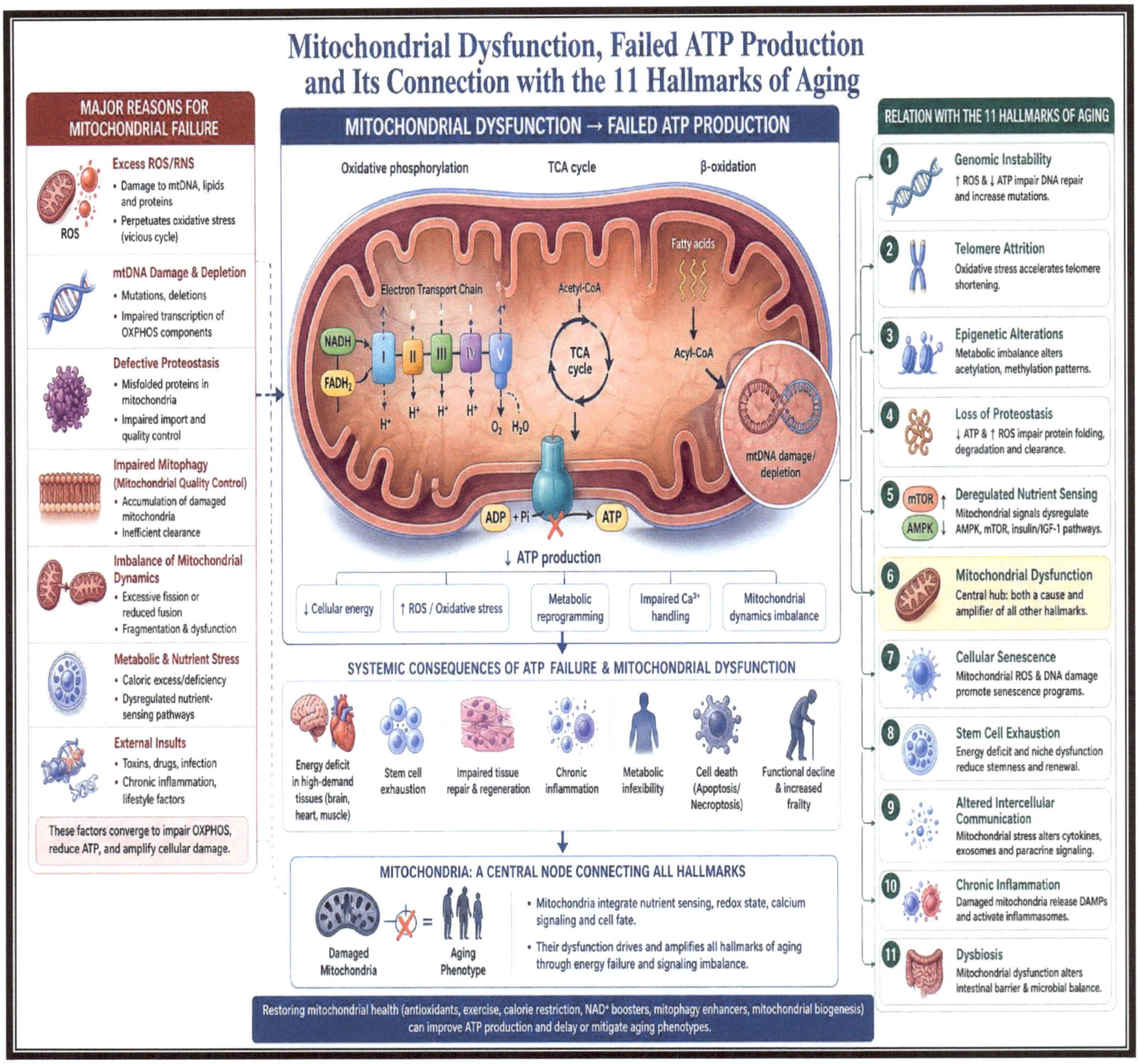

This diagram represents the major biological processes, often referred to as the Hallmarks of Aging, that contribute to aging at the cellular and molecular level. Each segment shows a key mechanism that leads to progressive decline in cell and tissue function.

1. Genomic Instability

- Refers to accumulation of DNA damage over time
- Causes: radiation, oxidative stress, replication errors
- Leads to:
    - Mutations
    - Cancer risk
    - Cell dysfunction

👉 DNA repair systems become less efficient with age

🧬 2. Telomere Shortening

- Telomeres protect chromosome ends
- With each cell division, they shorten

- When critically short:
  - Cells stop dividing (senescence)
  - Tissue regeneration declines

3. Compromised Autophagy

- Autophagy = "cell cleaning system"
- Removes damaged proteins and organelles

With aging:

- Autophagy decreases
- Cellular waste accumulates

👉 Leads to neurodegeneration and metabolic disorders

⚡ **4. Mitochondrial Dysfunction**

- Mitochondria produce ATP (energy)
- Aging leads to:
  - Reduced ATP production
  - Increased ROS (free radicals)

👉 Causes oxidative damage to DNA, proteins, and lipids

🧪 **5. Loss of Proteostasis**

- Proteostasis = protein balance (synthesis + folding + degradation)

With aging:

- Misfolded proteins accumulate
- Protein degradation systems fail

👉 Linked to diseases like Alzheimer's and Parkinson's

🌱 **6. Stem Cell Exhaustion**

- Stem cells repair and regenerate tissues

With aging:

- Stem cell number and function decline

👉 Leads to:

- Poor wound healing
- Organ degeneration

🔗 **7. Altered Intercellular Communication**

- Cells communicate via hormones, cytokines, signals

With aging:

- Communication becomes dysregulated
- Increased inflammatory signals

👉 Leads to "inflammaging" (chronic low-grade inflammation)

🧬 **8. Epigenetic Alterations**

Related to Epigenetics

- Changes in gene expression without altering DNA sequence
- Includes:
  - DNA methylation
  - Histone modification

👉 Leads to abnormal gene activation/silencing

⏳ **9. Cellular Senescence**

- Cells stop dividing but do not die
- Release harmful factors (SASP)

👉 Effects:

- Tissue damage
- Chronic inflammation

10. Nutritional Dysregulation

- Imbalance in nutrient sensing pathways

Key pathways affected:

- Insulin signaling
- mTOR
- AMPK

👉 Leads to:

- Metabolic syndrome
- Obesity
- Diabetes

🔁 **Integrated View (Very Important for Exams)**

These hallmarks are **interconnected**, not independent:

- Mitochondrial dysfunction → ↑ ROS → DNA damage
- DNA damage → cellular senescence
- Senescence → inflammation
- Inflammation → further damage

👉 This creates a **self-amplifying cycle of aging**

🧾 **Summary**

Aging is caused by multiple interconnected processes including DNA damage, telomere shortening, mitochondrial dysfunction, and impaired cellular repair systems, all of which lead to progressive decline in cell and organ function.

Mitochondria are essential for cellular energy production and metabolic regulation. Dysfunction of these organelles leads to impaired ATP generation, increased oxidative stress, and widespread cellular damage. Given their critical role in high-energy-demand organs, mitochondrial dysfunction is a major contributor to systemic diseases, particularly cardiovascular disorders.

📚 **Scientific References**

References: López-Otín C et al. Cell. 2013 & 2023; doi:10.1016/j.cell.2013.05.039; doi:10.1016/j.cell.2022.11.001; Nat Rev Mol Cell Biol. doi:10.1038/nrm.2017.88; Cell Metab. doi:10.1016/j.cmet.2016.08.003; Physiol Rev. doi:10.1152/physrev.00029.2015; Available from:

https://pmc.ncbi.nlm.nih.gov/articles/PMC3992297/,
https://pmc.ncbi.nlm.nih.gov/articles/PMC2360465/,
https://pmc.ncbi.nlm.nih.gov/articles/PMC8641024/,
https://pmc.ncbi.nlm.nih.gov/articles/PMC10044767/,
https://pmc.ncbi.nlm.nih.gov/articles/PMC3080271/.

Chapter-6

What is Telomere?

🧬 Telomeres: Definition, Structure, and Functional Significance

🔷 Definition

Telomeres are repetitive nucleotide sequences located at the **ends of chromosomes**, which protect genetic material from degradation and maintain chromosomal stability.

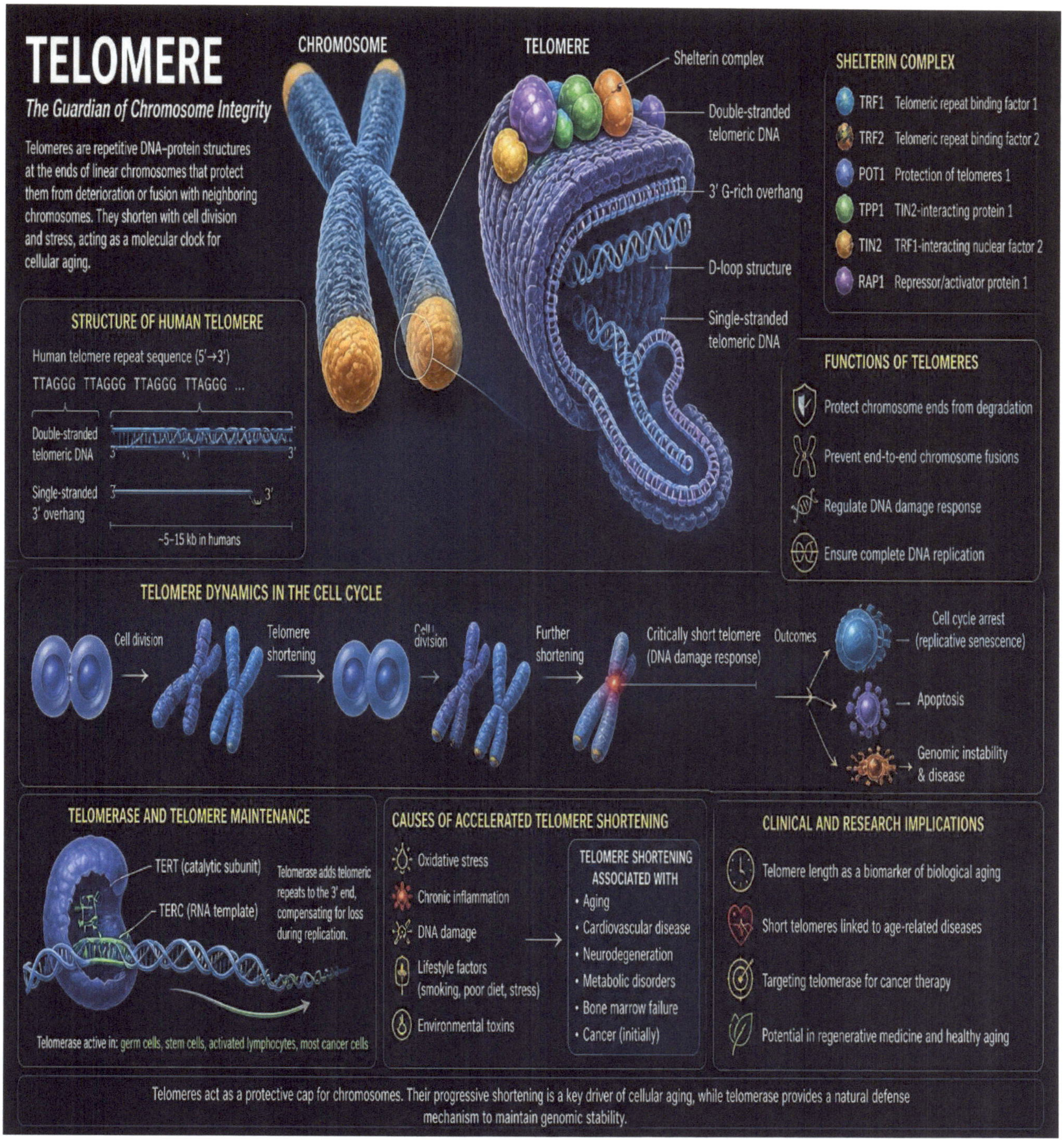

👉 In humans, the telomeric sequence is:

TTAGGG (repeated thousands of times)

🔷 **Basic Concept (Simple Understanding)**

👉 Telomeres act like the **"protective caps" of chromosomes**, similar to plastic tips at the ends of shoelaces.

Without telomeres:

- DNA would get damaged
- Chromosomes would fuse or degrade

🔷 **Structure and Location**

- Found at the **terminal ends of linear chromosomes**
- Associated with protective proteins (called the **shelterin complex**)
- Form a loop structure (**T-loop**) to protect DNA ends

🔷 **Function of Telomeres**

1. 🛡️ **Protection of Chromosomes**

- Prevent DNA ends from being recognized as damage
- Avoid chromosomal fusion and instability

2. 🔁 **Maintenance of Genetic Integrity**

- Ensure accurate DNA replication
- Prevent loss of important genes during cell division

3. ⏳ **Control of Cellular Lifespan**

- Telomeres shorten with each cell division
- Act as a **biological clock of aging**

👉 When critically short →

- Cell enters **senescence** or **apoptosis**

4. 🧬 **Regulation of Gene Expression**

- Telomere length influences nearby gene activity
- Known as **Telomere Position Effect (TPE)**

🔷 **Telomeres and DNA**

- Telomeres are **part of DNA** (non-coding repetitive sequences)
- They **do not code for proteins**
- Protect the coding regions of DNA from loss

👉 During DNA replication:

- DNA polymerase cannot fully replicate chromosome ends
- ➡️ This leads to **progressive telomere shortening**

🔷 **Telomeres and Chromosomes**

- Each chromosome has **two telomeres (one at each end)**
- They maintain **chromosome stability and integrity**

👉 Without telomeres:

- Chromosomes may fuse
- Genetic mutations increase
- Cancer risk rises

🔷 **Telomeres and Genes**

- Telomeres indirectly regulate genes
- Shortened telomeres → altered gene expression

👉 Effects:

- Cellular dysfunction
- Aging-related diseases

🔷 **Telomeres and Mitochondria**

There is a **strong bidirectional relationship**:

🔁 **Telomere → Mitochondria**

- Short telomeres activate stress pathways (e.g., p53)
- Leads to:
  - Reduced mitochondrial function
  - Decreased ATP production

🔁 **Mitochondria → Telomere**

- Mitochondria produce **Reactive Oxygen Species (ROS)**
- ROS damage telomeric DNA
- ➡️ Accelerates telomere shortening

In the past, scientists studied mitochondria and telomeres separately. But recent research shows that they are **closely connected and influence each other**.

- When mitochondria do not work properly, they can cause **telomeres to shorten**
- When telomeres are damaged, they can affect how mitochondria are formed and function

👉 This creates a **two-way relationship**, which plays an important role in aging and disease.

🔬 **Understanding Aging**

Over the last 30 years, research has shown that aging is not random—it is controlled by certain biological pathways that are shared across many living organisms.

Scientists have identified key processes called the **Hallmarks of Aging**, which explain how aging occurs in the body.

🧬 **Primary Causes of Aging**

Some of the most important causes include:

- **Genomic instability** (damage to DNA)
- **Telomere shortening** (loss of chromosome protection)
- **Epigenetic changes** (altered gene regulation)

👉 These processes are interconnected. For example:

Damage to telomeres can lead to DNA instability.

⚡ **Mitochondria and Aging**

Mitochondria are the "powerhouses" of the cell and produce energy. However, they also produce harmful molecules called **Reactive Oxygen Species (ROS)**.

- ROS can damage:
  - Mitochondrial DNA
  - Nuclear DNA

This damage can lead to:

- Mutations
- Cellular dysfunction
- Aging

👉 Earlier, scientists believed ROS were only harmful, but now we know:

- Small amounts of ROS can also activate protective mechanisms in the body

⏳ Telomere Shortening and Aging

Telomeres are protective caps at the ends of chromosomes.

- Each time a cell divides, telomeres become shorter
- When they become too short:
    - Cells stop dividing (senescence)
    - Aging increases

👉 Telomere length is very important for:

- Cell lifespan
- Overall health

⚠️ Factors That Speed Up Telomere Shortening

Telomeres shorten faster due to:

- Oxidative stress
- Smoking
- Obesity
- Cardiovascular risk factors

👉 Short telomeres are linked to:

- Heart disease
- Early death

🧡 Telomeres and Heart Disease

Recent studies show that:

- Shorter telomeres increase the risk of **coronary heart disease**
- They are also linked to **early mortality**

👉 This means telomere health is an important marker of overall aging and disease risk.

📄 Simple Summary

- Mitochondria and telomeres are closely connected
- Damage in one can affect the other
- Aging is driven by multiple linked processes like DNA damage, ROS, and telomere shortening
- Lifestyle factors can speed up these changes
- Maintaining telomere and mitochondrial health is important for longevity

Mitochondrial Dysfunction

↓

↑ ROS Production

↓

Telomere Damage

↓

Cellular Senescence

↓

↓ Mitochondrial Function

↓

More ROS Production

↓

Cycle Repeats

Telomeres Shortening with Age – Hallmark of Aging

Telomeres, the structures at the end of chromosomes, help to protect DNA from damage and allow chromosomes to replicate correctly during cell division.

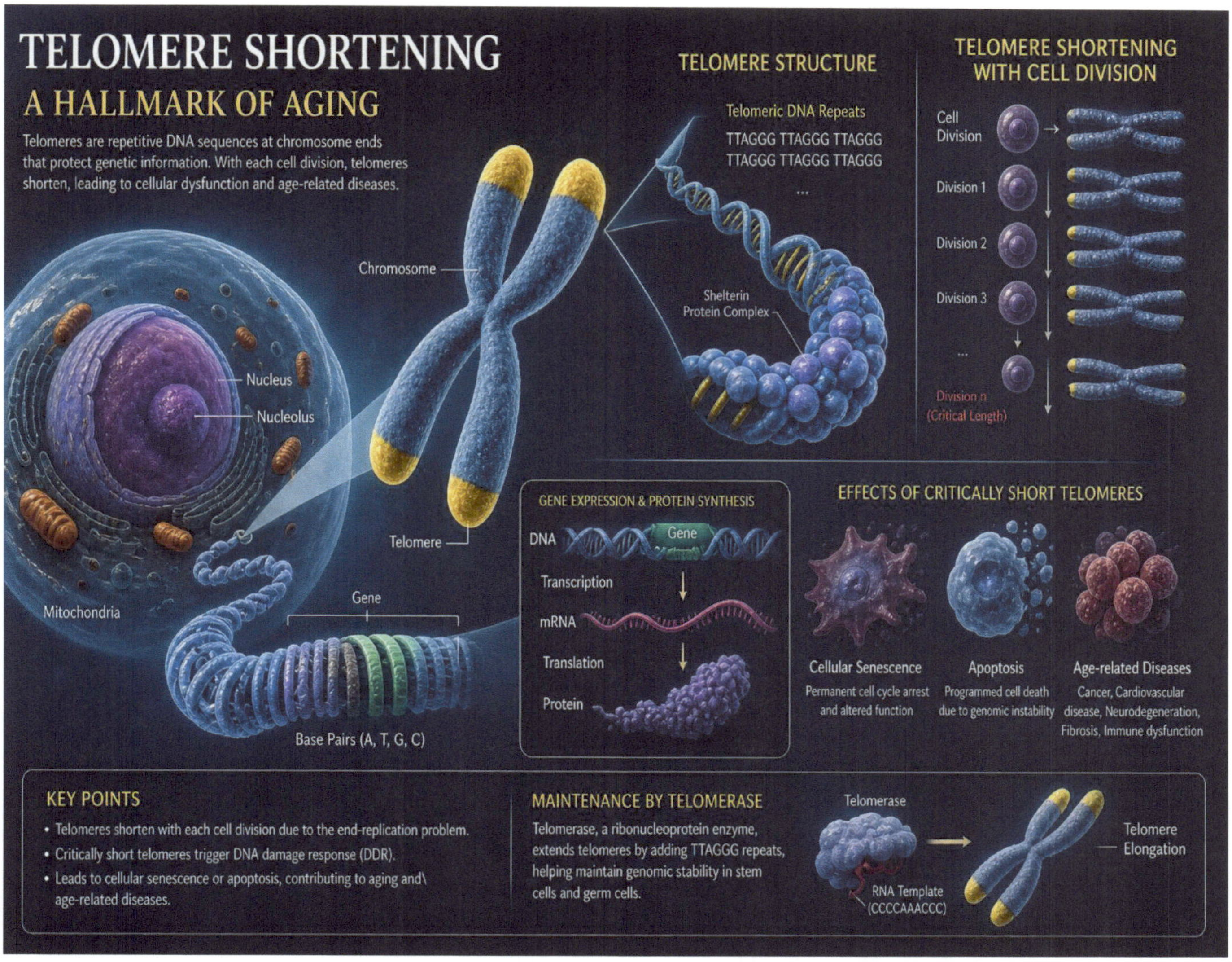

Telomeres are DNA–protein structures at the ends of chromosomes that protect the genome from degradation, unwanted recombination, and fusion. They are essential for maintaining genetic integrity. With each cell division, telomeric DNA shortens as part of the normal cellular process. When telomeres reach a critical length, cells enter senescence or undergo apoptosis. Telomere length can serve as a biological clock, influencing the lifespan of cells and organisms. Certain lifestyle factors may accelerate telomere shortening by causing DNA damage, which can impact overall health and longevity.

Accumulating evidence suggests that lifestyle factors influence health and lifespan by modulating telomere length. This review highlights the significance of telomeres in human health and aging, and summarizes lifestyle factors that may impact health and longevity by altering the rate of telomere shortening.

Recent studies indicate that telomere length, which is influenced by various lifestyle factors, affects the rate of aging and the onset of age-associated diseases.

Telomere length decreases with age. Progressive telomere shortening results in cellular senescence, apoptosis, or oncogenic transformation of somatic cells, thereby influencing health and lifespan.

Telomere Length, Lifestyle, and Aging

Telomeres play a critical role in determining cellular health, aging, and disease risk. Shorter telomeres are strongly associated with an increased incidence of diseases and reduced survival. As cells divide over time, telomeres gradually shorten, and when they become critically short, cells lose their ability to function properly, leading to aging and disease.

Importantly, the rate at which telomeres shorten is not fixed. It is influenced by lifestyle and environmental factors. Healthy choices such as balanced nutrition and regular physical activity can slow down telomere shortening, potentially delaying the onset of age-related diseases and increasing lifespan.

⚠️ Factors That Accelerate Telomere Shortening

Several lifestyle factors can speed up telomere shortening and negatively impact health, including:

- Smoking
- Obesity
- Physical inactivity
- Unhealthy diets

These factors increase oxidative stress and inflammation in the body, which damage DNA and accelerate telomere loss. Rapid telomere shortening is linked to the early development of many age-related conditions such as coronary heart disease, heart failure, diabetes, cancer, and osteoporosis.

For example, individuals with shorter telomeres in their white blood cells (leukocytes) have been shown to have up to a threefold higher risk of developing heart attacks. In older adults, shorter telomeres are also associated with significantly higher mortality rates.

🚬 Impact of Smoking and Obesity

Smoking has a particularly harmful effect on telomeres. It increases oxidative stress and accelerates telomere shortening, contributing to faster biological aging. Excessive telomere loss can lead to genomic instability, which increases the risk of cancer. In fact, many cancer cells are characterized by shortened telomeres.

Obesity also plays a major role in telomere shortening. It is associated with increased oxidative stress, inflammation, and DNA damage. Studies have shown that higher body mass index (BMI) and waist circumference are linked to increased levels of harmful molecules known as **Reactive Oxygen Species**, which damage DNA and accelerate telomere attrition.

🌍 Environmental and Psychological Factors

Environmental exposures, occupational hazards, and psychological stress also influence telomere length. Exposure to pollutants and harmful substances can accelerate telomere shortening.

Stress, in particular, has a significant biological impact. It triggers the release of stress hormones (glucocorticoids), which reduce the body's antioxidant defences. This leads to increased DNA damage and faster telomere shortening.

🥗 Role of Diet in Telomere Health

Diet plays a crucial role in maintaining telomere length and overall health. Nutritional patterns rich in antioxidants can help reduce oxidative stress and protect telomeres.

Studies have shown that diets high in omega-3 fatty acids are associated with slower telomere shortening. In contrast, low intake of antioxidants is linked to faster telomere loss. Antioxidants help neutralize harmful molecules and protect DNA from damage.

Benefits of Physical Activity

Regular physical activity helps maintain healthy telomeres by:

- Reducing body fat
- Improving metabolism
- Lowering oxidative stress
- Enhancing removal of cellular waste

These effects help preserve DNA integrity and slow down the aging process.

Telomeres, Aging, and Disease Risk

As telomeres shorten with age, cells gradually enter a state called senescence or undergo programmed cell death (apoptosis). Shortened telomeres are linked to genomic instability and increased cancer risk.

Research shows that older individuals with shorter telomeres have a significantly higher risk of death from cardiovascular and infectious diseases. Therefore, the rate of telomere shortening is a key factor that determines both healthspan and lifespan.

Lifestyle Strategies to Protect Telomeres

To slow aging and maintain telomere length, the following lifestyle strategies are recommended:

- Maintain a healthy, balanced diet
- Consume antioxidant-rich foods
- Engage in regular physical activity
- Manage stress through relaxation techniques
- Avoid smoking and excessive pollution exposure

Foods rich in antioxidants—such as fish (tuna, salmon, mackerel), seeds (flax, chia, sesame), fruits (berries, kiwi, grapes), vegetables (broccoli, sprouts, tomatoes), and beverages like green tea—help protect telomeres and support overall health.

Simple Summary

Telomere length is a key indicator of aging and health. Lifestyle factors such as diet, exercise, stress, and environmental exposure significantly influence the rate of telomere shortening, thereby affecting disease risk and lifespan.

Flowchart: Lifestyle → Telomere → Disease Pathway

LIFESTYLE FACTORS

| Smoking |

| Obesity |

| Physical Inactivity |

| Unhealthy Diet |

| Chronic Stress |

| Pollution/Environmental Toxins |

↓

↑ (ROS)

↓

Oxidative Stress & Inflammation

↓

DNA Damage

↓

Telomere Shortening (Attrition)

↓

Cellular Senescence/Apoptosis (Cell Aging)

↓

Genomic Instability

↓

ORGAN & SYSTEM DYSFUNCTION

↓

| Cardiovascular Disease |

| Type 2 Diabetes |

| Cancer |

| Neurodegenerative Disorders |

| Osteoporosis |

Key points

- Telomere length progressively decreases as individuals age.
- The rate at which telomeres shorten may serve as a biomarker for the pace of biological aging.
- Lifestyle factors including smoking, physical inactivity, obesity, psychological stress, and exposure to environmental pollution may accelerate telomere shortening, increase cancer risk, and hasten the aging process.
- Telomeres are structures located at the ends of chromosomes. Increasing evidence indicates that telomere length declines with age, a change now recognized as a hallmark of aging.
- Adherence to a plant-rich diet containing fiber, antioxidants, vitamins, and phytonutrients may contribute to longer telomere length.
- Engaging in regular physical activity and exercise reduces oxidative stress and inflammation, thereby protecting telomeres from damage.
- Consuming foods naturally rich in folate, rather than those fortified with synthetic folic acid, may support optimal telomere length.
- Elevated vitamin D levels are associated with longer telomeres and may contribute to the lengthening of previously shortened telomeres.
- Managing stress and maintaining healthy cortisol levels is important, as elevated levels can shorten telomeres and reduce lifespan.
- Biomarker tests related to telomere length include measurements of vitamin D, folate, and cortisol.

As telomeres become shorter, life expectancy may also decrease. Research has shown that individuals with shorter telomeres have a significantly higher risk of death, including about a 3-fold increase in deaths from heart disease and more than an 8-fold increase in deaths from infectious diseases. However, studies also suggest that certain lifestyle and biological approaches may help protect telomere length and, in some cases, even support its maintenance or improvement.

Category	Factors/Processes	What Happens in the Body	Final Impact
Unhealthy Lifestyle	Smoking, Obesity, Physical Inactivity, Poor Diet, Stress, Pollution	Increases harmful molecules like Reactive Oxygen Species	Triggers damage pathways
Oxidative Stress & Inflammation	Excess ROS, Chronic inflammation	Damages DNA, proteins, and cells	Cellular dysfunction begins
DNA Damage	Nuclear DNA + Mitochondrial DNA damage	Mutations and repair failure	Leads to genomic instability
Telomere Shortening	Loss of chromosome protection	Cells lose ability to divide properly	Accelerates aging
Cellular Response	Senescence (aging cells) or Apoptosis (cell death)	Reduced tissue regeneration	Organ decline
System-Level Effects	Impaired organ function	Reduced efficiency of body systems	Chronic health issues
Diseases	Heart disease, Diabetes, Cancer, Neurodegeneration, Osteoporosis	Increased disease risk	Reduced lifespan

Chapter-7

Cell Injury - Apoptosis, Necrosis, Autophagy, and Senescence

🧬 Cellular Damage and Cell Death in Aging

🔷 1. Introduction

Aging is characterized by the progressive accumulation of cellular and molecular damage, driven by both intrinsic and extrinsic stressors. This concept is central to multiple hallmarks of aging, including genomic instability, mitochondrial dysfunction, loss of proteostasis, and cellular senescence.

🔷 2. Sources of Cellular Stress

Cells are continuously exposed to diverse stressors that disrupt homeostasis:

- Hypoxia (low oxygen levels)
- DNA damage and replication errors
- Nutrient deprivation or metabolic imbalance
- Oxidative stress due to excess reactive oxygen species (ROS)

👉 These stressors collectively contribute to cellular dysfunction and aging progression.

🔷 3. Types of Cellular Damage

Cellular stress leads to multiple forms of macromolecular damage:

- DNA damage → mutations and genomic instability
- Protein misfolding → loss of proteostasis
- Lipid peroxidation → membrane dysfunction
- Mitochondrial damage → impaired ATP production and increased ROS

👉 Mitochondria are central to aging because they are both major sources and targets of ROS, creating a self-amplifying cycle of damage.

🔷 4. Role of Mitochondria in Cell Fate

Mitochondria regulate key cellular processes that determine cell survival:

- Apoptosis (programmed cell death)
- Autophagy (cellular recycling mechanism)
- Cellular senescence (permanent growth arrest)

👉 These processes are essential for maintaining tissue homeostasis and preventing accumulation of damaged cells.

🔷 5. Cell Death: Definition and Biological Significance

Cell death is a physiological process in which cells lose their functional integrity and are eliminated. In normal conditions, cell death is tightly regulated and balanced with cell division to maintain tissue health.

- Healthy human cells undergo a limited number of divisions (~50–60 cycles) before senescence or apoptosis
- Continuous cell turnover ensures replacement of damaged or aged cells

👉 Dysregulation of cell death contributes to aging and disease.

🔷 6. Types of Cell Death

6.1 Apoptosis (Programmed Cell Death)

- Controlled and energy-dependent process
- Eliminates damaged, aged, or unnecessary cells
- Maintains tissue homeostasis

📌 **Clinical relevance:**

- Reduced apoptosis → cancer
- Excess apoptosis → neurodegenerative diseases (e.g., Alzheimer's disease, Parkinson's disease)

6.2 Autophagy (Cellular Recycling)

- Degrades damaged organelles and proteins
- Activated during stress (e.g., starvation)
- Maintains cellular quality control

📌 Role in aging:

- Declines with age → accumulation of cellular waste
- Dysregulation contributes to metabolic and neurodegenerative diseases

6.3 Necrosis (Unregulated Cell Death)

- **Occurs due to acute injury or ischemia**
- **Leads to cell swelling, membrane rupture, and inflammation**
- **Results in irreversible tissue damage**

📌 **Examples:**

- **Gangrene**
- **Osteonecrosis**
- **Pulp necrosis (dental relevance)**

🔷 7. Causes of Cell Death

Cell death may occur due to:

- Cellular aging (replicative senescence)
- Irreparable DNA or protein damage
- Hypoxia and ischemia
- Exposure to toxins, infections, or radiation
- Metabolic and oxidative stress

🔷 8. Aging and Dysregulation of Cell Death

With aging:

- Apoptosis may be insufficient → accumulation of damaged cells → cancer
- Excessive apoptosis → tissue degeneration
- Autophagy declines → impaired cellular cleanup
- Necrosis increases → inflammation and tissue injury

👉 This imbalance contributes to age-related diseases and organ dysfunction.

🔷 9. Integration with Hallmarks of Aging

Hallmark	Role in Cell Death
Genomic instability	Triggers apoptosis
Mitochondrial dysfunction	ROS-induced damage
Loss of proteostasis	Protein aggregation
Cellular senescence	Growth arrest
Altered communication	Chronic inflammation

👉 **These hallmarks are interconnected and amplify cellular damage over time.**

🔷 10. Summary (High-Yield)

- Aging = accumulation of cellular damage
- Mitochondria play a central role via ROS and energy regulation
- Cell death is essential but must be tightly regulated
- Dysregulation leads to cancer, neurodegeneration, and tissue aging

🧬 Flowchart: Cellular Damage & Cell Death in Aging

AGING + CELLULAR STRESS

(Hypoxia | DNA Damage | Nutrient Imbalance | ROS)

↓

| Accumulation of Cellular |

| Damage |

↓

| Types of Molecular Damage |

| • DNA mutations (Genomic instability)|

| • Protein misfolding (Proteostasis ↓)|

| • Lipid peroxidation |

| • Mitochondrial damage |

↓

MITOCHONDRIAL DYSFUNCTION

(↑ ROS + ↓ ATP Production)

↓

| Cell Fate Decision Point |

↓

↓ ↓ ↓

APOPTOSIS AUTOPHAGY NECROSIS

(Programmed) (Recycling) (Uncontrolled)

↓ ↓ ↓

Removes Removes damaged Cell rupture +

damaged cells proteins/org. inflammation

↓ ↓ ↓

Homeostasis Cellular repair Tissue damage

↓

| Aging-Related Dysregulation|

↓

| • ↓ Apoptosis → Cancer |
| • ↑ Apoptosis → Neurodegeneration |
| • ↓ Autophagy → Waste accumulation |
| • ↑ Necrosis → Chronic inflammation |

↓

| Cellular Dysfunction |

↓

TISSUE DAMAGE & ORGAN DECLINE

↓

AGING + DISEASE

🔁 **Integrated Hallmark Link (Very High-Yield Add-on)**

Mitochondrial Dysfunction → ↑ ROS

↓

Genomic Instability → DNA Damage

↓

Cellular Senescence → Inflammation

↓

Altered Communication (Inflammaging)

↓

Further Cellular Damage

↓

🔄 Vicious Cycle of Aging

📚 **Scientific References**

- **Carlos López-Otín et al.,** ***Cell (2013)***
  - https://doi.org/10.1016/j.cell.2013.05.039
- **Carlos López-Otín et al.,** ***Cell (2023)***
  - https://doi.org/10.1016/j.cell.2022.11.001
- ***Nature Reviews Molecular Cell Biology*** **(Cell death & aging)**
  - https://doi.org/10.1038/nrm.2017.95
- ***Cell Metabolism*** **(Autophagy & metabolism)**
  - https://doi.org/10.1016/j.cmet.2018.03.012

- *Nature Reviews Molecular Cell Biology* **(Autophagy review)**
  - https://doi.org/10.1038/nrm.2017.22
- **Apoptosis and disease mechanisms**
  - https://pmc.ncbi.nlm.nih.gov/articles/PMC2117903/
- **Autophagy and aging**
  - https://pmc.ncbi.nlm.nih.gov/articles/PMC3612480/

Cellular Senescence – Hallmark of aging

The figure illustrates the major cellular stressors that drive the induction of cellular senescence, a state of irreversible cell cycle arrest. Key upstream triggers include mitochondrial dysfunction, endoplasmic reticulum (ER) stress, and increased production of Reactive Oxygen Species (ROS), all of which contribute to oxidative damage and disruption of cellular homeostasis. Additional inducers include telomere shortening, genomic DNA damage, hyperglycemia, insulin resistance, and chronic inflammatory signaling.

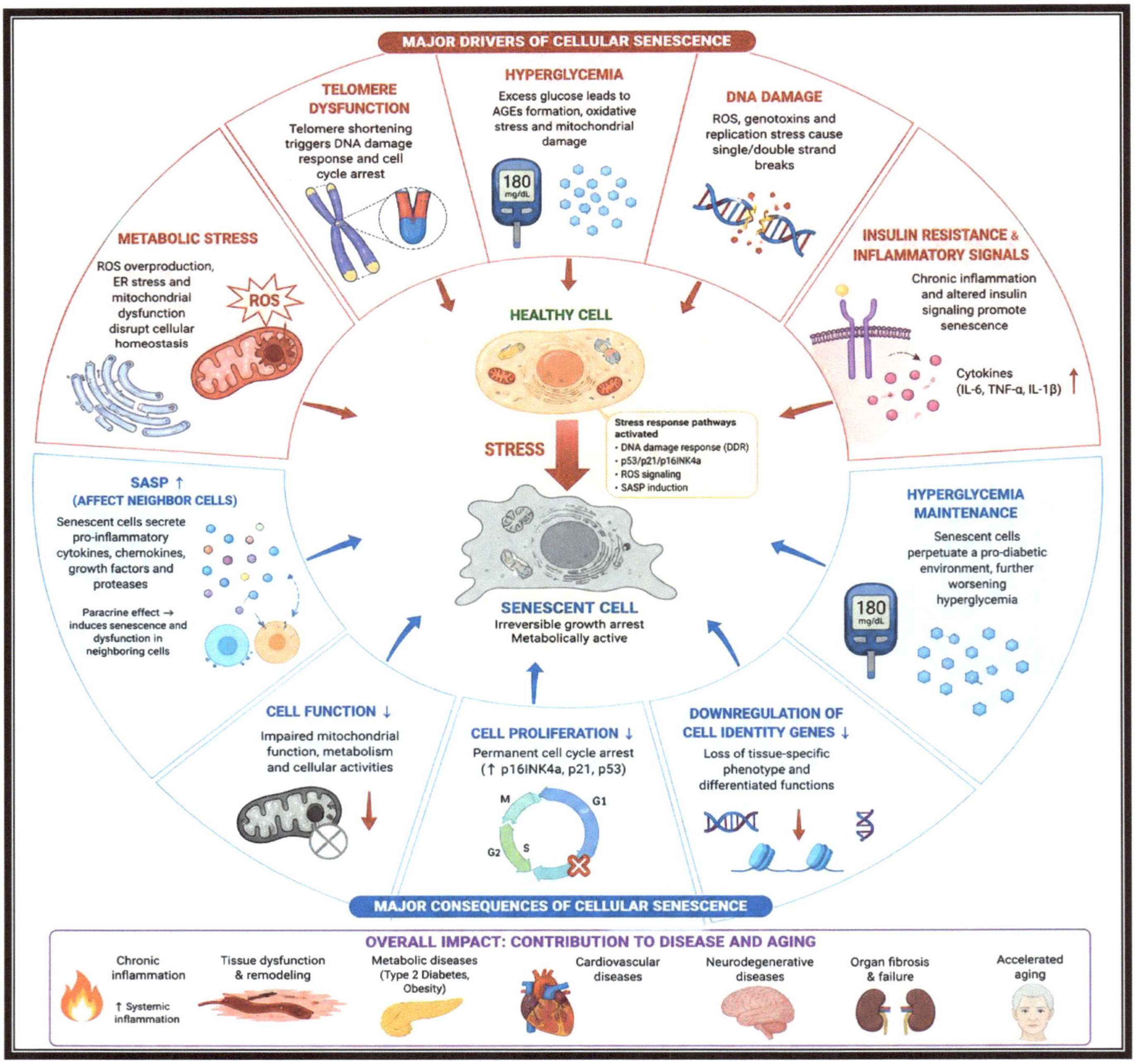

Hyperglycaemia, in particular, accelerates cellular senescence through multiple mechanisms, including increased oxidative stress, formation of advanced glycation end products (AGEs), and activation of pro-inflammatory pathways.

These processes are central to the pathogenesis of type 2 diabetes mellitus (T2DM), where senescent cells accumulate and contribute to metabolic dysfunction.

In response to severe or irreparable DNA damage, cells activate protective mechanisms such as apoptosis or cellular senescence. While apoptosis eliminates damaged cells, senescence prevents the proliferation of potentially harmful cells by inducing a stable and irreversible growth arrest. Importantly, senescent cells remain metabolically active despite losing their proliferative capacity.

A defining feature of senescent cells is the secretion of the **senescence-associated secretory phenotype (SASP)**, which consists of pro-inflammatory cytokines, chemokines, growth factors, and proteolytic enzymes. SASP factors can act in a paracrine manner, inducing senescence in neighbouring cells and amplifying tissue dysfunction through chronic inflammation.

Although cellular senescence plays beneficial roles in tumor suppression, wound healing, and tissue remodelling, its persistent accumulation is detrimental. Chronic senescence contributes to tissue degeneration, stem cell exhaustion, immune dysfunction, and the progression of age-related diseases.

In the cardiovascular and metabolic systems, senescence is strongly driven by mitochondrial dysfunction and associated oxidative and glycative stress. These processes promote telomere attrition, genomic instability, and impaired cellular function, thereby accelerating aging and increasing susceptibility to chronic diseases.

Hyperglycaemia, in particular, accelerates cellular senescence through multiple mechanisms, including increased oxidative stress, formation of advanced glycation end products (AGEs), and activation of pro-inflammatory pathways. These processes are central to the pathogenesis of type 2 diabetes mellitus (T2DM), where senescent cells accumulate and contribute to metabolic dysfunction.

In response to severe or irreparable DNA damage, cells activate protective mechanisms such as apoptosis or cellular senescence. While apoptosis eliminates damaged cells, senescence prevents the proliferation of potentially harmful cells by inducing a stable and irreversible growth arrest. Importantly, senescent cells remain metabolically active despite losing their proliferative capacity.

A defining feature of senescent cells is the secretion of the **senescence-associated secretory phenotype (SASP)**, which consists of pro-inflammatory cytokines, chemokines, growth factors, and proteolytic enzymes. SASP factors can act in a paracrine manner, inducing senescence in neighbouring cells and amplifying tissue dysfunction through chronic inflammation.

Although cellular senescence plays beneficial roles in tumor suppression, wound healing, and tissue remodelling, its persistent accumulation is detrimental. Chronic senescence contributes to tissue degeneration, stem cell exhaustion, immune dysfunction, and the progression of age-related diseases.

In the cardiovascular and metabolic systems, senescence is strongly driven by mitochondrial dysfunction and associated oxidative and glycative stress. These processes promote telomere attrition, genomic instability, and impaired cellular function, thereby accelerating aging and increasing susceptibility to chronic diseases.

Influencing factors:

- Chronological age, lifestyle habits, genetic inheritance, epigenetic changes, and psychosocial influences.

Types of senescence:

- In cardiovascular diseases, macromolecular damage leads to telomere length-dependent (replicative senescence) and length-independent (stress-induced premature senescence) senescence.

Cellular effects:

- Mitotic cardiovascular cells, such as endothelial and smooth muscle cells, undergo progressive telomere loss-based senescence, which is associated with cardiovascular disease phenotypes like atherosclerosis.

Potential implications:

- Atherosclerosis, heart rupture post-AMI (acute myocardial infarction), cardiac aging, abdominal aortic aneurysm, hypertension, heart regeneration, and cardiac remodelling.

Cellular senescence is a significant contributor to impaired bone strength, leading to conditions such as osteoporosis, fragility fractures, and sarcopenia.

Senescent cells in bone:

- Senescent osteoblasts demonstrate reduced mineralization capacity and impaired functional performance.
- Senescent osteoclasts display increased activity, resulting in bone loss and heightened risk of fragility fractures.
- Senescence-associated alterations in bone marrow stem cells lead to decreased osteogenic potential and compromised fracture healing.

Senescent alterations in muscle cells and satellite cells:

- Senescent muscle cells demonstrate reduced stem cell self-renewal capacity, changes in the intracellular microenvironment, and elevated protein degradation, all of which contribute to the development of sarcopenia.
- Cellular senescence impairs satellite cell maintenance and regeneration by sustaining p38 MAPK signaling and overexpressing p16INK4a.

Potential implications:

- A standardized set of senescence-associated factors and genes, called SenMayo, has been formulated to guide senotherapeutic therapies.

Cellular senescence plays a pivotal role in age-related disorders, including **Alzheimer's disease (AD) and Parkinson's disease (PD)**. CS is a potential contributor to age-associated inflammation in the brain, primarily in glial cells capable of replication.

AD pathophysiology:

- In Alzheimer's disease, senescent cells promote neuroinflammation by releasing pro-inflammatory cytokines, which activate microglia and sustain chronic inflammation.
- Senescent cells may disrupt clearance mechanisms, leading to the buildup of toxic protein aggregates.

PD pathophysiology:

- Parkinson's disease (PD) is defined by the degeneration of dopaminergic neurons, abnormal protein accumulation, neuroinflammation, mitochondrial dysfunction, oxidative stress, and cellular senescence.
- In Parkinson's disease, senescent cells secrete pro-inflammatory molecules, which contribute to persistent neuroinflammation and the progressive loss of dopaminergic neurons.

Impact on brain structure and function:

- Senescent glial cells and neurons lead to structural and functional alterations in the brain. Disruption of cell-to-cell contacts affects neuron-glia interactions, impacting neuronal ion levels and metabolic homeostasis.

Therapeutic considerations:

- Interventions targeting cellular senescence present a promising avenue to prevent cell loss and preserve brain functionality.

Senolytics, Senescent Cell Clearance, and Their Role in Aging

1. Introduction

Aging is associated with the accumulation of dysfunctional cells known as **senescent cells**. These cells no longer divide but remain metabolically active and secrete harmful inflammatory factors. Their progressive accumulation contributes to tissue dysfunction, chronic inflammation, and age-related diseases.

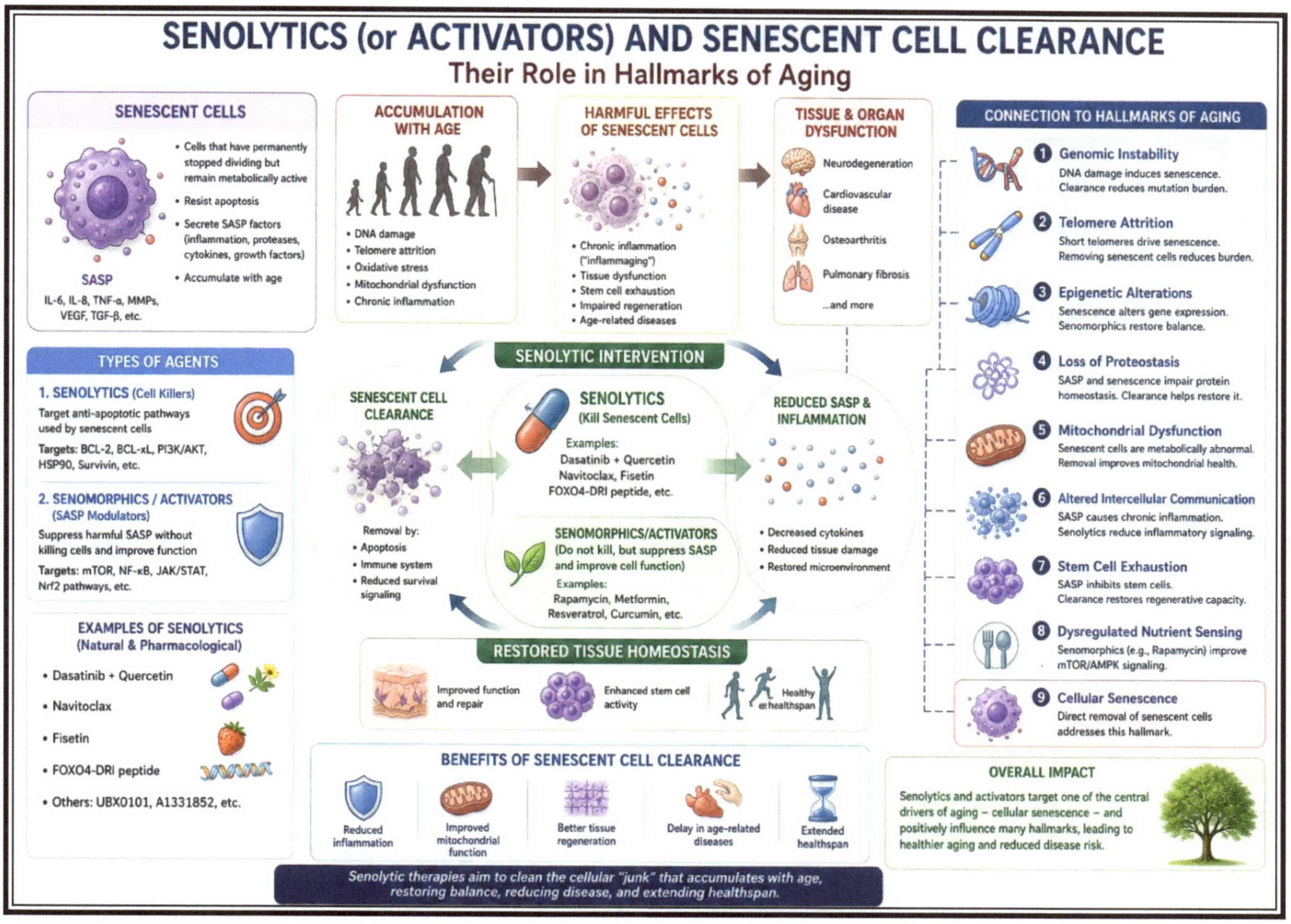

A modern therapeutic strategy targeting this process is the use of **senolytics** and related agents.

2. What are Senescent Cells?

Definition:

Senescent cells are cells that have permanently exited the cell cycle due to stress (e.g., DNA damage, telomere shortening, oxidative stress) but remain alive and metabolically active.

Key features:

- Irreversible growth arrest
- Resistance to apoptosis
- Secretion of harmful molecules (**SASP – Senescence-Associated Secretory Phenotype**)
- Accumulate with age

👉 **Impact:**

- Chronic inflammation ("inflammaging")
- Tissue degeneration
- Organ dysfunction

3. What are Senolytics?

Definition:

Senolytics are **agents that selectively eliminate senescent cells** without harming normal cells.

Mechanism:

Senescent cells survive by activating **anti-apoptotic pathways (SCAPs)**. Senolytics:

- Inhibit survival pathways (e.g., BCL-2 proteins)
- Induce apoptosis (programmed cell death)
- Reduce inflammatory signaling (SASP)

👉 In simple words:

Senolytics = "clean-up drugs" that remove aging (zombie) cells

4. What are Activators (Senomorphics/Senotherapeutics)?

Senotherapeutics represent a class of pharmacological agents and bioactive compounds that target cellular senescence, a biological state in which cells undergo permanent cell cycle arrest in response to stress but remain metabolically active. These senescent cells accumulate over time and secrete a range of pro-inflammatory and tissue-altering factors collectively known as the senescence-associated secretory phenotype (SASP), which contributes to aging and the development of chronic diseases.

Senotherapeutics are broadly classified into two major categories: senolytics and senomorphics (senostatics), based on their mechanism of action.

Senolytics are agents that selectively induce apoptosis in senescent cells while sparing normal, healthy cells. By targeting pro-survival pathways—commonly referred to as senescent cell anti-apoptotic pathways (SCAPs)—senolytics promote the clearance of these dysfunctional cells. This selective elimination has been associated with improvements in tissue function and may contribute to the attenuation of age-related physiological decline. Examples of senolytic agents include dasatinib, quercetin, fisetin, and navitoclax (ABT-263). Due to their targeted mechanism, senolytics are often administered intermittently, a strategy sometimes described as a "hit-and-run" approach.

In contrast, senomorphics do not eliminate senescent cells but instead modulate their phenotype, particularly by suppressing the deleterious effects of SASP. These agents act by inhibiting key inflammatory and signaling pathways such as NF-κB, mTOR, and JAK/STAT, thereby reducing the secretion of pro-inflammatory mediators and limiting tissue dysfunction. Common examples include metformin, rapamycin, ruxolitinib, and naturally occurring compounds such as apigenin and kaempferol. Senomorphics may be particularly useful in physiological contexts where senescent cells play beneficial roles, such as in wound healing and tissue repair.

There are two major categories:

1. Senolytics

- Kill senescent cells

2. Senomorphics (Activators/Modulators)

- Do NOT kill cells
- Reduce harmful secretions (SASP)
- Improve cell function

👉 Example:

- **Rapamycin, Metformin** → suppress SASP
- Improve cellular signaling rather than eliminating cells

5. Senescent Cell Clearance

Natural clearance:

- Immune system removes senescent cells
- Efficiency declines with age

Therapeutic clearance:

- Senolytics artificially remove accumulated cells

👉 Why clearance is important:

- Senescent cells accumulate over time
- They resist normal apoptosis
- They damage neighboring cells

👉 Result of clearance:

- Reduced inflammation
- Improved tissue repair
- Better organ function

Studies show that clearing senescent cells can improve healthspan and reduce disease burden.

6. Relation to Hallmarks of Aging

Senolytics are directly linked to multiple hallmarks:

Primary hallmark:

✔ **Cellular Senescence**

Secondary connections:

- **Genomic instability** → triggers senescence
- **Telomere attrition** → induces senescence
- **Mitochondrial dysfunction** → promotes SASP
- **Altered intercellular communication** → inflammation
- **Stem cell exhaustion** → impaired regeneration

👉 Key concept:

Senescent cells act as a "central driver" connecting multiple hallmarks of aging

7. Real-Life Examples of Senolytics

Pharmacological:

- Dasatinib + Quercetin (D+Q)
- Navitoclax
- FOXO4-DRI peptide

Natural compounds:

- Fisetin (found in strawberries)
- Quercetin (found in onions, apples)

👉 Research findings:

- Improved physical function in aged animals
- Reduced inflammation
- Potential benefits in:
    - Osteoarthritis
    - Cardiovascular disease
    - Neurodegeneration

8. Relation with Blood-Brain Barrier (BBB)

Important concept:

The **blood-brain barrier (BBB)** protects the brain from harmful substances.

Connection with senolytics:

1. **Brain aging involves senescent cells**
    - Found in neurons, astrocytes, microglia
    - Contribute to neurodegenerative diseases
2. **Senolytics must cross BBB**
    - To act on brain senescent cells
    - Not all compounds can do this
3. **Therapeutic potential in CNS**
    - Alzheimer's disease
    - Parkinson's disease
    - Cognitive decline

👉 Research insight:

Senotherapeutics are being developed specifically for the brain to restore function and reduce neurodegeneration.

9. Clinical and Research Significance

Benefits:

- Reduced inflammation
- Improved tissue regeneration
- Delayed age-related diseases
- Extended healthspan

Challenges:

- Safety concerns (off-target effects)
- Not all senescent cells are harmful
- Need for precise targeting
- Limited human clinical data

10. Simple Flow Diagram

Aging Stress → Senescent Cells ↑ → SASP ↑ → Inflammation ↑ → Tissue Damage ↑ → Disease

⬇️ (Intervention)

Senolytics → Senescent Cell Clearance → Reduced SASP → Improved Function

11. Conclusion

Senolytics represent a promising and emerging field in aging biology. By targeting one of the central hallmarks—**cellular senescence**—they offer a potential strategy to delay aging and prevent age-related diseases. However, further research is needed to establish safety, efficacy, and long-term outcomes in humans.

📚 Scientific References

📚 1. Cellular senescence (definition, features, SASP)

- https://www.ncbi.nlm.nih.gov/pmc/articles/PMC3836174
- 👉 **Core paper on senescence and SASP**
- https://www.ncbi.nlm.nih.gov/pmc/articles/PMC5503622
- 👉 **Senescence and aging overview**

- https://www.cell.com/fulltext/S0092-8674(11)00114-0
- 👉 **Classic paper defining SASP (Senescence-Associated Secretory Phenotype)**

🧬 **2. Senescent cells & aging (inflammaging, tissue dysfunction)**

- https://www.ncbi.nlm.nih.gov/pmc/articles/PMC4015650
- 👉 **Senescence drives aging and inflammation**
- https://www.nature.com/articles/nrm.2015.4
- 👉 **Senescence in tissue aging**

💊 **3. Senolytics (definition, mechanism, SCAPs)**

- https://www.ncbi.nlm.nih.gov/pmc/articles/PMC4475278
- 👉 **First major paper introducing senolytics concept**
- https://www.ncbi.nlm.nih.gov/pmc/articles/PMC6314897
- 👉 **Mechanisms of senolytics and SCAP pathways**

🧪 **4. Senotherapeutics (senolytics vs senomorphics)**

- https://www.ncbi.nlm.nih.gov/pmc/articles/PMC7067572
- 👉 **Classification of senotherapeutics**
- https://www.nature.com/articles/s41580-020-00314-1
- 👉 **Comprehensive review of senescence-targeting drugs**

🧫 **5. Senolytic drugs (Dasatinib, Quercetin, Navitoclax, Fisetin)**

- https://www.ncbi.nlm.nih.gov/pmc/articles/PMC4917649
- 👉 **Dasatinib + Quercetin (D+Q) study**
- https://www.ncbi.nlm.nih.gov/pmc/articles/PMC6128428
- 👉 **Fisetin as senolytic**
- https://www.ncbi.nlm.nih.gov/pmc/articles/PMC5564890
- 👉 **Navitoclax mechanism**

🔬 **6. Senescent cell clearance & health benefits**

- https://www.nature.com/articles/nature16932
- 👉 **Landmark study: clearing senescent cells improves lifespan/healthspan**
- https://www.ncbi.nlm.nih.gov/pmc/articles/PMC6363124
- 👉 **Effects of senescent cell removal**

👴 **7. Hallmarks of aging (link to senescence)**

- https://www.cell.com/fulltext/S0092-8674(13)00645-4
- 👉 **Original Hallmarks of Aging paper**
- https://www.cell.com/fulltext/S0092-8674(22)01377-0
- 👉 **Updated hallmarks (2023)**

🧠 **8. Senescence & brain/BBB/neurodegeneration**

- https://www.ncbi.nlm.nih.gov/pmc/articles/PMC6770068
- 👉 **Senescence in brain aging**
- https://www.ncbi.nlm.nih.gov/pmc/articles/PMC7268927
- 👉 **Senolytics in neurodegenerative diseases**

🧪 **9. Senomorphics (rapamycin, metformin, JAK inhibitors)**

- https://www.ncbi.nlm.nih.gov/pmc/articles/PMC6814613
- 👉 **Rapamycin & SASP**
- https://www.ncbi.nlm.nih.gov/pmc/articles/PMC5943638

- 👉 **Metformin and aging**

📊 10. Clinical relevance & future perspectives

- https://www.ncbi.nlm.nih.gov/pmc/articles/PMC7484808
- 👉 **Clinical translation of senolytics**
- https://www.nature.com/articles/s41591-019-0501-0
- 👉 **Human trials of senolytics**

Baker DJ et al. Clearance of senescent cells delays ageing. Nature.

Kirkland JL et al. Senolytics: targeting aging cells.

Chapter-8

Autophagy and Clearance of Pathogens

Autophagy, Mitophagy, and Mitochondrial Biogenesis: Integrated Regulators of Cellular Homeostasis and Aging

1. Introduction: Cellular Quality Control and Survival Mechanisms

Cells are constantly exposed to metabolic stress, environmental insults, and internal damage. To maintain survival and optimal function, they rely on highly regulated quality control systems. Among these, autophagy represents a fundamental adaptive process that ensures cellular integrity by degrading and recycling damaged intracellular components.

Autophagy is not merely a degradation pathway; rather, it is a dynamic survival mechanism that integrates metabolism, stress responses, immunity, and aging biology. Its dysregulation has been implicated in a wide spectrum of diseases, including neurodegeneration, metabolic disorders, cancer, and cardiovascular diseases.

2. Concept of Autophagy: A Cellular Recycling and Quality Control System

Autophagy (literally meaning "self-eating") is a lysosome-mediated catabolic process through which cells:

- Remove damaged organelles
- Eliminate misfolded or aggregated proteins
- Recycle intracellular components

This process ensures:

- Maintenance of cellular homeostasis
- Efficient energy utilization
- Protection against cellular stress

From a functional perspective, autophagy acts as both:

- A recycling system → providing substrates for energy and biosynthesis
- A quality control system → preventing accumulation of toxic cellular debris

3. Molecular Mechanism of Autophagy

Autophagy is orchestrated by a group of proteins known as autophagy-related genes (ATGs).

Stepwise Process

1. Initiation
    - Triggered by stress signals such as nutrient deprivation or hypoxia
    - Activation of autophagy signaling pathways
2. Formation of Autophagosome
    - Double-membrane vesicles (autophagosomes) engulf damaged cellular components
3. Fusion with Lysosome
    - Autophagosomes fuse with lysosomes to form autolysosomes
4. Degradation and Recycling
    - Lysosomal enzymes degrade contents into basic molecules
    - These are reused for:
        - Energy production
        - Synthesis of new cellular components

4. Triggers and Regulation of Autophagy

Autophagy is activated primarily under conditions of cellular stress, including:

- Nutrient deprivation
- Hypoxia
- Oxidative stress
- Cellular damage

Physiological Inducers

- Caloric restriction
- Fasting
- Physical exercise

These conditions activate energy-sensing pathways such as:

- AMP-activated protein kinase (AMPK) → promotes autophagy
- mTOR inhibition → removes suppression of autophagy

5. Autophagy in Aging and Longevity

Autophagy plays a central role in healthy aging.

Key Observations

- Autophagic activity declines with age
- Reduced autophagy leads to:
    - Accumulation of damaged proteins and organelles
    - Increased oxidative stress
    - Cellular dysfunction

Impact on Aging

- Contributes to:
    - Neurodegenerative diseases
    - Metabolic disorders
    - Immune decline

Thus, autophagy is considered a protective anti-aging mechanism.

6. Autophagy and Immunity

Autophagy also functions as an important component of the innate immune system:

- Eliminates intracellular pathogens (bacteria, viruses)
- Regulates inflammatory signaling
- Maintains immune cell function

However, both excessive activation and impaired autophagy can be detrimental:

- Hyperactivation → cellular damage
- Inhibition → accumulation of pathogens and toxic materials

🔬 7. Mitochondria–Autophagy Axis

7.1 Mitochondrial Function in Cellular Physiology

Mitochondria are essential for:

- ATP production via oxidative phosphorylation (OXPHOS)
- Regulation of apoptosis
- Calcium homeostasis
- Generation of reactive oxygen species (ROS)

They are central to both bioenergetics and signaling pathways.

7.2 Mitophagy: Selective Removal of Damaged Mitochondria

Mitophagy is a specialized form of autophagy that specifically targets dysfunctional mitochondria.

Triggers of Mitophagy

- Loss of mitochondrial membrane potential
- Excess ROS production
- mtDNA damage
- Hypoxia or nutrient stress

Functions of Mitophagy

- Eliminates damaged mitochondria
- Prevents excessive ROS generation
- Maintains mitochondrial quality

Clinical Relevance

Defective mitophagy is associated with:

- Neurodegenerative disorders (e.g., Parkinson's disease)
- Metabolic dysfunction
- Accelerated aging

7.3 Bidirectional Relationship: Mitochondria and Autophagy

The interaction between mitochondria and autophagy is reciprocal:

Autophagy → Mitochondria

- Removes dysfunctional mitochondria
- Maintains mitochondrial quality

Mitochondria → Autophagy

- Regulate autophagy through:
    - ROS signaling
    - Energy status (ATP levels)
    - Metabolic intermediates

👉 Dysfunction in either system disrupts cellular homeostasis and promotes disease.

8. Mitochondrial Biogenesis: Generation of New Mitochondria

8.1 Definition and Importance

Mitochondrial biogenesis is the process by which cells:

- Increase mitochondrial number
- Replace damaged mitochondria
- Adapt to metabolic demands

This process is essential for:

- Energy homeostasis
- Cellular adaptation to stress

8.2 Key Molecular Regulator: PGC-1α

The central regulator of mitochondrial biogenesis is:

👉 PGC-1α (Peroxisome proliferator-activated receptor gamma coactivator-1 alpha)

Mechanism

PGC-1α activates:

- Nuclear respiratory factors (NRF-1, NRF-2)
- Mitochondrial transcription factor A (TFAM)

This leads to:

- Replication of mitochondrial DNA (mtDNA)
- Increased mitochondrial protein synthesis

8.3 Role of AMPK

AMPK acts as a cellular energy sensor:

- Activated during low energy states
- Stimulates PGC-1α → promotes mitochondrial biogenesis

Aging Connection

- AMPK activity declines with age
- Leads to reduced mitochondrial biogenesis and function

🔄 9. Balance Between Mitophagy and Biogenesis

Cellular health depends on a dynamic balance between:

- Mitophagy → removal of damaged mitochondria
- Biogenesis → generation of new mitochondria

Homeostasis Model

Mitochondrial Damage

↓

Mitophagy (Removal)

↓

Mitochondrial Biogenesis (Replacement)

↓

Healthy Mitochondrial Pool

↓

Optimal Cellular Function

Imbalance Leads To

- Accumulation of dysfunctional mitochondria
- Increased oxidative stress
- Development of:
    - Metabolic diseases
    - Neurodegeneration
    - Cardiovascular disorders

🧠 10. Clinical and Pathophysiological Implications

Dysregulation of the autophagy–mitochondria axis contributes to:

- Type 2 diabetes mellitus
- Alzheimer's disease
- Parkinson's disease
- Cardiovascular diseases
- Aging-related decline

📚 Scientific References

References: López-Otín C et al. Cell. 2013 & 2023; doi:10.1016/j.cell.2013.05.039; doi:10.1016/j.cell.2022.11.001; Nat Rev Mol Cell Biol. doi:10.1038/nrm.2017.22; Cell. doi:10.1016/j.cell.2011.01.036; Nat Rev Immunol. doi:10.1038/nri3532; Cell Metab. doi:10.1016/j.cmet.2011.06.012; Available from: https://pmc.ncbi.nlm.nih.gov/articles/PMC3612480/, https://pmc.ncbi.nlm.nih.gov/articles/PMC2862365/, https://pmc.ncbi.nlm.nih.gov/articles/PMC3992297/, https://pmc.ncbi.nlm.nih.gov/articles/PMC2360465/, https://pmc.ncbi.nlm.nih.gov/articles/PMC3080271/, https://pmc.ncbi.nlm.nih.gov/articles/PMC8641024/.

🧬 Ketosis and Autophagy: Metabolic Adaptation and Implications in Aging

◆ 1. Concept of Ketosis

Ketosis is a **metabolic state** in which the body shifts from glucose-based energy metabolism to **fat-derived energy utilization**. Under normal conditions, glucose derived from dietary carbohydrates serves as the primary energy source.

However, during **low carbohydrate availability (fasting or ketogenic diet)**:

- Glycogen stores become depleted
- Insulin levels decrease
- Lipolysis is activated

➡️ This leads to increased production of **ketone bodies** (β-hydroxybutyrate, acetoacetate) in the liver, which serve as alternative energy substrates for the brain and peripheral tissues.

◆ 2. Ketogenic Diet (KD)

The ketogenic diet is a **high-fat, low-carbohydrate dietary intervention** that induces ketosis.

Composition:

- **Fat:** 70–80%
- **Protein:** 10–20%
- **Carbohydrates:** 5–10%

Mechanism:

- Reduces glucose availability
- Promotes fat oxidation
- Increases ketone production

Common dietary sources include:

- Fats: oils, butter, nuts
- Proteins: meat, fish, eggs
- Minimal carbohydrates (restricted grains, fruits)

◆ 3. Ketosis and Autophagy (High-Yield Link)

Ketosis is closely linked to **autophagy activation**, a key process in the **hallmarks of aging**.

Mechanistic Link:

- ↓ Nutrient availability → ↓ mTOR activity
- ↑ AMP/ATP ratio → ↑ AMPK activation
- Result → **Induction of autophagy**

👉 Autophagy enhances:

- Removal of damaged proteins
- Clearance of dysfunctional mitochondria (mitophagy)
- Cellular repair and survival

📌 Thus, ketosis mimics a **"low nutrient state"**, promoting longevity-associated pathways.

🔷 4. Physiological and Clinical Benefits

Metabolic Effects:

- Weight loss (especially visceral fat)
- Improved insulin sensitivity

Neurological Benefits:

- Reduced seizures in epilepsy
- Potential benefit in neurodegenerative disorders such as Alzheimer's disease

Cardiometabolic Effects:

- Reduced triglycerides
- Increased HDL cholesterol
- Improved metabolic syndrome

Cellular Effects:

- Reduced inflammation
- Enhanced mitochondrial efficiency
- Increased energy stability

🔷 5. Role in Aging (Hallmark Integration)

Ketosis influences multiple hallmarks of aging:

Hallmark	Effect of Ketosis
Nutrient sensing	↓ mTOR, ↑ AMPK
Mitochondrial dysfunction	Improved efficiency
Loss of proteostasis	↑ Autophagy
Inflammation	↓ Chronic inflammation

👉 Overall effect: **promotes cellular resilience and longevity pathways**

🔷 6. Adverse Effects and Limitations

Common side effects include:

- "Keto flu" (fatigue, headache)
- Dehydration
- Constipation
- Halitosis ("keto breath")

Long-term risks:

- Hyperlipidemia
- Kidney stones
- Reduced bone density

🔷 7. Ketosis vs Diabetic Ketoacidosis (DKA)

Feature	Ketosis	DKA
Ketone level	Mild ↑	Severe ↑
Blood pH	Normal	Acidic
Cause	Diet/fasting	Insulin deficiency
Risk	Safe	Life-threatening

👉 DKA is a medical emergency commonly associated with uncontrolled diabetes.

◆ 8. Summary

- Ketosis = fat-based metabolism with ketone production
- Activates **AMPK and autophagy**, inhibits **mTOR**
- Provides metabolic and neuroprotective benefits
- Plays a role in **healthy aging mechanisms**
- Must be distinguished from pathological ketoacidosis

Scientific References

- Cell Metabolism (Ketosis & metabolism)
- https://doi.org/10.1016/j.cmet.2017.06.018
- Nature Reviews Molecular Cell Biology (Autophagy & mTOR)
- https://doi.org/10.1038/nrm.2017.22
- Cleveland Clinic (Clinical ketosis overview)
- https://my.clevelandclinic.org/health/articles/ketosis
- Annual Review of Nutrition (Ketogenic diet review)
- https://doi.org/10.1146/annurev-nutr-071816-064902
- Cell (Hallmarks of aging)
- https://doi.org/10.1016/j.cell.2013.05.039

Autophagy, Fasting, and Ketosis in Aging — Mechanisms and Therapeutic Implications

◆ 1. Introduction

Aging is characterized by the progressive decline in cellular repair, metabolic flexibility, and stress resistance. Among the most important adaptive processes influencing aging are autophagy, fasting, and ketosis.

These processes are evolutionarily conserved survival mechanisms that:

- Enhance cellular repair
- Improve metabolic efficiency
- Reduce accumulation of cellular damage

Understanding their interconnection provides insight into **how lifestyle and metabolism influence aging biology**.

◆ 2. Autophagy: The Cellular Recycling System

Definition:

Autophagy is a lysosome-mediated degradation process that removes:

- Damaged organelles
- Misfolded proteins
- Cellular debris

Types:

- Macroautophagy
- Microautophagy
- Chaperone-mediated autophagy

Function:

- Maintains cellular homeostasis
- Prevents toxic accumulation
- Supports longevity

🔷 3. Fasting: A Metabolic Switch

Definition:

Fasting is the voluntary or physiological absence of caloric intake leading to metabolic adaptation.

Phases of fasting:

1. **Fed state** → glucose metabolism
2. **Post-absorptive state** → glycogen use
3. **Fasting state** → fat breakdown
4. **Prolonged fasting** → ketosis

Key Effects:

- ↓ Insulin
- ↑ Glucagon
- ↑ AMPK activation
- ↓ mTOR signaling

👉 These changes **activate autophagy**

🔷 4. Ketosis: The Alternative Energy State

Ketosis is a metabolic state in which the body shifts from using glucose (sugar) as its primary energy source to using ketone bodies, which are produced from the breakdown of fats in the liver.

Ketosis is a metabolic state where the body produces ketone bodies:

- Beta-hydroxybutyrate (BHB)
- Acetoacetate

Trigger:

- Prolonged fasting
- Low carbohydrate intake

Function:

- Provides energy to brain and muscles
- Reduces oxidative stress
- Improves mitochondrial efficiency

🧠 Simple Explanation

Normally, your body runs on **glucose** from carbohydrates.

But when carbohydrate intake is low (or during fasting), the body:

1. Uses stored glucose (glycogen) first
2. Then starts breaking down fat
3. The liver converts fat into **ketone bodies**
4. These ketones become the **main fuel**, especially for the brain

👉 This state is called **ketosis**

⚡ Why is Ketosis Important?

- Provides **alternative energy** for the brain
- Helps in **fat burning**
- May reduce **oxidative stress**
- Linked with **autophagy activation**

🔷 5. Molecular Link: Autophagy, Fasting, and Ketosis

Core signaling pathways:

1. mTOR (Mechanistic Target of Rapamycin)

- Inhibits autophagy
- Active in fed state

2. AMPK (Energy Sensor)

- Activates autophagy
- Active during fasting

🔷 6. Role in Hallmarks of Aging

Hallmark	Effect
Loss of proteostasis	Autophagy removes damaged proteins
Mitochondrial dysfunction	Mitophagy improves function
Deregulated nutrient sensing	Fasting restores balance
Cellular senescence	Reduces accumulation of damaged cells
Stem cell exhaustion	Enhances regeneration

🔷 7. Autophagy and Longevity

Evidence:

- Caloric restriction extends lifespan
- Fasting mimicking diets improve healthspan
- Autophagy activation linked to longevity genes

Mechanisms:

- Reduced oxidative stress
- Improved protein quality control
- Enhanced metabolic efficiency

🔷 Conclusion

Autophagy, fasting, and ketosis form a **powerful interconnected network** that regulates cellular health and aging. By modulating nutrient sensing pathways, these processes enhance repair mechanisms, reduce damage accumulation, and improve metabolic resilience.

They represent a key bridge between **lifestyle interventions and molecular aging biology**, making them highly relevant for both research and clinical practice.

📚 Scientific References

1. Mizushima N. Autophagy: process and function (*Cell*)
2. Longo VD. Fasting and longevity (*Cell Metabolism*)
3. Madeo F et al. Caloric restriction and aging (*Nature Reviews*)
4. Newman JC et al. Ketogenic metabolism (*Cell Metabolism*)
5. López-Otín C et al. Hallmarks of Aging (*Cell*)

OMAD and Autophagy – AMPK pathway activation

Fasting or OMAD (One meal a day) triggers a powerful cleanup crew in your cells called autophagy. This process sweeps away damaged parts, recycling them into fresh energy and vital building blocks. As a result, your body enjoys healthier aging, a stronger metabolism, less inflammation, and more efficient cellular repair. By triggering autophagy through fasting, you may shield yourself from age-related diseases, boost insulin sensitivity, and keep inflammation at bay.

The primary benefits of autophagy include cellular cleanup and recycling, which contribute to anti-aging, increased longevity, and disease prevention by removing toxic proteins and damaged cellular components.

Autophagy also enhances metabolic health, such as improved insulin sensitivity and weight regulation, supports brain function by providing protection against neurodegenerative diseases like Alzheimer's and Parkinson's, strengthens the immune system, and reduces inflammation.

This process maintains cellular health, supplies energy during periods of stress, and protects against chronic conditions, thereby improving overall cellular renewal and function.

A growing body of evidence indicates that intermittent fasting or calorie restriction can induce adaptive autophagy and extend the longevity of eukaryotic cells.

Cellular stress resulting from energy scarcity signals cells to activate autophagy, a process in which old and dysfunctional components are broken down and recycled for fuel and cellular renewal.

Ketosis occurs when glucose stores are depleted, prompting the body to shift to fat as its primary energy source. This metabolic state further promotes autophagy.

The One Meal A Day (OMAD) dietary approach significantly influences cellular energy-sensing pathways, resulting in the activation of AMP-activated protein kinase (AMPK) and the induction of autophagy.

Once activated, **AMP-activated protein kinase (AMPK)** inhibits the mechanistic Target of Rapamycin Complex 1 (mTORC1). The mTORC1 pathway typically promotes cell growth and prevents the breakdown of cellular components when nutrients are abundant, such as after a large meal.

Note - The OMAD diet often leads to hunger, fatigue, irritability, headaches, and dizziness due to fluctuations in blood glucose levels. Individuals may also experience nutrient deficiencies, digestive issues, reduced metabolic rate, or elevated cholesterol and blood pressure. This dietary approach is not suitable for everyone, particularly those who are pregnant, breastfeeding, managing diabetes, have a history of eating disorders, or live with chronic illnesses.

Research indicates that consuming only one meal per day may elevate blood pressure and cholesterol levels, particularly when that meal consists of highly processed or high-carbohydrate foods. Additional risks associated with fasting include shakiness and physical weakness.

Nutrient deficiencies represent a significant concern, as it is challenging to obtain all essential vitamins and minerals in a single meal. Over time, this can result in fatigue or compromised immune function. Digestive issues, such as bloating or gastrointestinal discomfort, may also arise from consuming a large volume of food in one sitting.

Glycation, Advanced Glycation End Products (AGEs), and Impaired Autophagy in Aging

🔬 What is Glycation?

Definition:

Glycation is a non-enzymatic biochemical process in which reducing sugars, such as glucose or fructose, react with proteins, lipids, or nucleic acids to form unstable intermediate compounds that subsequently undergo complex rearrangements to generate advanced glycation end products (AGEs). This spontaneous reaction is driven by elevated circulating glucose levels and occurs progressively with aging.

Unlike enzymatic modifications, glycation is uncontrolled and leads to structural and functional alterations of biomolecules. The accumulation of AGEs contributes to protein cross-linking, impaired cellular function, increased oxidative stress, and activation of inflammatory pathways. As a result, glycation is strongly associated with tissue stiffness, chronic inflammation, and the pathogenesis of age-related diseases, including diabetes, cardiovascular disorders, and neurodegenerative conditions such as Alzheimer's disease.

Fasting and caloric restriction may help mitigate glycation by reducing circulating glucose levels, improving insulin sensitivity, and activating cellular repair mechanisms such as autophagy. These effects collectively decrease the formation and accumulation of AGEs, thereby contributing to improved metabolic and cellular health.

👉 **Glycation is not a hallmark of aging by itself**, but it is **strongly connected to multiple hallmarks**, especially:

1. Loss of Proteostasis

- Glycation damages proteins → misfolding
- Leads to accumulation of dysfunctional proteins

2. Disabled Autophagy

- Glycated proteins become harder to degrade
- Impaired autophagy → accumulation of AGEs

3. Mitochondrial Dysfunction

- AGEs increase ROS production
- Damages mitochondrial proteins

4. Altered Intercellular Communication

- AGEs bind to RAGE receptors
- Trigger inflammation ("inflammaging")

⚠️ **What is Glycation and Why It Is Detrimental**

Glycation is detrimental because it **irreversibly damages essential biological molecules**, especially proteins, and the body has limited ability to repair or remove these modifications.

👉 **Mostly harmful in biological systems**

Why it is bad:

- Alters protein structure
- Reduces enzyme activity
- Causes protein cross-linking
- Increases oxidative stress
- Triggers chronic inflammation

🔥 **What are AGEs (Advanced Glycation End Products)?**

AGEs are:

- Irreversibly modified proteins/lipids
- Accumulate with age
- Strong drivers of:
    - Diabetes complications
    - Cardiovascular disease
    - Neurodegeneration

⛔ **Why Glycation Increases with Age**

- Higher blood glucose exposure over time
- Reduced detoxification capacity
- Decline in proteostasis
- Reduced autophagy
- Increased oxidative stress

🧪 **Does Fasting Help Reduce Glycation?**

👉 **Yes — indirectly and significantly**

Mechanisms:

1. Reduced Glucose Availability

- Less circulating sugar → less glycation reaction

2. Activation of Autophagy

- Fasting → activates autophagy
- Removes glycated/damaged proteins

3. Improved Insulin Sensitivity

- Reduces glucose spikes
- Slows AGE formation

4. Reduced Oxidative Stress

- Less ROS → slower AGE formation

🔁 **Flow Chart (Chain Reaction)**

High Glucose/Aging

↓

Non-enzymatic Glycation

↓

Formation of AGEs

↓

Protein Cross-Linking & Damage

↓

Loss of Proteostasis

↓

↓ Autophagy Efficiency

↓

Accumulation of Damaged Proteins

↓

Mitochondrial Dysfunction + ROS ↑

↓

Inflammation (RAGE activation)

↓

Cellular Dysfunction & Aging

🔄 **Fasting Intervention Flow**

Fasting/Caloric Restriction

↓

↓ Blood Glucose Levels

↓

↓ Glycation Rate

↓

↑ Autophagy Activation

↓

Removal of Damaged/Glycated Proteins

↓

Improved Proteostasis

↓

Reduced Inflammation & Oxidative Stress

↓

Slower Aging Progression

Scientific References

1. National Center for Biotechnology Information. (2020). *Advanced glycation end products*. Retrieved from
2. Singh, R., et al. (2014). *Advanced glycation end-products: A review*. Retrieved from
3. Uribarri, J., et al. (2010). *Glycation and aging*. Retrieved from
4. Ott, C., et al. (2014). *Role of advanced glycation end products in cellular signaling*. Retrieved from
5. Stadtman, E. R. (2006). *Protein oxidation and aging*. Retrieved from
6. Rubinsztein, D. C., et al. (2011). *Autophagy and aging*. Retrieved from
7. López-Otín, C., et al. (2013). *The hallmarks of aging*. Retrieved from
8. Mizushima, N., & Komatsu, M. (2011). *Autophagy: Renovation of cells and tissues*. Retrieved from
9. de Cabo, R., & Mattson, M. P. (2019). *Effects of intermittent fasting on health and aging*. Retrieved from
10. Li, J., et al. (2012). *Advanced glycation end products and Alzheimer's disease*. Retrieved from

Disabled Autophagy – Hallmark of Aging

Disabled Autophagy as a Hallmark of Aging

Autophagy is a tightly regulated intracellular degradation system that maintains cellular homeostasis by recycling damaged organelles, misfolded proteins, and other cytoplasmic components. In young, healthy cells, this process operates efficiently as a quality-control and adaptive survival mechanism. However, with aging, autophagic activity becomes progressively impaired—this decline is now widely recognized as a core feature of biological aging.

1. Conceptual Framework: Why Autophagy Matters in Aging

Autophagy functions as a "cellular renewal system." It balances biosynthesis with degradation, ensuring that cellular components remain functional. Aging disrupts this balance, leading to accumulation of cellular damage. Importantly, autophagy is not merely a waste-disposal pathway—it is deeply integrated with metabolic sensing, stress responses, and longevity pathways.

2. Molecular Basis of Declining Autophagy

a. Dysregulation of Nutrient-Sensing Pathways

Key signaling pathways that regulate autophagy become altered with age:

- **mTOR (mechanistic Target of Rapamycin):** Chronically activated in aging, suppresses autophagy initiation.
- **AMPK (AMP-activated protein kinase):** Reduced activation diminishes autophagic induction during energy stress.
- **Insulin/IGF-1 signaling:** Hyperactivity inhibits autophagic flux.

b. Impaired Autophagic Machinery

There is reduced expression and function of essential autophagy-related genes (ATGs), leading to:

- Inefficient autophagosome formation
- Defective cargo recognition
- Reduced lysosomal fusion

c. Lysosomal Dysfunction

Even when autophagosomes form, degradation fails due to:

- Decline in lysosomal acidity
- Reduced activity of hydrolases
- Accumulation of indigestible material (e.g., lipofuscin)

3. Types of Autophagy Affected in Aging

- **Macroautophagy:** General bulk degradation declines significantly.
- **Mitophagy:** Selective removal of damaged mitochondria is impaired, leading to mitochondrial dysfunction and ROS accumulation.
- **Chaperone-mediated autophagy (CMA):** Reduced substrate recognition due to decreased LAMP-2A receptor levels.

4. Cellular Consequences

a. Proteostasis Collapse

Accumulation of misfolded and aggregated proteins contributes to neurodegenerative diseases such as Alzheimer's and Parkinson's.

b. Mitochondrial Dysfunction

Failure of mitophagy leads to:

- Increased oxidative stress
- Reduced ATP production
- Activation of apoptotic pathways

c. Cellular Senescence

Damaged components trigger stress responses that push cells into a senescent state, characterized by irreversible growth arrest and pro-inflammatory secretions (SASP).

d. Stem Cell Exhaustion

Autophagy is essential for stem cell maintenance; its decline impairs regenerative capacity.

5. System-Level Impact

At the tissue and organismal level, defective autophagy contributes to:

- Chronic inflammation ("inflammaging")
- Metabolic disorders (e.g., insulin resistance)
- Increased susceptibility to age-related diseases

6. Experimental and Clinical Correlations

- Genetic enhancement of autophagy (e.g., ATG overexpression) extends lifespan in model organisms.
- Pharmacological agents like rapamycin, spermidine, and caloric restriction mimic autophagy activation and show longevity benefits.
- Human studies correlate reduced autophagic markers with aging tissues and degenerative diseases.

7. Integrative Perspective

Disabled autophagy should not be viewed in isolation but as part of an interconnected network of aging hallmarks. It interacts with:

- Genomic instability
- Epigenetic alterations

- Loss of proteostasis
- Deregulated nutrient sensing

Thus, impaired autophagy acts both as a **driver** and an **amplifier** of aging processes.

8. Key Takeaway for Advanced Understanding

Rather than a simple "decline in degradation," disabled autophagy represents a **systems-level failure of cellular renewal**, where defective clearance, impaired signaling, and reduced adaptability converge. This transforms autophagy from a protective mechanism into a bottleneck that accelerates cellular and organismal aging.

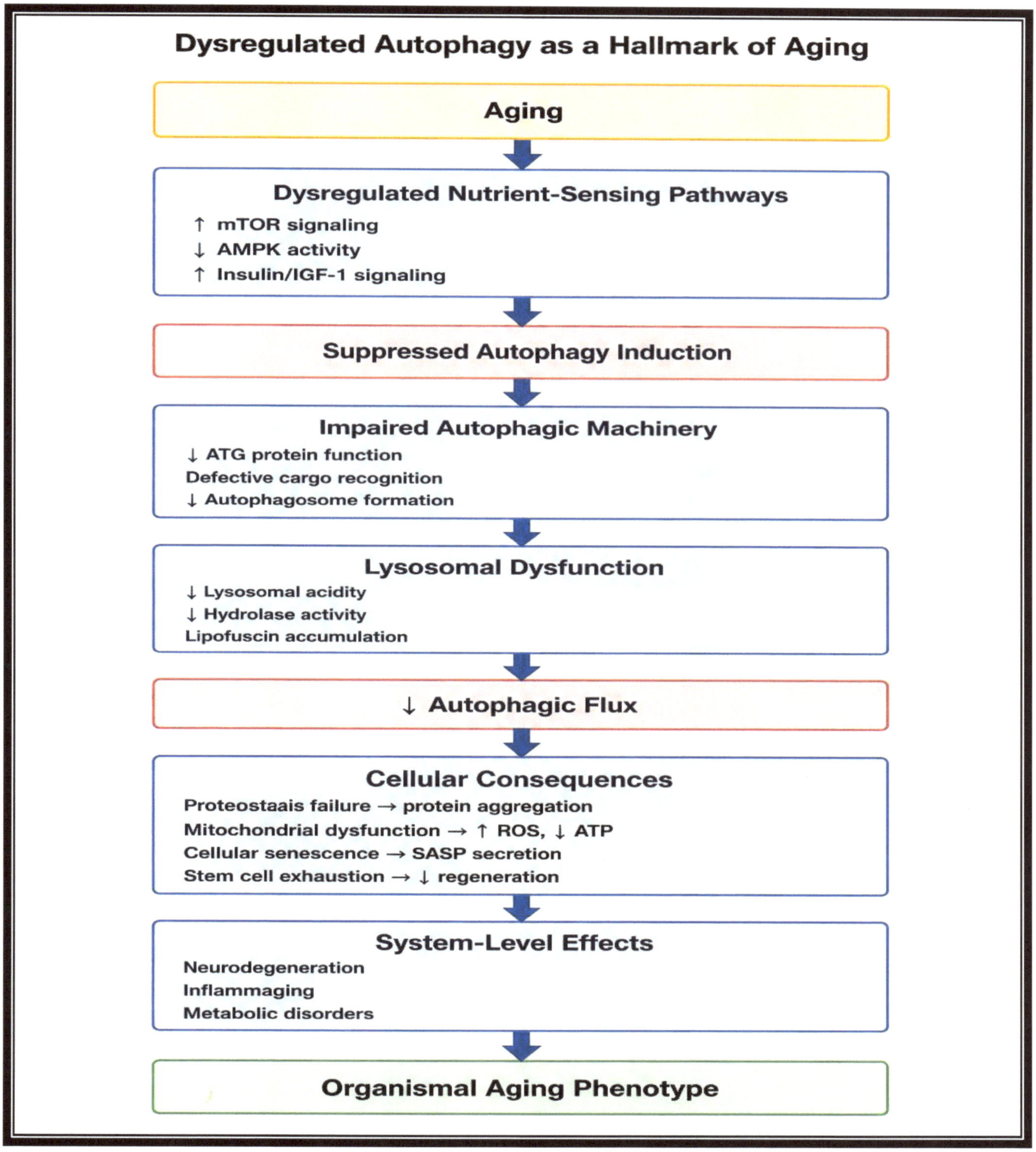

mTOR vs Autophagy: Mutual Inhibition

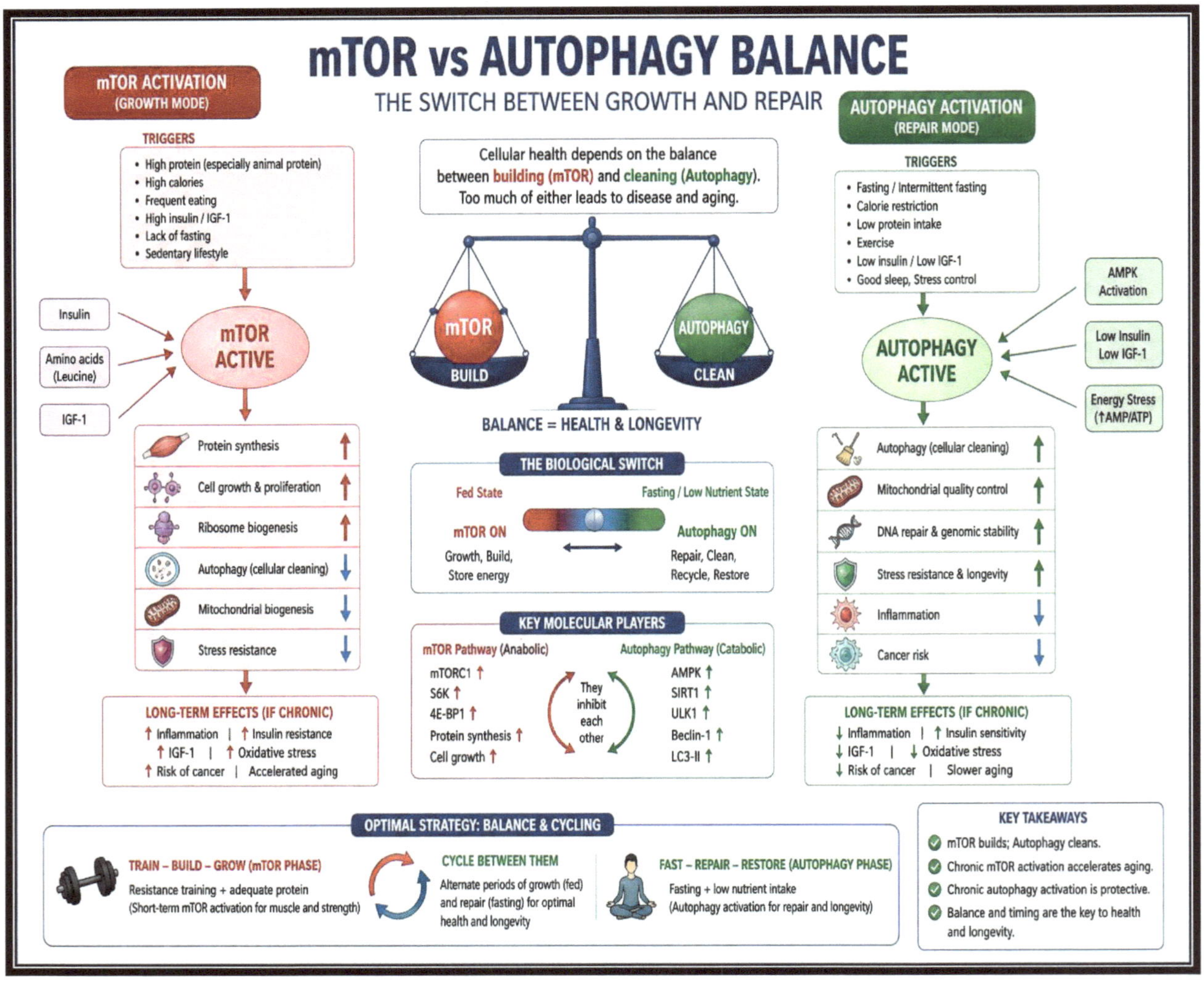

mTOR (growth pathway) and **Autophagy (repair pathway)** cannot be fully active at the same time.

👉 When one is ON → the other is OFF

🟠 **1. How mTOR Inhibits Autophagy**

🔬 **Mechanism:**

mTORC1 directly inhibits **ULK1** (key autophagy initiator protein)

Without ULK1 → autophagy cannot start

👉 Pathway:

High nutrients → ↑ mTOR → ⛔ ULK1 → ❌ Autophagy

Analogy:

🏗️ Construction (mTOR) is ON

🧹 Cleaning crew (autophagy) is blocked

👉 “Don’t clean, keep building”

🟢 **2. How Autophagy Pathways Inhibit mTOR**

🔬 **Mechanism:**

AMPK (energy sensor) inhibits mTOR

AMPK activates **TSC2** → suppresses mTOR

Also activates **ULK1** → starts autophagy

👉 Pathway:

Low energy/fasting → ↑ AMPK → ⛔ mTOR → ✅ Autophagy

🧹 **Analogy:**

🔋 Efficient battery detected

🛑 Stop construction

🧹 Start cleaning & repair

👉 "Pause growth, fix the system"

⚖️ **Why This Mutual Inhibition Exists**

🧠 **Biological Logic:**

Cells must choose:

Condition	Priority
Plenty nutrients	Growth (mTOR)
Stress/low energy	Repair (Autophagy)

👉 Running both together would be:
❌ Energy inefficient
❌ Biologically conflicting

⚠️ **Clinical Insight (High Yield)**

Chronic mTOR ON →

Cancer risk ↑

Aging ↑

Chronic autophagy ON →

Muscle loss ⚠️

👉 Balance is key

🔥 **3. ↑ Cancer Risk (In Some Contexts)**

🔬 **What happens biologically:**

Cancer =
👉 **Uncontrolled cell growth**

Now connect:

↑ IGF-1 → stimulates proliferation

↑ mTOR → promotes growth

↓ Autophagy → damaged cells NOT removed

👉 Perfect environment for: mutated cells to survive + grow

⚠️ Chronic autophagy ON →

Muscle loss ⚠️

👉 Balance is key

📚 Scientific References

(Autophagy, Fasting, AMPK, Aging)

1. Autophagy & Aging (Hallmark Concept)

- Carlos López-Otín et al., *Cell (2013)*
- https://doi.org/10.1016/j.cell.2013.05.039
- Updated Hallmarks (includes autophagy relevance)
- https://doi.org/10.1016/j.cell.2022.11.001

2. Fasting, Caloric Restriction & Autophagy

- Nature Reviews Molecular Cell Biology
- https://doi.org/10.1038/nrm.2016.28
- Cell Metabolism (Fasting & longevity)
- https://doi.org/10.1016/j.cmet.2019.02.018
- New England Journal of Medicine (Intermittent fasting review)
- https://doi.org/10.1056/NEJMra1905136

3. AMPK–mTOR Pathway & Autophagy

- Nature (AMPK–mTOR signaling)
- https://doi.org/10.1038/nature11872
- Cell Research
- https://doi.org/10.1038/cr.2013.86

4. Autophagy Mechanism & Cellular Homeostasis

- Nature (Autophagy overview – Yoshinori Ohsumi work)
- https://doi.org/10.1038/nature15371
- Nature Reviews Molecular Cell Biology
- https://doi.org/10.1038/s41580-018-0008-6

5. Autophagy, Neuroprotection & Disease

- Lancet Neurology
- https://doi.org/10.1016/S1474-4422(15)00038-4
- Cell Stem Cell
- https://doi.org/10.1016/j.stem.2017.11.010

6. Ketosis & Metabolic Switching

- Cell Metabolism
- https://doi.org/10.1016/j.cmet.2015.09.001
- Cleveland Clinic
- https://my.clevelandclinic.org/health/articles/24003-ketosis

7. Clinical Risks of OMAD/Fasting

- American Journal of Clinical Nutrition
- https://doi.org/10.1093/ajcn/87.4.961
- National Institutes of Health
- https://www.nia.nih.gov/health/intermittent-fasting

📚 🔬 Open-Access (PMC Articles)

- https://pmc.ncbi.nlm.nih.gov/articles/PMC3106288/
- https://pmc.ncbi.nlm.nih.gov/articles/PMC5783752/
- https://pmc.ncbi.nlm.nih.gov/articles/PMC6520897/
- https://pmc.ncbi.nlm.nih.gov/articles/PMC7996517/

Chapter-9

What is Epigenetics?

🔷 1. Definition of Epigenetics

Epigenetics refers to **heritable and reversible changes in gene expression that occur without alteration in the DNA sequence**.

👉 In simple terms:

- DNA = "genetic code"
- Epigenetics = "switches that turn genes ON or OFF"

These modifications regulate **when, where, and how genes are expressed**, thereby determining cellular identity and function.

🔷 2. Epigenetics as a Hallmark of Aging

Epigenetic alterations are one of the key hallmarks of aging. Over time, cells undergo:

- **Aberrant DNA methylation patterns**
- **Histone modifications**
- **Chromatin remodelling changes**

👉 These changes lead to:

- Dysregulated gene expression
- Reduced cellular repair
- Increased susceptibility to disease

🔷 3. Core Epigenetic Mechanisms

3.1 DNA Methylation

- Addition of a **methyl group (CH_3)** to DNA
- Typically silences gene expression

👉 Function:

- Controls gene activity
- Maintains cellular identity

📌 Aging Effect:

- Global hypomethylation + site-specific hypermethylation
- Leads to genomic instability and disease

3.2 Histone Modification

- Chemical changes to histone proteins
- Alters chromatin structure

👉 Result:

- DNA becomes more or less accessible for transcription

3.3 Non-coding RNA Regulation

- miRNAs regulate gene expression post-transcriptionally

🔷 4. Role of MTHFR and Folate Cycle

The **MTHFR gene** plays a central role in epigenetics.

Mechanism:

- Converts folate → **methyl folate (active form)**
- Produces **S-adenosylmethionine (SAM)**
- SAM acts as the **universal methyl donor**

👉 Importance:

- Supports DNA methylation
- Maintains epigenetic stability

📌 Dysfunction →

- Impaired methylation
- Increased disease risk (cardiovascular, neurological)

🔷 5. Epigenetics and Cellular Regeneration

Epigenetics regulates:

- **Cell proliferation**
- **Differentiation and dedifferentiation**
- **Tissue repair mechanisms**

👉 Key Concept:

Cells can be "reprogrammed" into a **more youthful or stem-like state**, enhancing regeneration.

📌 Example:

- Induced pluripotent stem cells (iPSCs)

🔷 6. Lifestyle Modulation of the Epigenome

Epigenetic patterns are **highly dynamic and modifiable** by environmental factors.

6.1 Diet

- Mediterranean diet (fruits, vegetables, healthy fats)
- Contains epigenetic modulators (polyphenols, flavonoids)

👉 Examples:

- Curcumin (turmeric)
- Catechins (green tea)

6.2 Physical Activity

- Improves DNA methylation patterns
- Enhances mitochondrial function

6.3 Stress and Sleep

- Chronic stress → accelerates epigenetic aging
- Adequate sleep → maintains epigenomic stability

6.4 Environmental Exposure

- Toxins (pollution, pesticides, plastics)
- Negatively affect gene regulation

6.5 Sunlight and Vitamin D

- Vitamin D regulates >200 genes
- Influences immune and metabolic pathways

6.6 Caloric Restriction & Fasting

- Activates longevity pathways
- Modifies epigenetic marks
- Promotes healthy aging

🔷 7. Nutrigenomics: Definition and Concept

Nutrigenomics is the study of **interaction between nutrients and genes**.

👉 It answers two key questions:

11. How do genes affect nutrient metabolism?
12. How do nutrients influence gene expression?

🔷 8. Mechanism of Nutrigenomics

- Nutrients act as **signaling molecules**
- Modify epigenetic marks (methylation, histones)
- Influence metabolic pathways

👉 Example:

- Diet can activate or suppress genes linked to obesity, diabetes, or cancer

🔷 9. Personalized Medicine and Nutrigenomics

- Genetic testing (blood/saliva)
- Customized diet plans
- Targeted disease prevention

📌 Clinical relevance:

- Obesity
- Metabolic syndrome
- Cancer risk

🔷 10. Epigenetics vs Nutrigenomics (High-Yield Table)

Feature	Epigenetics	Nutrigenomics
Definition	Gene regulation without DNA change	Interaction of diet & genes
Focus	Environment & gene expression	Nutrients & gene response
Mechanism	DNA methylation, histones	Nutrient signaling
Application	Aging, disease regulation	Personalized nutrition

👉 Simple analogy:

- Epigenetics = **control system**
- Nutrigenomics = **diet influencing that control system**

🔷 11. Integration with Hallmarks of Aging

Epigenetics interacts with multiple hallmarks:

Hallmark	Epigenetic Role
Genomic instability	DNA repair gene regulation
Mitochondrial dysfunction	Metabolic gene control
Loss of proteostasis	Protein synthesis regulation
Cellular senescence	Gene silencing
Nutrient sensing	Diet–gene interaction

👉 Leads to a **self-amplifying aging cycle**

🔷 12. Summary (Exam-Oriented)

- Epigenetics = reversible regulation of gene expression
- DNA methylation is a key mechanism
- MTHFR & folate cycle are essential for methylation
- Lifestyle significantly influences epigenetic aging
- Nutrigenomics enables personalized medicine
- Both are central to **healthy aging and disease prevention**

📚 Scientific References

- Carlos López-Otín et al., *Cell (2013)*
- https://doi.org/10.1016/j.cell.2013.05.039
- Nature Reviews Molecular Cell Biology (Epigenetics review)
- https://doi.org/10.1038/nrm.2016.59
- Nature Reviews Genetics (DNA methylation)
- https://doi.org/10.1038/nrg.2017.80
- Annual Review of Nutrition (Nutrigenomics)
- https://doi.org/10.1146/annurev-nutr-071816-064902
- National Institutes of Health
- https://www.genome.gov/about-genomics/fact-sheets/Epigenomics-Fact-Sheet
- Epigenetics and aging (PMC)
- https://pmc.ncbi.nlm.nih.gov/articles/PMC3581015/

Genome, Epigenome, and Phenotype: Understanding the Flow of Biological Information

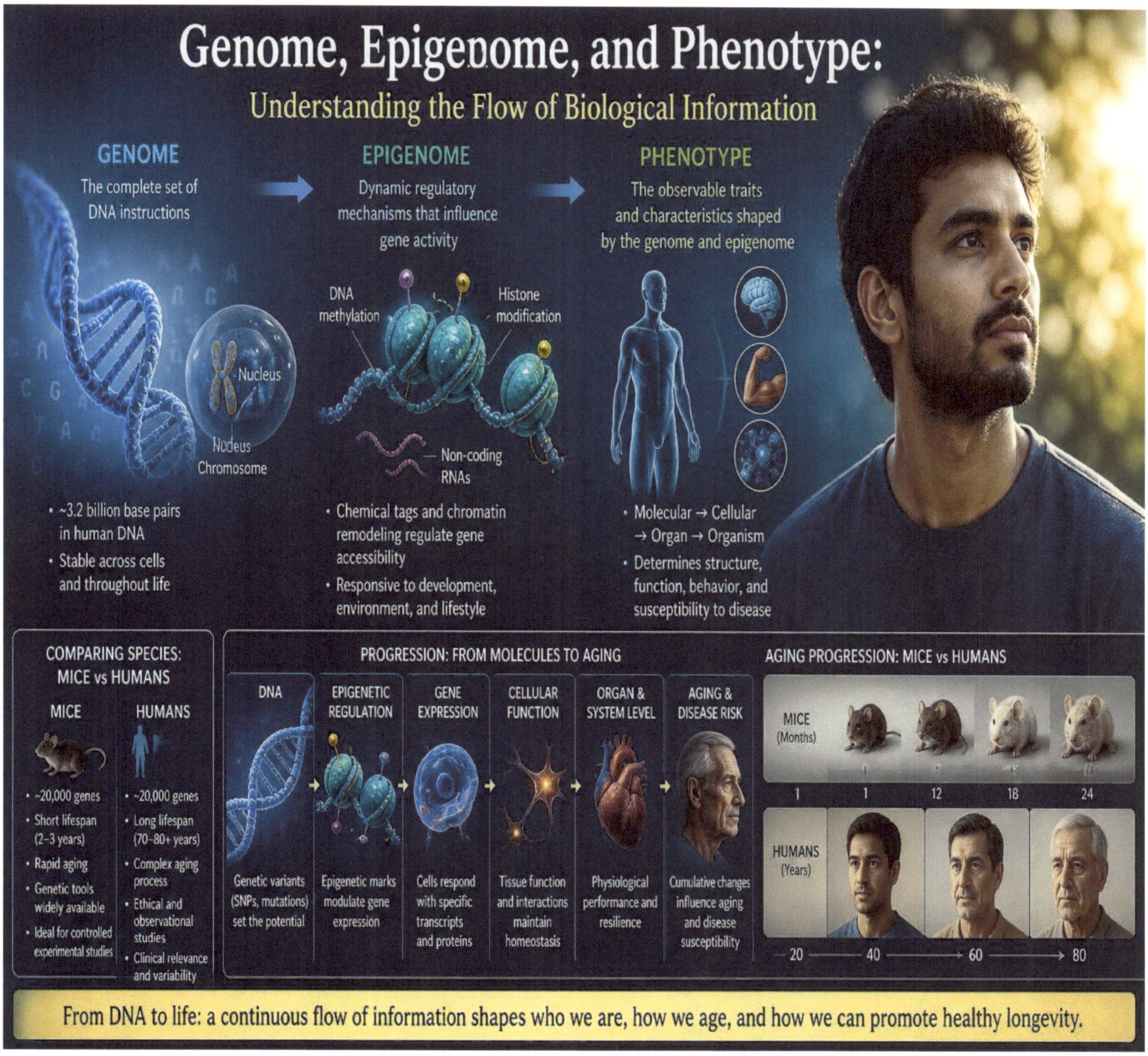

To understand epigenetics and its role in aging, it is important to first distinguish between three closely related concepts: the genome, the epigenome, and the phenotype.

1. Genome

The **genome** refers to the complete set of genetic material (DNA) present in an organism. It contains all the genes that provide instructions for building and maintaining the body.

The concept of the genome was comprehensively mapped through efforts such as the Human Genome Project, which helped identify and sequence human DNA.

👉 Key idea:

The genome is relatively **stable** and does not change significantly over an individual's lifetime (except for mutations).

2. Epigenome

The **epigenome** consists of chemical modifications that regulate how genes are turned "on" or "off" without altering the underlying DNA sequence.

These modifications include:

- DNA methylation
- Histone modification
- Chromatin remodelling

Epigenetic changes are influenced by:

- Diet and nutrition
- Environmental exposures
- Stress and lifestyle

👉 Key idea:

The epigenome is **dynamic and responsive**, and plays a central role in the **hallmarks of aging**, particularly epigenetic alterations.

3. Phenotype

The **phenotype** refers to the observable characteristics of an individual, such as physical traits, biochemical properties, and physiological functions.

Phenotype is shaped by:

- Genetic factors (genome)
- Epigenetic regulation (epigenome)
- Environmental influences

👉 Key idea:

Phenotype is the **final outcome**—what we actually see as the result of interactions between genes and environment.

Connecting the Three

A simple way to understand their relationship:

- **Genome → provides the blueprint**
- **Epigenome → controls how the blueprint is used**
- **Phenotype → represents the final outcome**

This relationship is central to understanding aging, as environmental and lifestyle factors can modify the epigenome over time, leading to changes in gene expression and ultimately influencing health, disease, and longevity.

🧠 Meaning of "Clinical Phenotypes"

📘 Simple Definition

Clinical phenotypes are the observable signs, symptoms, and characteristics of a disease as seen in a patient.

🔬 Break It Down

🧬 Genotype

- Genetic makeup (DNA)
- Not directly visible

👁 Phenotype

- What is expressed or observed
- Includes physical traits + biological Behavior

🩺 Clinical Phenotype

👉 What a doctor actually **sees, measures, or diagnoses**

🧾 **Examples**

🧠 **Example 1: Fatigue**

- **Underlying biology:** NAD^+ ↓, mitochondrial dysfunction
- **Clinical phenotype:**

  👉 Low energy, tiredness, poor stamina

🧴 **Example 2: Skin Aging**

- **Underlying biology:** DNA repair ↓, oxidative stress ↑
- **Clinical phenotype:**

  👉 Wrinkles, dull skin, slow healing

🧠 **Example 3: Metabolic Syndrome**

- **Underlying biology:** Insulin resistance, cortisol ↑
- **Clinical phenotype:**

  👉 Belly fat, high sugar, high BP

🧠 **Example 4: Neurodegeneration**

- **Underlying biology:** Neuronal damage, NAD^+ ↓
- **Clinical phenotype:**

  👉 Memory loss, cognitive decline

👉 So:

Clinical phenotype = final visible outcome of all internal biological processes

Clinical phenotypes represent the observable manifestations of underlying molecular and cellular dysfunction in the human body.

💡 **Even Simpler**

Clinical phenotype = what the patient feels and what the doctor sees.

📊 **Diagram: From Genotype → Phenotype → Clinical Phenotype**

🧬 ***"From DNA to Disease Manifestation"***

GENOTYPE
(Genetic Blueprint – DNA)
A, T, C, G sequence
Encodes biological potential

↓

Influenced by:
Nutrition | Stress | Environment
Hormones | Lifestyle | Aging

↓

EPIGENOME
(Regulatory Layer)
"Librarian/Volume Knob"
Controls gene expression

↓

PHENOTYPE
(Biological Function)
Protein synthesis
Cellular behavior
Metabolism & repair

↓

When Homeostasis is Maintained:
⚖️ Balanced Function
↓
HEALTHY STATE

When Homeostasis is Lost:
↓

CELLULAR DYSFUNCTION
Mitochondria ↓
DNA Repair ↓
Inflammation ↑

↓

CLINICAL PHENOTYPE
(Observable Outcomes)
Fatigue
Skin Aging/Pigmentation
Hair Fall
Metabolic Syndrome
Cognitive Decline

🧠 **Mini Interpretation**

Genetic information (genotype) provides the biological blueprint, while the epigenome regulates how this information is expressed. The resulting phenotype reflects cellular function. When homeostasis is disrupted, these changes manifest as clinical phenotypes—the observable signs and symptoms of disease.

GENOTYPE (DNA)
↓
EPIGENOME (Control System)
↓
PHENOTYPE (Cell Function)
↓
HOMEOSTASIS ⚖️/IMBALANCE
↓
CLINICAL PHENOTYPE (Disease)

Epigenetic Alterations – Hallmark of Aging

🧬 Epigenetics and Mitochondrial Function in Health, Aging, and Disease

🔬 Epigenetic Regulation of Gene Expression

Epigenetic alterations refer to heritable and reversible changes in gene expression that occur without any modification in the underlying DNA sequence. These changes take place primarily within the cell nucleus and involve chemical modifications of DNA and associated histone proteins, thereby regulating chromatin structure and transcriptional activity.

Key sites of epigenetic modification include:

- **CpG islands**, where DNA methylation occurs
- **Histone tails**, where post-translational modifications such as acetylation and methylation take place

These epigenetic marks are dynamic and can be influenced by environmental factors, diet, aging, and embryonic development, enabling cells to adapt gene expression profiles in response to internal and external stimuli.

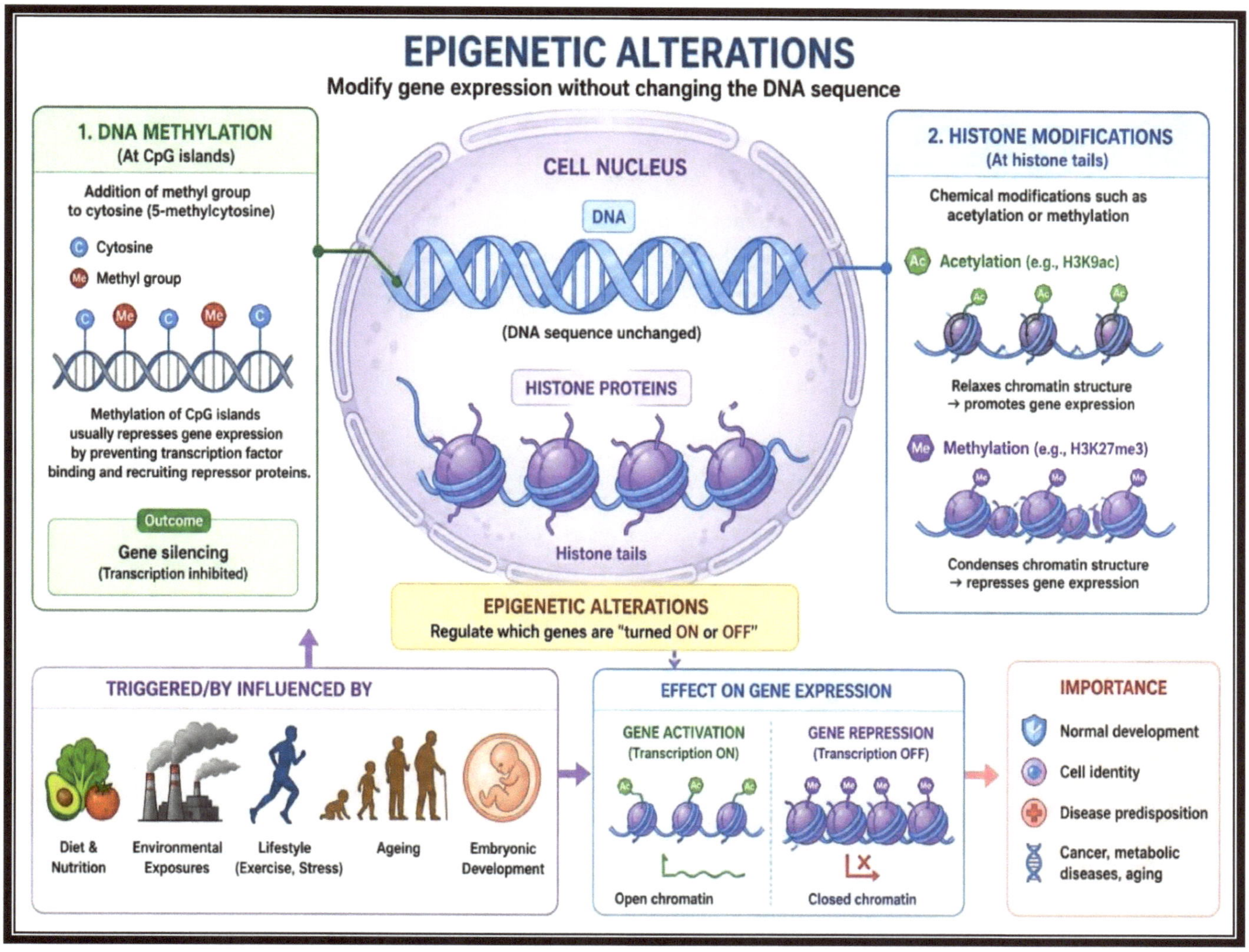

Major Epigenetic Mechanisms

Epigenetic regulation can be broadly classified into three major mechanisms:

1. **DNA Methylation**

   This involves the addition of a methyl group to cytosine residues, primarily at CpG dinucleotides, catalysed by DNA methyltransferases (DNMTs). DNA methylation generally leads to transcriptional repression by inhibiting transcription factor binding and recruiting repressor complexes.

2. **Histone Modifications**

   post-translational modifications of histone proteins—including acetylation, methylation, phosphorylation, and ubiquitination—alter chromatin structure and regulate gene accessibility. For example:

   - Histone acetylation → chromatin relaxation → gene activation
   - Histone methylation → context-dependent activation or repression

3. **Non-coding RNAs (ncRNAs)**

   Regulatory RNAs such as microRNAs (miRNAs) and long non-coding RNAs (lncRNAs) modulate gene expression at transcriptional and post-transcriptional levels.

Mitochondria: Structure and Functional Significance

Mitochondria are essential organelles responsible for multiple cellular processes, including:

- ATP production through oxidative phosphorylation
- Regulation of cellular metabolism
- Maintenance of metal ion homeostasis
- Control of apoptosis and cell survival

A unique feature of mitochondria is the presence of their own genome (mitochondrial DNA, mtDNA), located within the mitochondrial matrix and distinct from nuclear DNA.

🔁 Epigenetics–Mitochondria Crosstalk

Recent evidence highlights a bidirectional interaction between epigenetic regulation and mitochondrial function:

🔹 Epigenetic Influence on Mitochondria

Epigenetic modifications regulate the expression of nuclear genes encoding mitochondrial proteins, thereby affecting:

- Mitochondrial biogenesis
- Oxidative phosphorylation efficiency
- ATP production

Altered epigenetic patterns can lead to mitochondrial dysfunction, contributing to:

- Neurodegenerative disorders
- Metabolic diseases
- Circadian rhythm disturbances
- Cancer

🔹 Mitochondrial Influence on Epigenetics

Mitochondria regulate the availability of key metabolic intermediates required for epigenetic enzymes, including:

- ATP
- Acetyl-CoA
- NAD^+
- α-ketoglutarate

These metabolites act as cofactors or substrates for chromatin-modifying enzymes, thereby directly influencing epigenetic states and gene transcription.

🧡 Epigenetics, Mitochondria, and vascular disease

The interaction between environmental factors, epigenetic signaling, and mitochondrial metabolism plays a crucial role in vascular health. Dysregulation of this axis contributes to altered vascular phenotype and increased cardiovascular risk.

Environmental exposures across the lifespan induce epigenetic modifications in chromatin, leading to reprogramming of gene expression and functional adaptation. However, maladaptive epigenetic changes can impair mitochondrial function and promote vascular pathology.

Mitochondrial Epigenetics and Inflammation

Mitochondria play a central role in regulating inflammatory responses. Epigenetic modifications affecting mitochondrial function can influence inflammation in both aging and cancer.

A key concept is **"inflammaging"**, a chronic, low-grade inflammatory state associated with aging.

Contributing mechanisms include:

- Increased oxidative stress
- Alterations in mtDNA copy number
- Release of mitochondrial DNA into the cytosol

These factors activate immune signaling pathways and disrupt cellular homeostasis.

Epigenetic modifications involved in mitochondrial regulation include:

- DNA methylation of mtDNA
- Post-translational modifications of mitochondrial proteins
- Regulation by mitochondrial and nuclear non-coding RNAs

Role in Cancer and Aging

Epigenetic remodelling of mitochondrial pathways contributes to tumorigenesis by:

- Promoting abnormal cell proliferation
- Altering immune responses
- Supporting tumor microenvironment development

Mitochondria also regulate inflammatory signaling by modulating:

- Reactive oxygen species (ROS)
- Metabolic intermediates

Thus, mitochondria are often considered **key regulators of the inflammatory response**.

Inflammation and Disease Progression

Inflammation, although essential for immune defence, can become pathological when chronic. It plays a significant role in:

- Cancer progression
- Atherosclerosis
- Type 2 diabetes
- Alzheimer's disease
- Rheumatoid arthritis
- Aging

Various factors such as infections, obesity, smoking, environmental toxins, and alcohol consumption can trigger inflammatory responses.

Epigenetic Changes in mtDNA

Epigenetic modifications of mitochondrial DNA include:

- DNA methylation and hydroxymethylation
- Changes in mtDNA replication and transcription

These alterations contribute to mitochondrial dysfunction and are associated with multiple disease states.

Summary

Epigenetic mechanisms act as critical regulators of gene expression without altering DNA sequence. Their dynamic interaction with mitochondrial function plays a central role in cellular metabolism, inflammation, aging, and disease. Disruption of this finely tuned system leads to mitochondrial dysfunction, altered gene expression, and increased susceptibility to metabolic, cardiovascular, and neurodegenerative diseases.

The "Backup Copy" Theory of Aging and Epigenetic Information Loss

Aging may not simply reflect permanent damage to DNA, but rather a loss of the epigenetic instructions that control cellular function. Crucially, cells are believed to retain a hidden "backup copy" of these original instructions, which can potentially be restored to recover youthful behavior.

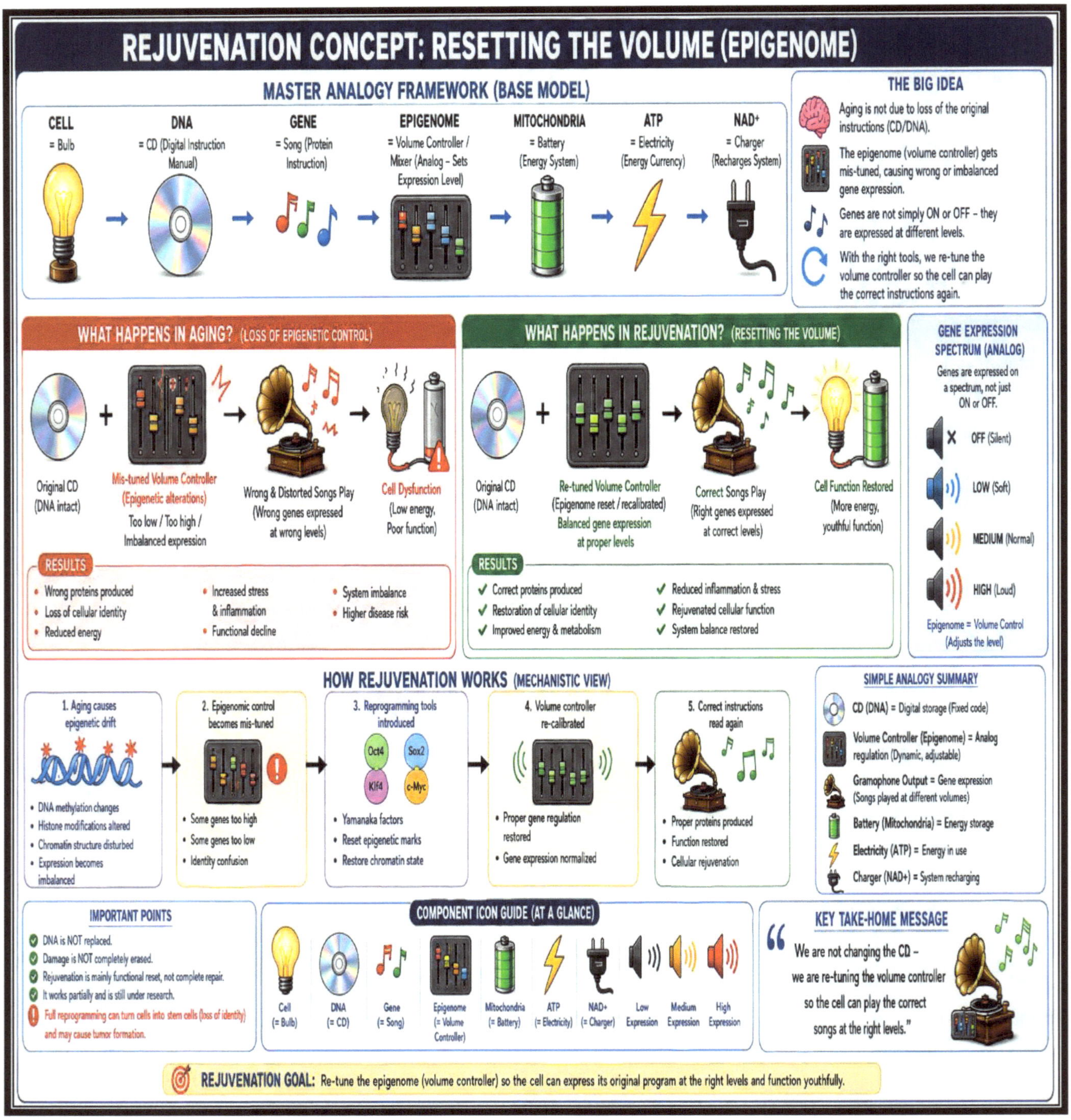

Master Analogy Framework (Base Model)

- Cell = Bulb - Represents overall cellular function and output
- DNA (Genome) = Digital CD (Original Instruction Manual- fixed sequence)

  Fixed sequence: ATCG = code, a stable, digital-like storage system encoding genetic instructions

  Mutation = scratched CD ❌

- Gene = Song 🎵 (protein instruction) - Individual functional units of DNA that encode specific proteins
- Mitochondria = Battery 🔋 (energy source) - Primary energy-generating system
- ATP = Electricity ⚡ (usable cellular energy)
- NAD^+ = Charger 🔌 (recharges system) - Maintains energy metabolism and redox balance
- Epigenetics = Remote 🎚️ (controls which gene/song plays) or Volume Controller/Mixer 🎚️🔊

👉 **DNA = digital-like**

👉 **Epigenome = analog (volume control, not just remote like ON/OFF 🎚️❌)**

Epigenetics = Volume knob 🎚️

Low expression = 🔈

Medium expression = 🔉

High expression = 🔊

🎵 **Gene Expression**

- Correct genes = Right songs 🎶✅ **or Loud music** 🔊
- Wrong genes = Wrong songs 🔊❌ **or No music** 🔇
- Gene activation = Song playing ▶️
- Gene silencing = Song paused ⏸️

⚙️ **Functional States of the Cell**

🟢 Healthy/Young Cell

- Healthy cell = Bright glowing bulb 💡✨
- High energy = Full battery 🔋 + strong light 💡
- Efficient metabolism = Smooth music 🎶 (correct songs)

🟠 **Aging/Dysfunctional Cell**

- Low energy = Dim bulb 💡⚫
- Energy failure = Fused battery 🔋❌
- Cell dysfunction = Flickering bulb 💡⚡
- Severe damage = Dead bulb 💡❌

🎚️ **Epigenetics (Control System)**

Normal epigenetics = Well-tuned volume controller 🎚️✅
(Balanced gene expression at appropriate levels)

Epigenetic damage = Mis-tuned volume controller 🎚️⚠️
(Some genes overexpressed 🔊/others under expressed 🔈)

Epigenetic drift = Gradual loss of tuning/signal distortion 🎚️📉📈
(Progressive imbalance in gene expression with aging)

Reprogramming (Rejuvenation) = Re-calibration of volume controller 🎚️🔄
(Restoration of optimal gene expression levels)

🎼 **CD/Gramophone System (Information Flow)**

- DNA intact = Clean CD 💿✨
- DNA damage = Scratched CD 💿❌
- Cell reading DNA or Cell output = CD playing ▶️ or Music from Gramophone 🎶
- Correct output = Clear music 🎶
- Wrong output = Distorted noise 🔊❌

🔋 Energy System Expansion

- High ATP = Bright electricity ⚡⚡
- Low ATP = Weak current ⚡❌
- Energy failure = Power cut ⚡🚫

🧹 Cell Maintenance System

- Autophagy = Cleaning system 🧹
- Efficient autophagy = Clean room 🧼✨
- Failed autophagy = Garbage accumulation 🗑️❌

🔥 Damage & Stress

- Free radicals = Rust ⚡
- Oxidative stress = Corrosion spreading 🧪
- Inflammation = Slow fire 🔥
- Chronic inflammation = Continuous burning 🔥♨️

🧟 Cell Fate

- Senescent cells = Zombie cells 🧟
- Apoptosis = Programmed shutdown ⛔
- Healthy turnover = Replacement system 🔄

👷 Repair System

- Stem cells = Repair engineers 👷
- Stem cell exhaustion = No engineers 🚫👷

🧬 Aging vs Rejuvenation Summary

🟠 Aging

Volume control mis-tuned 🎚️⚠️
(Gene expression becomes imbalanced — some genes too high 🔊, others too low 🔈)

Distorted gene expression output 🎶🔊❌
(Incorrect proteins produced due to improper expression levels)

Reduced cellular performance 💡⚫
(Dim or unstable functional output)

Declining energy capacity 🔋⚠️
(Mitochondrial inefficiency and reduced ATP production)

Disrupted cellular signaling/output 🔊⚠️
(Loss of harmony in cellular processes)

🟢 Rejuvenation

Volume controller re-tuned 🎚️🔄
(Epigenetic balance restored across genes)

Correct gene expression levels 🎶🔊🔉🔈
(Right genes expressed at appropriate intensity)

Efficient cellular output 🎶✅
(Accurate protein synthesis and function)

High cellular energy state ⚡🔋✅
(Improved mitochondrial function and ATP production)

Healthy cell function 💡 ✨
(Bright, stable, and optimal performance)

💾 **Backup Copy Concept**

👉 **Backup Copy = Original "Clean CD"** 💿 ✨
(Genetic information largely remains intact and preserved)

With aging → CD remains mostly intact, but reading becomes impaired 🎚 ⚠️
(Epigenetic miscalibration affects how instructions are interpreted)

Music (cell function) becomes distorted 🎶🔊❌
(Due to improper regulation of gene expression, not complete loss of information)

👉 **Key Issue:**

Volume control is mis-tuned 🎚 ⚠️

Gene expression becomes imbalanced (🔊 overexpression/ 🔈 under expression)

🔬 **What Happens in Aging?**

Epigenetic control becomes progressively mis-tuned 🎚 ⚠️
(Gene expression regulation loses precision and balance)

Gene expression becomes imbalanced 🎶🔊 🔈
(Some genes are overexpressed 🔊 while others are under expressed 🔈)

Cellular function becomes inefficient and disorganized ⚙️ ⚠️
(Loss of coordinated activity and functional stability)

🔬 **1. Genomic Instability**

Concept:

DNA damage accumulates over time due to environmental and internal stress.

Analogy:

- **DNA CD** 💿 **gets scratched and damaged**
- Instructions become unreadable

👉 Result:

- Wrong proteins
- Cell malfunction

🎚 **2. Epigenetic Alterations**

Gene regulation becomes progressively **dysregulated and imbalanced**, rather than simply turning on or off.

Analogy (Analog Control Model)

Volume controller becomes mis-tuned 🎚 ⚠️
(Loss of precise control over gene expression levels)

Gene expression becomes imbalanced 🎶🔊 🔈
(Some genes are overexpressed 🔊 while others are under expressed 🔈)

👉 **Cellular identity becomes unstable**
(Cells lose their specialized function and regulatory precision)

🔋 **3. Mitochondrial Dysfunction**

Concept:

Reduced energy production + increased ROS

Analogy:

- **Battery 🔋 becomes weak**
- Bulb 💡 flickers

👉 Low energy + more "rust" (damage)

🧹 **4. Loss of Proteostasis**

Concept:

Protein folding and clearance fail

Analogy:

- **Factory produces defective products 🏭❌**
- Garbage not removed

👉 Junk accumulates in cell

🧬 **5. Telomere Attrition**

Concept:

DNA ends shorten with each division

Analogy:

- **DNA protection caps 🧬 get worn out**

👉 Cell stops dividing

⚙️ **6. Deregulated Nutrient Sensing**

mTOR Signaling Pathway

Concept:

Cells misinterpret nutrient signals

Analogy:

- **Fuel system ⛽ becomes confused**
- Either:
    - too much growth
    - or poor energy usage

👉 System imbalance

🧟 **7. Cellular Senescence**

Concept:

Cells stop dividing but don't die

Analogy:

- **Zombie cells 🧟**
- Not working but releasing toxic signals

👉 Harm nearby cells

🔥 **8. Inflammaging**

Inflammaging

Concept:

Chronic low-grade inflammation

Analogy:

- **Slow fire 🔥 inside body**

👉 Continuous damage

👷 **9. Stem Cell Exhaustion**

Concept:

Reduced repair capacity

Analogy:

- **Repair engineers 👷 retire or decrease**

👉 Damage not fixed

📡 **10. Altered Intercellular Communication**

Concept:

Cells stop communicating properly

Analogy:

- **Messages 📩 between cells get distorted**

👉 System-wide dysfunction

💾 **11. Disabled Macroautophagy**

Autophagy

Concept:

Cellular cleaning declines

Analogy:

- **Cleaning system 🧹 stops working**

👉 Waste accumulates

🧬 **12. Dysbiosis (Microbiome Aging)**

Gut Microbiome

Concept:

Gut bacteria imbalance

Analogy:

- **Internal ecosystem 🌱 becomes unhealthy**

👉 Affects immunity, metabolism

🧠 **13. Integrated "Backup Copy" Concept**

(Advanced Concept – David Sinclair Model)

Analogy:

- **Original CD 💿 still exists as backup copy**
- Problem = remote 🎛 misreads instructions

👉 Reset epigenetic control → cell becomes young again

🔄 **Rejuvenation Concept**

👉 Using special tools (like Yamanaka factors):

- We **reset the remote** 🎛
- Cell starts reading the **original clean CD** 💿 again

Yamanaka Factors

These are 4 key proteins:

- Oct4
- Sox2

- Klf4
- c-Myc

👉 **Their role:**

- Reset epigenetic marks
- Restore youthful gene expression

What Rejuvenation Does

Instead of:
❌ fixing every damaged protein/DNA

We:
✔️ reset the **control system (epigenetics)**

👉 Result:

- Cell "remembers" its original function
- Starts behaving like a younger cell

⚠️ **Important Clarification (VERY IMPORTANT)**

- DNA is NOT replaced
- Damage is NOT fully erased
- It's mainly **functional reset**, not complete repair

👉 That's why:

- It works partially
- Still under research

👉 **Using Yamanaka factors:**

Step-by-step:

1. **Reset the Remote** 📱
   - Epigenetic marks corrected
   - Gene control restored
2. **Read the Original CD** 💿 **Again**
   - Correct genes activated
   - Proper proteins produced

👉 Result:

- Cell behaves younger again ✨

"Aging is not because the instruction manual is lost, but because the cell forgets how to read it properly — and the 'backup copy' helps restore the original instructions."

"We are not changing the CD — we are fixing the remote so the cell can play the correct instructions again."

📚 **Scientific References**

Yamanaka Factors & Reprogramming

Induction of Pluripotent Stem Cells – Shinya Yamanaka (Original Paper)

https://www.cell.com/cell/fulltext/S0092-8674(06)00976-7

Partial Reprogramming and Aging Reversal

https://www.nature.com/articles/s41586-020-2975-4

Sinclair (Cell, 2023) for backup copy theory

DNA Methylation and the Methylation Cycle in Health and Disease

Overview of DNA Methylation

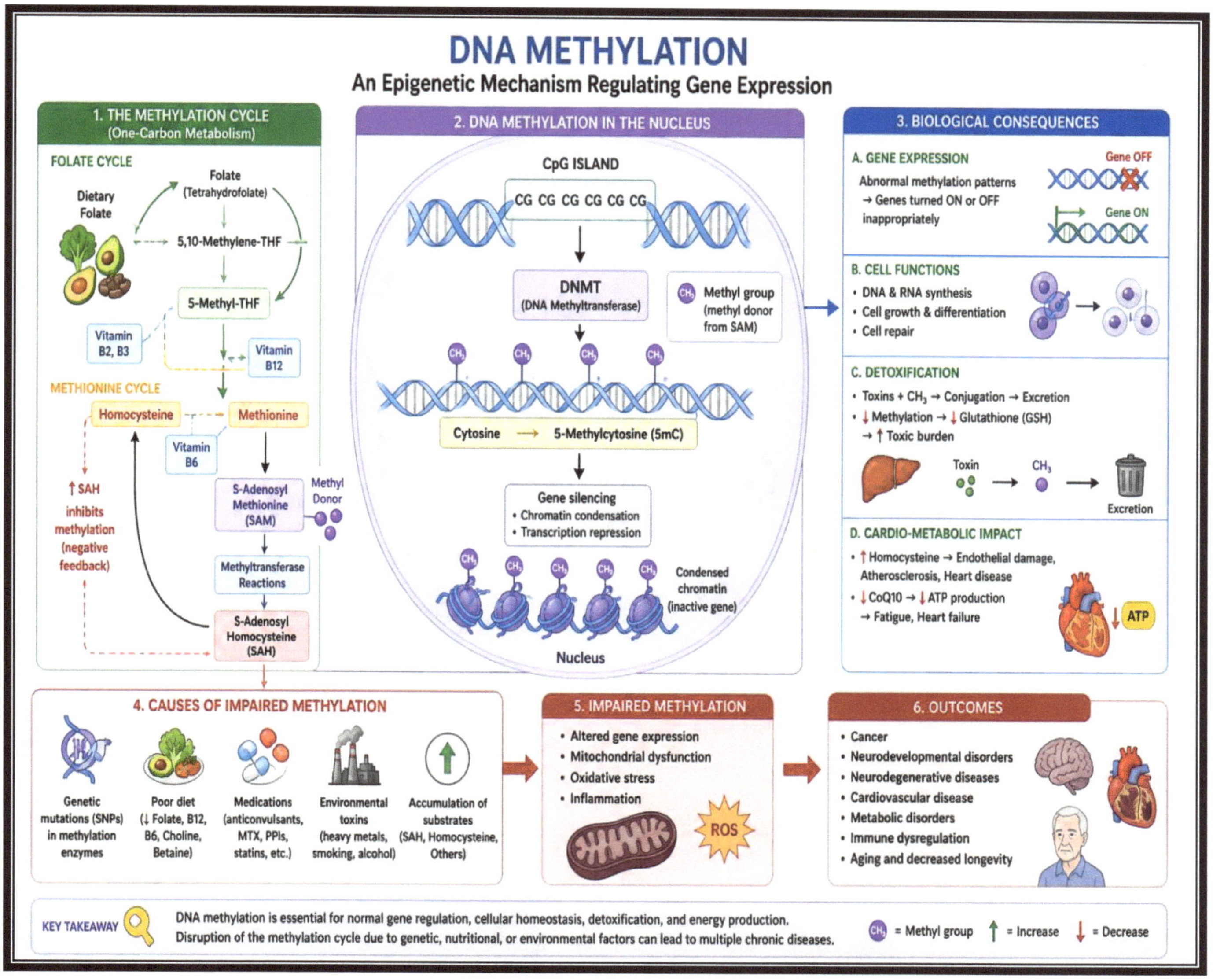

DNA methylation is a key epigenetic mechanism involving the transfer of a methyl group (–CH_3) to cytosine residues, primarily at CpG dinucleotides, catalyzed by DNA methyltransferases (DNMTs). This process regulates gene expression without altering the underlying DNA sequence, typically leading to transcriptional repression.

Methylation is part of a broader one-carbon metabolism pathway, which integrates folate and methionine cycles to maintain cellular homeostasis.

Consequences of Impaired Methylation

Defective methylation can disrupt multiple physiological systems:

1. Altered Gene Expression

- Aberrant DNA and RNA expression patterns
- Increased susceptibility to chronic diseases, including cancer

2. Neurotransmitter Imbalance

- Impaired synthesis and regulation of neurotransmitters
- Associated with psychiatric disorders and neurodevelopmental conditions

3. Impaired Detoxification

- Reduced ability to eliminate toxins, including heavy metals
- Accumulation of harmful metabolites

Regulation of the Methylation Cycle

Efficient methylation depends on the availability of:

- Methyl donors (e.g., folate, vitamin B12)
- Cofactors (e.g., vitamin B6, riboflavin)
- Functional enzymes

The cycle is tightly regulated. Accumulation of intermediate substrates can lead to **negative feedback inhibition**, diverting metabolites into alternative pathways and potentially generating toxic byproducts.

Causes of Methylation Dysfunction

Methylation may be impaired due to:

- **Genetic polymorphisms (SNPs)** affecting key enzymes
- Deficiency of essential vitamins and cofactors
- Drug interactions interfering with metabolic pathways
- Exposure to environmental toxins (e.g., heavy metals)
- Inadequate intake of methyl donors (e.g., methylfolate, methylcobalamin)
- Accumulation of metabolic intermediates within the cycle

Role of Methylation in Cellular Processes

1. Cell Repair

Methylation is essential for RNA synthesis and cellular signaling. During stress, impaired methylation reduces the cell's ability to respond and repair damage effectively.

This is particularly critical in the nervous system, which has high RNA turnover and metabolic demand.

2. Cell Synthesis and Proliferation

Methylation is required for nucleotide synthesis (DNA and RNA building blocks).

Tissues with rapid turnover—such as:

- Bone marrow
- Immune cells (RBCs and WBCs)
- Neural tissue

are especially vulnerable to methylation defects.

3. Detoxification

Methylation contributes to detoxification by facilitating the conjugation and elimination of toxins.

A major consequence of impaired methylation is reduced levels of Glutathione, which plays a central role in:

- Neutralizing reactive oxygen species
- Regenerating antioxidants (vitamins C and E)
- Detoxifying heavy metals and xenobiotics
- Regulating immune responses (cytokine production, lymphocyte activity)
- Supporting DNA synthesis and repair

Methylation and Cardiovascular Disease

Disruption of the methylation cycle can impair the conversion of homocysteine to methionine, leading to **hyperhomocysteinemia**, a well-established risk factor for cardiovascular disease.

Additionally, impaired methylation may reduce levels of Coenzyme Q10 (CoQ10), which is essential for mitochondrial energy production. Low CoQ10 levels are associated with:

- Cardiomyopathy
- Congestive heart failure

Notably, statins—commonly used lipid-lowering drugs—can further decrease CoQ10 levels, potentially exacerbating mitochondrial dysfunction.

Methylation and Energy Metabolism

Methylation plays a crucial role in mitochondrial function by:

- Supporting CoQ10 synthesis
- Regulating fatty acid oxidation

Impaired methylation can compromise cellular energy production, contributing to chronic conditions such as:

- Chronic fatigue syndrome
- Fibromyalgia
- Chronic pain syndromes

Summary

DNA methylation is a fundamental epigenetic process essential for gene regulation, detoxification, cell repair, and energy metabolism. Disruption of the methylation cycle—due to genetic, nutritional, or environmental factors—can lead to widespread metabolic dysfunction and is implicated in numerous chronic diseases, including cardiovascular disorders, neurodegeneration, and fatigue syndromes.

Scientific References

DNA methylation & epigenetics

- https://www.ncbi.nlm.nih.gov/books/NBK26829
- https://www.nature.com/articles/nrg201659

One-carbon metabolism (folate–methionine cycle)

- https://www.ncbi.nlm.nih.gov/pmc/articles/PMC2782876
- https://www.ncbi.nlm.nih.gov/books/NBK2260

Methylation in cancer & gene expression

- https://www.ncbi.nlm.nih.gov/pmc/articles/PMC3762382
- https://www.nature.com/articles/nrc201780

Neuropsychiatric & brain function

- https://www.ncbi.nlm.nih.gov/pmc/articles/PMC4728667
- https://pubmed.ncbi.nlm.nih.gov/23306145

Glutathione & detoxification

- https://www.ncbi.nlm.nih.gov/pmc/articles/PMC4684116
- https://www.ncbi.nlm.nih.gov/books/NBK279396

Vitamins & cofactors

- https://ods.od.nih.gov/factsheets/Folate-HealthProfessional
- https://ods.od.nih.gov/factsheets/VitaminB12-HealthProfessional
- https://ods.od.nih.gov/factsheets/VitaminB6-HealthProfessional

Genetic polymorphisms (MTHFR etc.)

- https://www.ncbi.nlm.nih.gov/pmc/articles/PMC5655818

🧡 **Cardiovascular (homocysteine)**

- https://www.ncbi.nlm.nih.gov/pmc/articles/PMC2672135
- https://www.ahajournals.org/doi/10.1161/CIRCULATIONAHA.109.192703

⚡ **CoQ10 & mitochondria**

- https://www.ncbi.nlm.nih.gov/pmc/articles/PMC5452224
- https://www.ncbi.nlm.nih.gov/pmc/articles/PMC3096178

🔋 **Energy metabolism & fatigue**

- https://www.ncbi.nlm.nih.gov/pmc/articles/PMC6363527
- https://pubmed.ncbi.nlm.nih.gov/26731066

What Is Methylation?

Methylation: Concept, Mechanism, and Clinical Importance

🔬 What is Methylation?

Methylation is a **fundamental biochemical process** in the human body in which a small chemical group called a **methyl group (–CH_3)** is added to other molecules.

👉 This process happens **billions of times per second in every cell**, making it essential for life.

Think of methylation as a **"molecular switch"**:

- It can **turn genes ON or OFF**
- It helps control how cells function, grow, and respond to stress

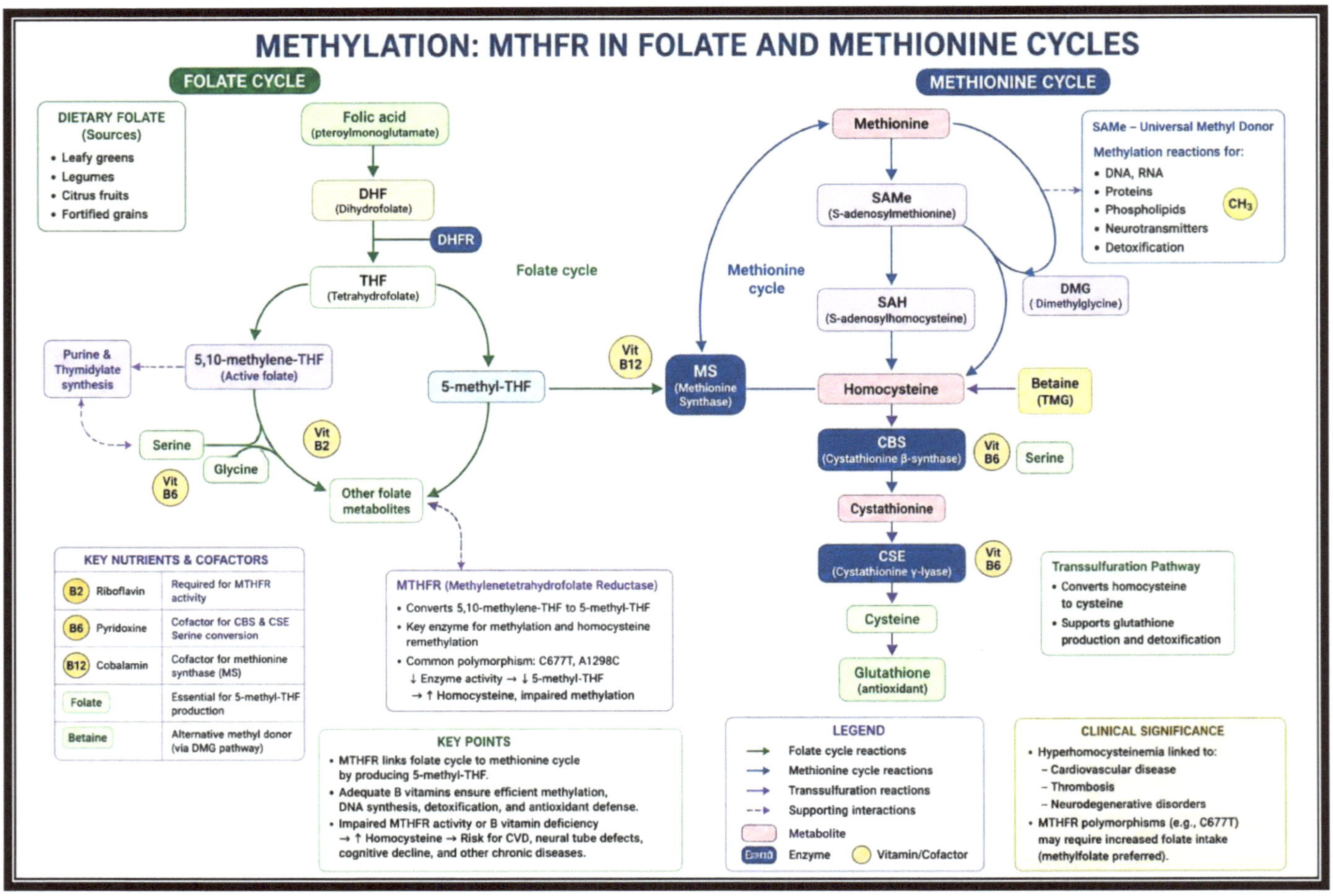

What Is MTHFR?

Why is Methylation Important?

Methylation plays a central role in many vital physiological processes:

1. Gene Regulation

- Controls **gene expression** without changing DNA sequence
- Ensures genes work at the right time and in the right amount

2. DNA Synthesis and Repair

- Required for **formation of DNA and RNA**
- Helps in **repairing damaged DNA**

3. Detoxification

- Adds methyl groups to toxins → makes them easier to remove
- Helps eliminate:
    - Heavy metals
    - Environmental toxins
- Supports production of Glutathione → key detox molecule

4. Cardiovascular Protection

- Regulates levels of homocysteine
- High homocysteine → inflammation + vascular damage

5. Energy Production

- Supports mitochondrial function
- Required for synthesis of:
    - Coenzyme Q10
- Essential for ATP production

6. Nervous System Function

- Helps in neurotransmitter production
- Maintains **myelin sheath (nerve insulation)**

7. Immune Function & Inflammation Control

- Reduces oxidative stress (free radicals)
- Regulates inflammatory pathways

8. Hormonal and Metabolic Regulation

- Helps in:
    - Cholesterol metabolism
    - Hormone synthesis
    - Histamine regulation

Role of the MTHFR Gene

The MTHFR enzyme is a key enzyme in methylation.

Function:

- Converts folate into its **active form (5-methyl-THF)**
- This active folate is required to:
    - Convert homocysteine → methionine
    - Continue the methylation cycle

👉 If MTHFR is not working properly → methylation slows down

🔁 The Methylation Cycle (Step-by-Step)

The methylation cycle involves **4 key molecules**:

1. Methionine

- An amino acid obtained from diet

2. S-adenosylmethionine (SAM)

- The **main methyl donor** in the body
- Gives methyl groups to other molecules

3. S-adenosylhomocysteine (SAH)

- Formed after SAM donates methyl group

4. Homocysteine

- A critical intermediate
- Can either:
    - Be recycled → methionine
    - Or go to detox pathway → cysteine → glutathione

Cycle Summary

Methionine

↓

SAM (methyl donor)

↓

SAH

↓

Homocysteine

↓

↙ ↘

Methionine Cysteine → Glutathione

(recycle) (detox pathway)

🧪 Role of Vitamins (Cofactors)

Methylation depends heavily on B vitamins:

Vitamin	Role
Folate (B9)	Provides methyl groups
Vitamin B12	Converts homocysteine → methionine
Vitamin B6	Helps detox pathway (homocysteine → cysteine)
Riboflavin (B2)	Supports MTHFR enzyme

👉 Important: These must be in **active forms**:

- Folate → 5-MTHF
- B12 → methylcobalamin
- B6 → pyridoxal-5-phosphate

⚠️ What Happens if Methylation is Impaired?

▼ Causes:

- MTHFR gene mutations (SNPs)
- Vitamin deficiencies
- Poor diet
- Toxins (heavy metals)
- Certain medications

▼ Effects:

🧬 Cellular Level:

- Poor DNA repair
- Altered gene expression

🧠 Neurological:

- Neurotransmitter imbalance
- Mood disorders

❤️ Cardiovascular:

- ↑ Homocysteine → heart disease

⚡ Metabolic:

- ↓ Energy production
- Mitochondrial dysfunction

🧹 Detox:

- ↓ Glutathione
- ↑ toxin accumulation

🧠 Clinical Importance

Methylation defects are linked to:

- Cardiovascular disease
- Neurodegenerative disorders
- Cancer
- Chronic fatigue syndrome
- Autism spectrum disorders
- Metabolic syndrome

📘 Summary

Methylation is a vital biochemical process that regulates gene expression, detoxification, energy production, and cellular repair. The MTHFR enzyme plays a central role in maintaining this cycle by activating folate. Disruption of methylation due to genetic, nutritional, or environmental factors can lead to widespread metabolic and clinical disorders.

🧬 Methylation, Methionine Metabolism, and MTHFR Gene Mutations: Clinical Implications in Cellular Function and Disease

Methylation is a fundamental biochemical process that plays a central role in cellular metabolism, gene regulation, detoxification, and overall physiological homeostasis. One of the key outcomes of methylation is the formation of active folate (methyl folate or 5-methyltetrahydrofolate), which is the biologically usable form of vitamin B9 required for critical cellular reactions.

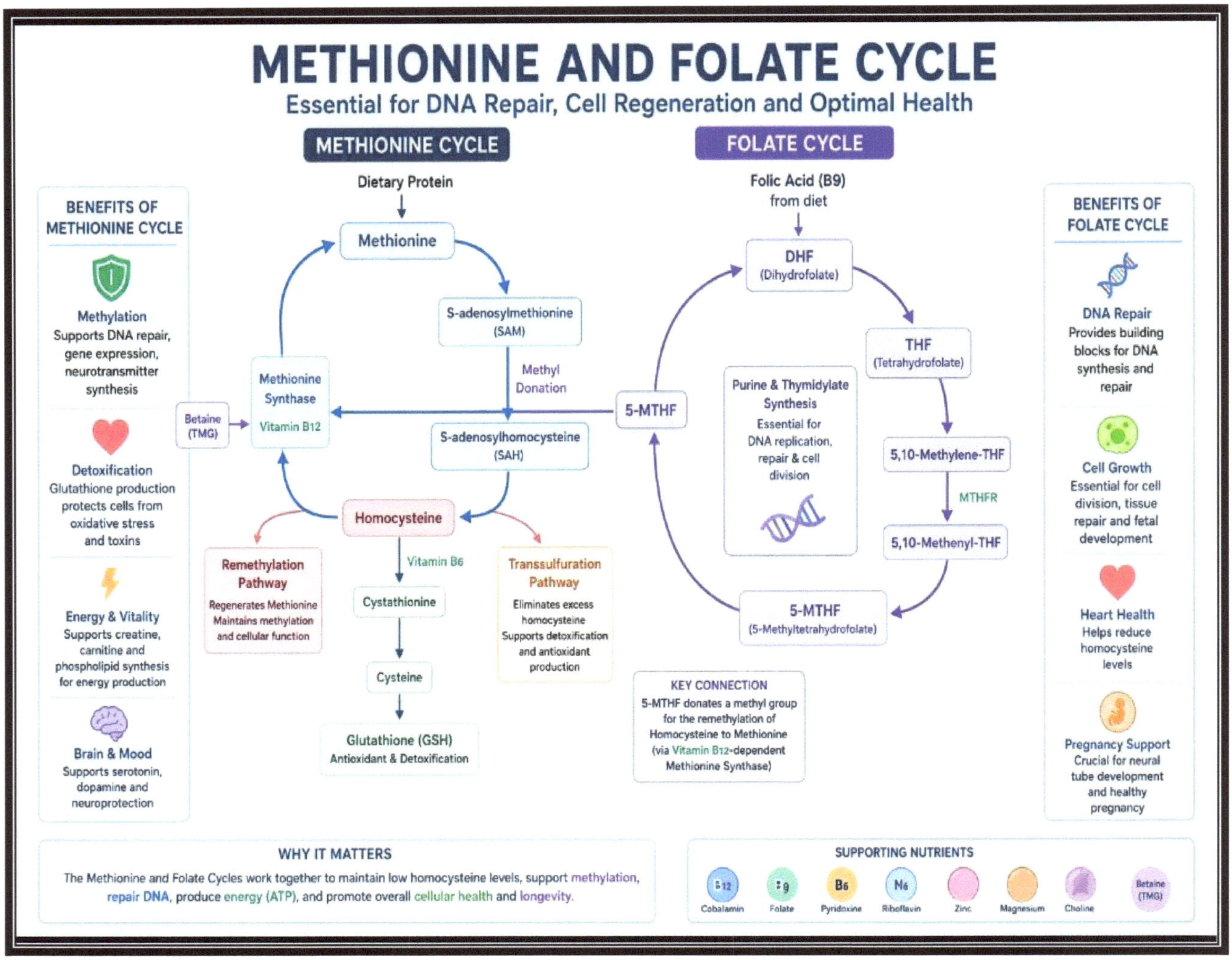

At the core of this pathway lies methionine, an essential sulfur-containing amino acid. Methionine serves multiple vital functions beyond protein synthesis. It acts as a precursor for S-adenosylmethionine (SAM), the universal methyl donor, and contributes significantly to detoxification processes. Through its sulfur group, methionine supports the neutralization and elimination of toxic substances, including heavy metals such as lead. Additionally, it plays roles in reducing histamine levels, supporting antioxidant defences, facilitating estrogen metabolism, and maintaining normal cellular growth and repair.

🧬 MTHFR Gene and Its Functional Significance

The MTHFR enzyme is a key regulatory enzyme in the methylation cycle. It catalyses the conversion of folate into its active form (5-methyl-THF), which is required for the remethylation of homocysteine to methionine.

A mutation in the MTHFR gene results in a **single nucleotide polymorphism (SNP)** that reduces the efficiency of this enzyme. As a result, there is:

- Decreased production of active folate
- Impaired methylation capacity
- Accumulation of homocysteine
- Reduced synthesis of critical biomolecules

Clinical Consequences of MTHFR Mutation

Defective methylation due to MTHFR polymorphisms has widespread systemic effects:

🧠 Neurological and Neuropsychiatric Effects

- Cognitive impairment, memory loss
- Fatigue, weakness, neuropathy

- Increased risk of neurodevelopmental disorders
- Psychiatric conditions such as depression, anxiety, OCD, bipolar disorder, and schizophrenia

Immune and Inflammatory Dysfunction

- Impaired immune response
- Increased susceptibility to autoimmune diseases
- Chronic inflammatory states

Cellular and Genetic Effects

- Impaired DNA and RNA synthesis and repair
- Reduced protein production and cellular turnover
- Increased genomic instability → higher cancer risk

Cardiovascular and Metabolic Effects

- Elevated homocysteine → endothelial damage
- Increased risk of:
    - Stroke
    - Coronary artery disease
    - Thrombosis
- Lipid dysregulation → cholesterol deposition in vessels

Detoxification Impairment

- Reduced production of Glutathione
- Accumulation of:
    - Heavy metals
    - Environmental toxins

Hormonal and Endocrine Effects

- Disruption of estrogen metabolism
- Thyroid, adrenal, and pituitary dysfunction
- Increased risk of metabolic diseases such as diabetes

Neurodegenerative and Systemic Disorders

- Increased susceptibility to:
    - Alzheimer's disease
    - Multiple sclerosis
    - Autism spectrum disorders
    - Crohn's disease

Folic Acid vs. Folate: Clinical Relevance

Although often used interchangeably, **folate** and **folic acid** are not identical:

- **Folate**: Naturally occurring, biologically active form found in foods
- **Folic acid**: Synthetic form that requires enzymatic conversion (via MTHFR) to become active

In individuals with MTHFR mutations:

- Conversion of folic acid is inefficient
- Leads to **functional folate deficiency**, even if intake is adequate

Role of B-Complex Vitamins

The methylation cycle is highly dependent on B vitamins as cofactors:

- Vitamin B9 (folate) → methyl donor
- Vitamin B12 → remethylation of homocysteine

- Vitamin B6 → trans-sulfuration pathway
- Vitamin B2 → supports MTHFR enzyme

Deficiency or improper activation of these vitamins can significantly impair methylation efficiency.

Conceptual Summary

Methylation is a central biochemical pathway linking nutrient metabolism with gene regulation, detoxification, and cellular repair. The MTHFR enzyme plays a pivotal role in maintaining this cycle by generating active folate. Genetic variations in MTHFR can disrupt methylation, leading to widespread metabolic, neurological, cardiovascular, and immunological consequences. Understanding these mechanisms is essential for developing targeted nutritional and therapeutic interventions.

Vitamin B9 (Folate and Folic Acid): Clinical and Biochemical Overview

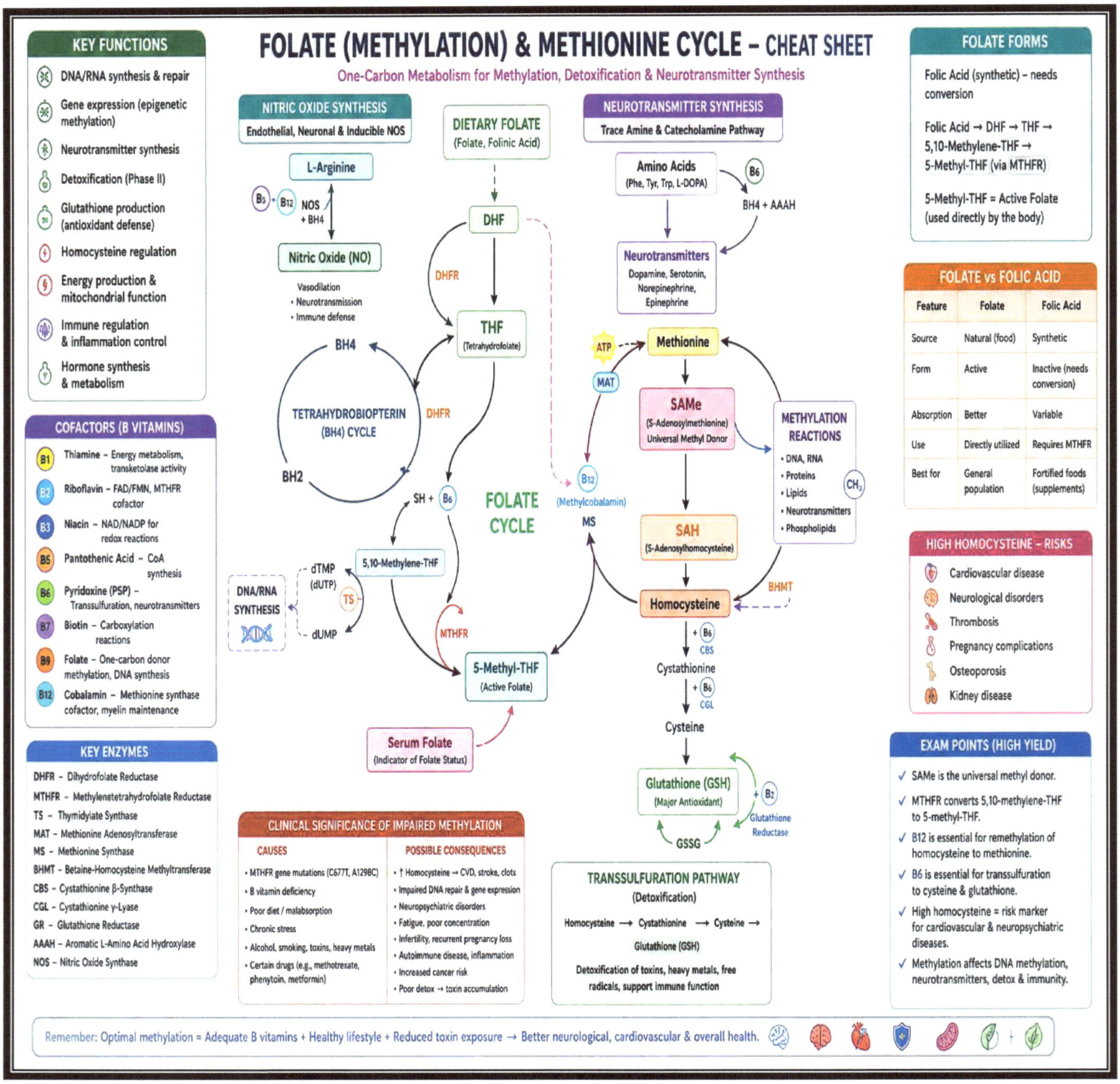

1. Introduction to Vitamin B9

Vitamin B9 is an essential water-soluble vitamin that naturally exists in the form of **folate**. It plays a critical role in **one-carbon metabolism**, which is fundamental for:

- DNA synthesis and repair
- Cell division and growth
- Methylation reactions

Due to its central role in rapidly dividing tissues, vitamin B9 is particularly important in **pregnancy, hematopoiesis, and cellular regeneration**.

2. Clinical Consequences of Folate Deficiency

Deficiency of vitamin B9 can lead to multiple systemic effects:

Cardiovascular Risk

- Low folate levels impair the remethylation of homocysteine to methionine
- This leads to **elevated homocysteine levels (hyperhomocysteinemia)**
- Associated with increased risk of:
    - Atherosclerosis
    - Ischemic heart disease
    - Stroke

Pregnancy and Fetal Development

- Folate is essential for proper **neural tube development**
- Deficiency during early pregnancy can result in:
    - Neural tube defects (e.g., spina bifida, anencephaly)

Cancer Risk

- **Low dietary folate** is associated with impaired DNA repair and genomic instability → increased cancer risk
- However, **excess folic acid supplementation** may:
    - Promote growth of pre-existing malignant cells
    - Be associated with increased risk of certain cancers (e.g., prostate cancer)

  👉 This highlights the importance of **balanced folate status rather than excess supplementation**

3. What is Folate? (Natural Form)

Folate refers to a group of naturally occurring vitamin B9 compounds found in food.

Key Features

- Derived from the Latin word *"folium"* (leaf)
- Rich sources:
- Leafy green vegetables
- Legumes
- Fruits

Metabolic Activation

- Dietary folate is converted in the body into its active form:
- 👉 **5-methyltetrahydrofolate (5-MTHF)**
- This active form participates directly in:
    - DNA synthesis
    - Methylation cycle

4. What is Folic Acid? (Synthetic Form)

Folic acid is the **synthetic, oxidized form of vitamin B9**, commonly used in:

- Nutritional supplements
- Fortified foods (e.g., flour, cereals)

Key Characteristics

- Chemically stable
- Requires metabolic conversion to become active

5. Differences in Metabolism: Folate vs Folic Acid

Folate (Natural Form)

- Easily converted to **5-MTHF**
- Directly usable by the body

Folic Acid (Synthetic Form)

- Requires conversion via:
    - Dihydrofolate reductase (DHFR)
- Conversion occurs mainly in the **liver**

Clinical Issue

- Conversion can be:
    - Slow
    - Inefficient (especially in individuals with genetic variants like MTHFR)

👉 Result:

- Accumulation of **unmetabolized folic acid** in circulation
- Potential metabolic and clinical implications

6. Integration with Methylation Cycle

Vitamin B9 plays a central role in the **methylation pathway**:

Folate → 5-MTHF → donates methyl group → Homocysteine → Methionine → SAMe

👉 This supports:

- DNA methylation
- Neurotransmitter synthesis
- Detoxification

7. Key Take-Home Points (Exam-Oriented)

- Folate = natural form of vitamin B9
- Folic acid = synthetic form requiring activation
- Active form = **5-MTHF**
- Deficiency → ↑ homocysteine, anemia, developmental defects
- Excess folic acid → potential adverse effects (controversial)
- Central role in **DNA synthesis and methylation**

8. Simple Conceptual Summary

Think of vitamin B9 as a **"biochemical builder and regulator"**:

- It helps build DNA
- It regulates gene expression through methylation
- It maintains cardiovascular and neurological health

👉 But balance is critical:

- Too little → deficiency disorders
- Too much (synthetic form) → possible dysregulation

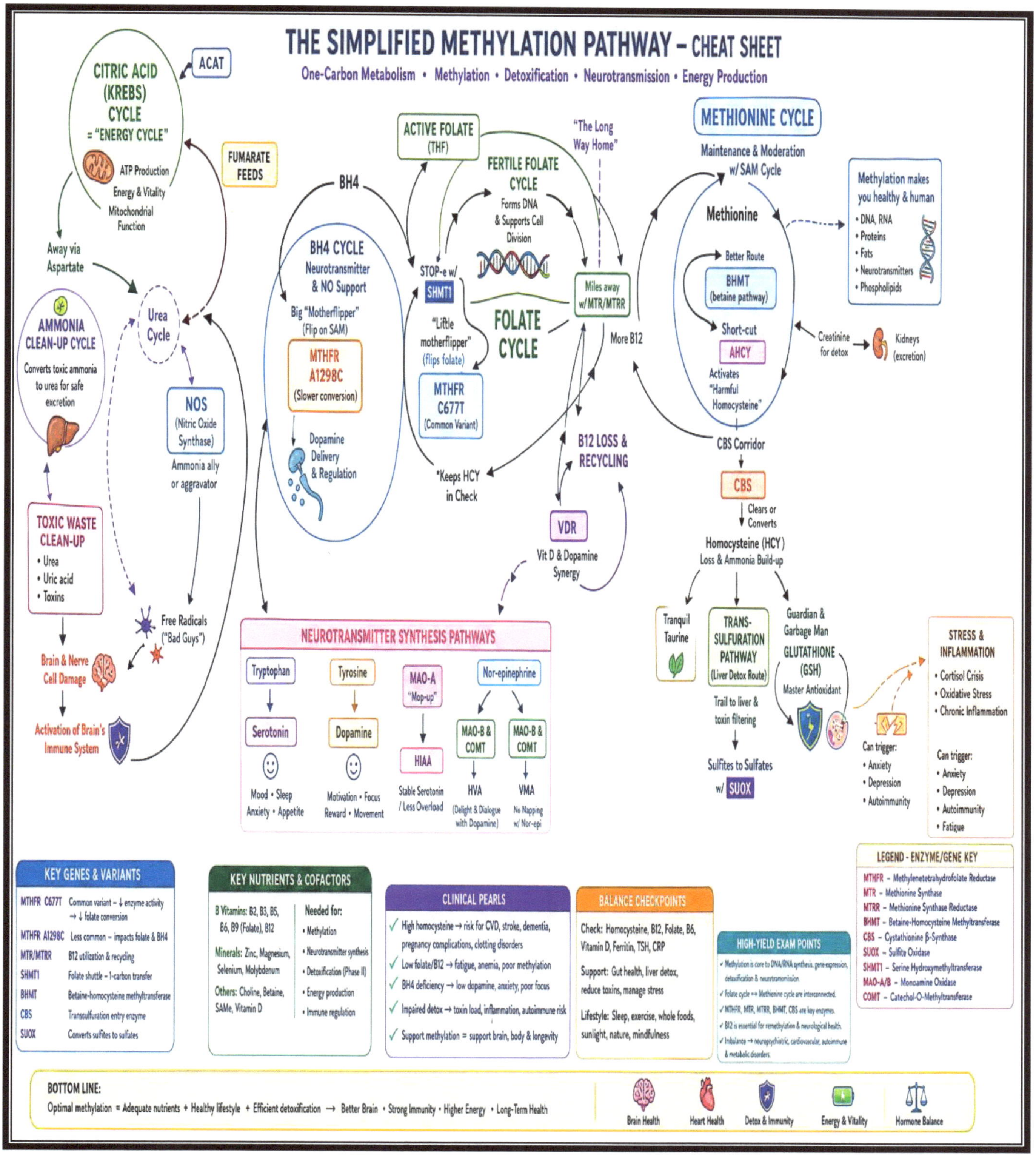

Methylation Balance and DNA Methylation in Health and Disease

1. Understanding Methylation Balance (Over-methylation Concept)

Methylation is a fundamental biochemical process in which the body transfers a **methyl group (–CH_3)** to different molecules. This process regulates **gene expression, neurotransmitters, detoxification, and cellular repair**.

For optimal health, methylation must remain **balanced**—neither too low nor too high.

What is Over-methylation?

Over-methylation occurs when there is an **excess availability of methyl groups** in the body. This may happen due to:

- High intake of methyl-donating supplements (e.g., folic acid, methylfolate, methyl-B12)
- Altered enzyme activity in the methylation cycle
- Imbalance in neurotransmitter metabolism

How Over-methylation Affects the Body

Excess methylation can **over-activate certain biochemical pathways**, especially those involved in **brain chemistry and gene regulation**.

Neurological & Psychological Effects

- Anxiety and overthinking
- Poor sleep or insomnia
- Brain fog and low mental clarity
- Depression or paranoia
- ADHD-like symptoms

👉 Mechanism:

Over-methylation can alter levels of key neurotransmitters such as **serotonin, dopamine, and norepinephrine**, leading to imbalance in mood and cognition.

Physical Symptoms

- Fatigue
- Sensitivity to light, chemicals, or foods
- Dry eyes and dry mouth
- Digestive disturbances
- Skin issues

👉 These symptoms arise due to **altered detoxification pathways and cellular signaling**.

Clinical Insight

- Over-methylation is often described as a state of **"excess calm but poor drive"**, in contrast to under-methylation, which is linked to irritability and inflammation.
- Evidence is still evolving, but clinically, maintaining **methylation balance** is key rather than simply increasing methyl donors.

2. DNA Methylation: A Core Epigenetic Mechanism

What is DNA Methylation?

DNA methylation is a type of **epigenetic modification** where a methyl group is added to DNA (usually at **CpG sites**).

👉 Important:

- It **does NOT change the DNA sequence**
- It **changes gene expression (ON/OFF regulation)**

Physiological Role

DNA methylation is essential for:

- Regulation of gene activity
- Embryonic development
- Genomic stability
- X-chromosome inactivation
- Suppression of harmful or unnecessary genes

3. When DNA Methylation Goes Wrong (Dysregulation)

DNA methylation can be **beneficial or harmful**, depending on where and how it occurs.

A. Hypermethylation (Too Much Methylation)

- Leads to **gene silencing**
- Problematic when it silences **tumor suppressor genes**

Example

- **BRCA1 gene**
    - Normally repairs DNA damage
    - When methylated → gene is silenced → ↑ cancer risk (breast & ovarian)
- **CDKN2A gene**
    - Controls cell cycle progression
    - Methylation → loss of control → uncontrolled cell growth

👉 Result: Increased risk of **cancer progression**

B. Hypomethylation (Too Little Methylation)

- Leads to **gene overactivation**
- Can activate **oncogenes (cancer-promoting genes)**

👉 Result:

- Genomic instability
- Increased mutation rate
- Cancer development

4. DNA Methylation and Disease Connection

Cancer

- Tumor suppressor genes → **silenced by hypermethylation**
- Oncogenes → **activated due to hypomethylation**
- Leads to uncontrolled cell proliferation

Cardiovascular Disease

- Abnormal methylation affects genes involved in:
    - Inflammation
    - Lipid metabolism
    - Vascular function

Neurodegenerative Disorders

- Altered methylation affects:
    - Neuronal survival
    - Synaptic function
    - Memory pathways

Examples: Alzheimer's disease, Parkinson's disease

5. Integrating Methylation with Cellular Function

Methylation is tightly linked with:

- **Folate cycle**
- **Methionine cycle**
- **Homocysteine metabolism**
- **Neurotransmitter synthesis**
- **Detoxification pathways**

👉 Imbalance in methylation leads to:

- Altered gene expression
- Impaired detoxification
- Neurotransmitter imbalance
- Increased oxidative stress

6. Key Concept

- Methylation = **transfer of CH_3 group → regulates gene expression**
- DNA methylation = **epigenetic silencing mechanism**
- Over-methylation → **neurotransmitter imbalance + cognitive symptoms**
- Hypermethylation → **tumor suppressor gene silencing**
- Hypomethylation → **oncogene activation**
- Balance is crucial for:
    - Brain function
    - Detoxification
    - Cardiovascular health
    - Cancer prevention

7. Simple Narrative Flow

Think of methylation as a **"biochemical switch system"** in the body:

- When properly balanced → genes function normally, brain works efficiently, toxins are cleared
- When excessive → brain becomes overstimulated or dysregulated
- When defective → harmful genes may activate, leading to disease

At the DNA level, methylation acts like a **dimmer switch**:

- Too much dimming → important protective genes turn OFF
- Too little dimming → harmful genes turn ON

🧬 What is Under-Methylation (Hypomethylation)?

Under-methylation means the body has **too few methyl groups ($–CH_3$)** available for important biochemical processes.

👉 In simple terms:

"The body is not able to methylate enough."

This leads to **reduced activity of methylation-dependent pathways**, affecting:

- Gene regulation
- Neurotransmitter balance
- Detoxification
- DNA repair

⚙️ Why Does Under-Methylation Occur?

🔹 **Nutritional Causes**

- Deficiency of:
    - Vitamin B9 (folate)
    - Vitamin B12
    - Vitamin B6
- Low intake of methyl donors (methionine, choline)

◆ **Genetic Causes**

- Mutations in enzymes like:
    - **MTHFR**
    - Methionine synthase

👉 These reduce efficiency of the methylation cycle

◆ **Other Causes**

- Chronic stress
- Toxin exposure
- Poor diet
- Chronic illness

How Under-Methylation Affects the Body

1. Neurotransmitter Imbalance

Low methylation → ↓ production of:

- Serotonin
- Dopamine

👉 Leads to:

- Depression
- Low motivation
- Anxiety (different from over-methylation type)

2. Gene Expression Problems

- Inadequate DNA methylation → genes may be **inappropriately active**
- Can contribute to:
    - Cancer (oncogene activation)
    - Inflammation

3. Detoxification Impairment

- Poor methylation → ↓ glutathione production
- Toxins accumulate

👉 Leads to:

- Fatigue
- Chemical sensitivity

4. High Homocysteine Levels

- Methionine cycle slows down
- Homocysteine builds up

👉 Increases risk of:

- Cardiovascular disease
- Stroke

⚠️ Common Symptoms of Under-Methylation

🧠 Psychological

- Depression
- Low mood
- Low motivation
- Poor focus

💪 Physical

- Fatigue
- Poor detoxification
- Allergies
- Chronic inflammation

🧬 Cellular

- Impaired DNA repair
- Increased oxidative stress

Under vs Over Methylation

Feature	Under-Methylation	Over-Methylation
Methyl groups	Low	Excess
Mood	Depression	Anxiety
Energy	Low	Variable
Sleep	Often poor	Often poor
Neurotransmitters	Low serotonin/dopamine	Imbalanced/excess activity
Homocysteine	High	Normal/low

Mechanism (Simple Flow)

Low Folate/B12 → ↓ Methylation → ↓ SAMe → Poor methyl transfer →

- Neurotransmitter imbalance
- DNA instability
- ↑ Homocysteine
- Disease risk

🎯 Key Points

- Under-methylation = **reduced methyl donor availability**
- Leads to:
- ↑ Homocysteine
- ↓ neurotransmitters
- ↓ detox capacity
- Strongly linked to:
- Depression
- Cardiovascular disease
- Aging-related disorders

🧠 **Simple Analogy**

Think of methylation as a **"switch system" for your body**:

- Under-methylation = **not enough switches turned ON/OFF properly**
- 👉 Result: confusion in cellular function

📚 **Scientific References**

1. General Overview of Methylation

DNA Methylation (Overview – NIH/NCBI)

https://www.ncbi.nlm.nih.gov/books/NBK26829/

Epigenomics Fact Sheet – NIH

https://www.genome.gov/about-genomics/fact-sheets/Epigenomics-Fact-Sheet

🧬 Methylation & One-Carbon/Methionine Cycle

2. One-Carbon Metabolism & Methylation Cycle

One-Carbon Metabolism and Methylation (Review)

https://www.ncbi.nlm.nih.gov/pmc/articles/PMC2790188/

Methionine Metabolism – NCBI Bookshelf

https://www.ncbi.nlm.nih.gov/books/NBK558922/

🧬 MTHFR Gene & Clinical Significance

3. MTHFR Gene Function

MTHFR Gene – MedlinePlus Genetics

https://medlineplus.gov/genetics/gene/mthfr/

4. MTHFR Mutation & Disease Risk

MTHFR Polymorphisms and Disease (Review)

https://www.ncbi.nlm.nih.gov/pmc/articles/PMC6613097/

🧡 Homocysteine & Cardiovascular Risk

5. Homocysteine and Disease

Homocysteine Studies – American Heart Association

https://www.ahajournals.org/doi/10.1161/CIRCULATIONAHA.109.192705

🧠 DNA Methylation & Epigenetics

6. DNA Methylation Mechanism

DNA Methylation in Human Disease

https://www.ncbi.nlm.nih.gov/pmc/articles/PMC2790189/

7. Epigenetics & Gene Regulation

What is Epigenetics? – CDC

https://www.cdc.gov/genomics/disease/epigenetics.htm

🧬 Folate, Folic Acid & Vitamin B9

8. Folate Metabolism

Folate Fact Sheet – NIH Office of Dietary Supplements

https://ods.od.nih.gov/factsheets/Folate-HealthProfessional/

9. Folate vs Folic Acid

Folic Acid and Neural Tube Defects – CDC

https://www.cdc.gov/ncbddd/folicacid/about.html

🧹 Glutathione & Detoxification

10. Glutathione Role

Glutathione in Health and Disease

https://www.ncbi.nlm.nih.gov/pmc/articles/PMC4684116/

🧠 Neurotransmitters & Methylation

11. Methylation & Brain Function

Methylation and Neuropsychiatric Disorders

https://www.ncbi.nlm.nih.gov/pmc/articles/PMC3752900/

🧬 Cancer & DNA Methylation

12. Hypermethylation & Cancer

DNA Methylation and Cancer

https://www.ncbi.nlm.nih.gov/pmc/articles/PMC3743358/

⚠️ **Important Clarification (Scientific Accuracy)**

✔️ **Supported by science:**

- Methylation regulates gene expression ✔️
- MTHFR affects folate metabolism ✔️
- Homocysteine link to cardiovascular risk ✔️
- DNA methylation involved in cancer ✔️

⚠️ **Less strongly established/evolving:**

- "Over-methylation vs under-methylation" as clinical categories → **not universally accepted in mainstream medicine**
- Direct causal claims for:
    - ADHD
    - OCD
    - Autism (complex, multifactorial conditions)

👉 These are **areas of ongoing research**, not definitive conclusions.

📘 **Summary**

Your material aligns well with:

- **Biochemistry (one-carbon metabolism)**
- **Epigenetics (DNA methylation)**
- **Clinical nutrition (folate, B vitamins)**

The references above come from:

- **NIH/NCBI**
- **CDC**
- **Peer-reviewed journals**

Digital Genome and Analog Epigenome: A Systems View of Biological Information

🧬 **What is "ATCG digital marking" on DNA?**

✅ **Scientifically correct idea:**

DNA is made of four bases:

- **A** (Adenine)
- **T** (Thymine)
- **C** (Cytosine)
- **G** (Guanine)

👉 These form a **sequence-based code**

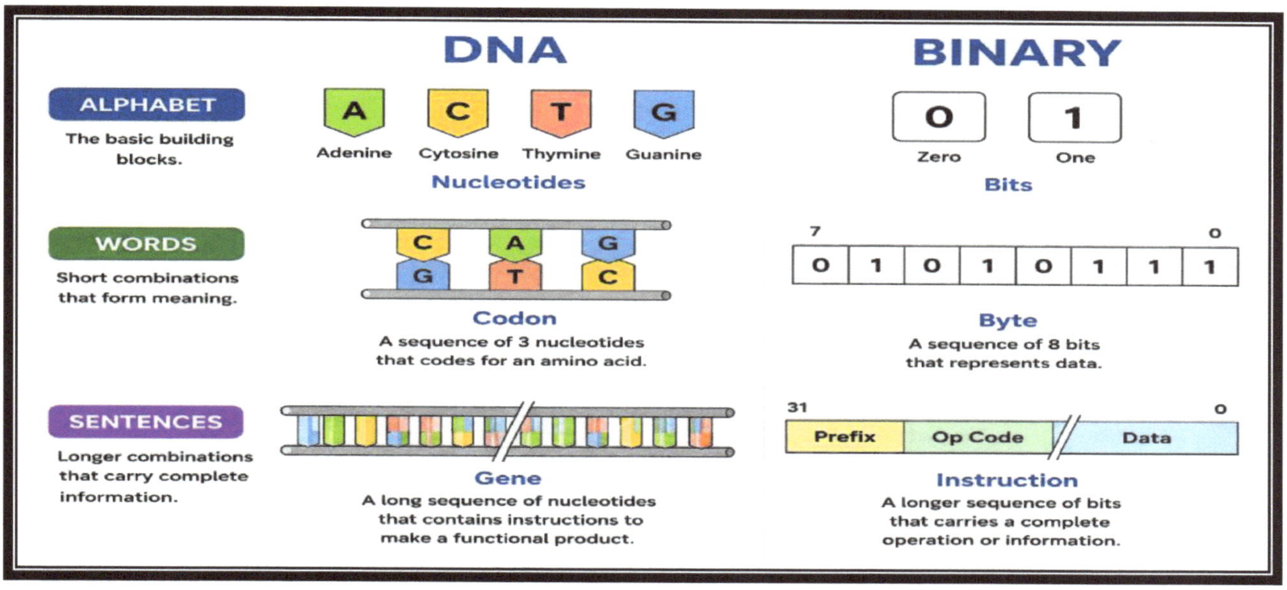

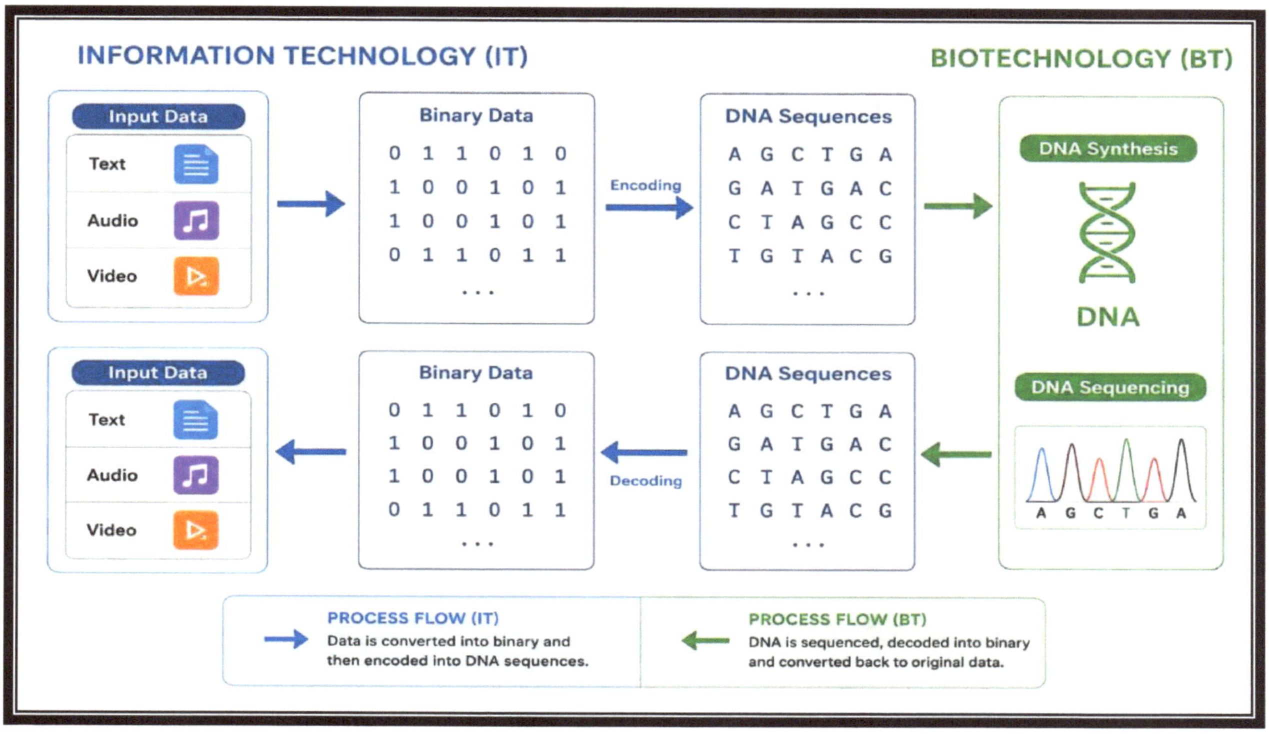

💡 **Why people call it "digital"**

- It behaves like a **discrete code (like binary in computers)**
- Information is stored in **exact sequences**
- Example:
  - ATCG ≠ TAGC (order matters)

✅ So this statement is valid:

"DNA stores biological information in a digital-like sequence using A, T, C, and G."

✅ **Scientifically correct concept:**

Epigenome = **chemical modifications ON DNA or histones**

Examples:

- DNA methylation
- Histone acetylation
- Chromatin remodelling

💡 **Why people call it "analog"**

Because:

- It's not just ON/OFF
- It's **gradual and reversible**
- It changes based on:
  - Diet
  - environment
  - stress
  - aging

✅ **So this statement is acceptable:**

"While DNA stores information in a digital sequence, the epigenome regulates gene expression in a more dynamic, analog-like manner."

🧠 **Correct Scientific Framing**

Feature	DNA	Epigenome
Type	Digital-like	Analog-like
Role	Stores code	Regulates expression
Stability	Stable	Dynamic
Change	Rare	Frequent

Digital vs Analog Biology

DNA provides the blueprint, while the epigenome determines how, when, and to what extent that blueprint is used.

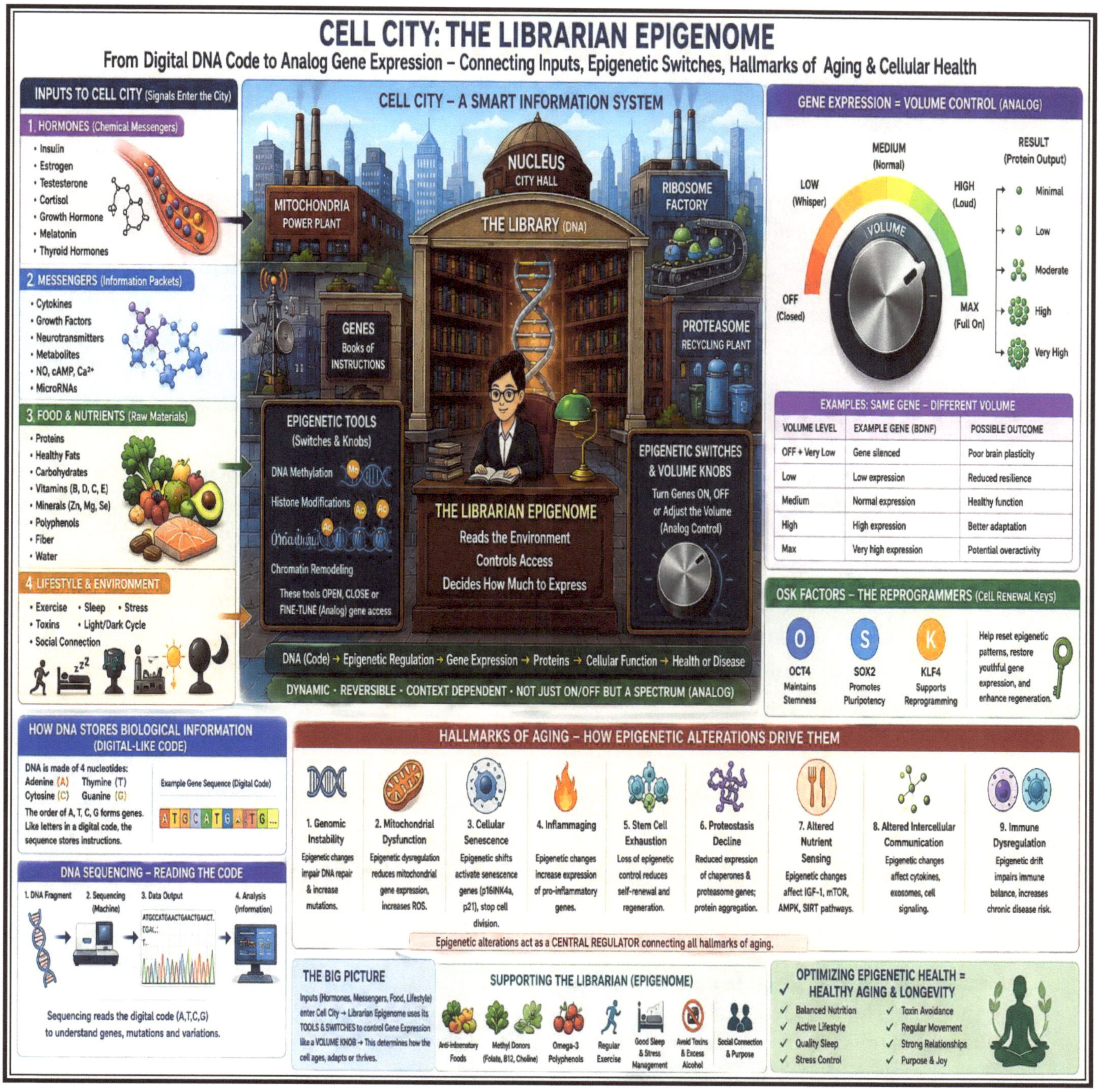

🔁 Flow

DNA (Code)

↓

Epigenetic Signals

↓

Gene Expression

↓

Protein Production

↓

Cell Function

Clinical Relevance

Examples:

- Cancer → epigenetic dysregulation
- Metabolic disease → gene expression changes

Scientific Boundaries

While environmental and nutritional factors can influence epigenetic regulation, these effects are complex, variable, and not fully predictable at an individual level.

Digital Genome and Analog-Like Epigenome: A Systems View of Biological Information in Aging

Introduction

Biological systems can be understood, in part, as information-processing systems. At the core of this system lies deoxyribonucleic acid (DNA), which encodes the genetic instructions required for cellular structure and function. However, the expression of this information is not static. It is dynamically regulated by a complex layer of biochemical modifications collectively referred to as the epigenome.

A useful conceptual framework is to view DNA as a **digital-like information system**, where genetic instructions are stored in discrete nucleotide sequences, and the epigenome as an **analog-like regulatory system**, where gene expression is modulated in a graded and context-dependent manner. While this analogy is not literal, it provides a helpful model for understanding how genetic information is both stored and regulated.

This chapter explores the relationship between the genome and epigenome, their roles in aging, and the implications for health and disease.

DNA as a Digital-Like Information System

DNA is composed of four nucleotides:

- Adenine (A)
- Thymine (T)
- Cytosine (C)
- Guanine (G)

These nucleotides form a sequence that encodes genetic information. The order of these bases determines the synthesis of proteins through transcription and translation.

The term "digital-like" is used to describe DNA because:

- Information is stored in **discrete units (nucleotides)**
- The sequence is **highly specific and stable**
- Small changes (mutations) can lead to significant functional consequences

For example, a single nucleotide substitution can alter an amino acid in a protein, potentially affecting its structure and function.

Thus, DNA provides a relatively stable **biological blueprint** that is inherited across generations.

The Epigenome as an Analog-Like Regulatory Layer

In contrast to the relatively stable genome, the epigenome consists of **chemical modifications** that influence gene expression without altering the underlying DNA sequence.

Major epigenetic mechanisms include:

- **DNA methylation** (addition of methyl groups to cytosine residues)
- **Histone modifications** (acetylation, methylation, phosphorylation)
- **Chromatin remodelling** (structural changes affecting DNA accessibility)

These modifications regulate whether genes are:

- Actively transcribed
- Silenced
- Expressed at varying levels

The epigenome is often described as "analog-like" because:

- Gene expression is **not simply on or off**, but exists on a spectrum
- It is **dynamic and reversible**
- It responds to environmental inputs such as nutrition, stress, toxins, and aging

Importantly, the epigenome does not encode genetic information but **modulates how genetic information is used**.

Integration of Genome and Epigenome

A simplified representation of biological information flow is:

DNA (sequence information) → Epigenetic regulation → Gene expression → Protein synthesis → Cellular function

In this framework:

- DNA provides the **instructions**
- The epigenome determines **when, where, and how much** those instructions are executed

This layered regulation allows cells with identical DNA to exhibit vastly different functions, as seen in differentiation of tissues such as neurons, hepatocytes, and immune cells.

🧠 **The Core Truth**

👉 **Genes are rarely just ON or OFF**
👉 Most genes are expressed at **different levels (a spectrum)**

In reality:

- Genes can be:
- Very low expression
- Moderate
- High
- Expression changes continuously

👉 Better analogy:
Volume knob 🎚️ (not a switch)

⚖️ **So Both Statements Are True**

Statement	Meaning	When to Use
"ON/OFF"	**Simplified extreme states**	**Basic teaching**
"Spectrum"	**Real biological Behavior**	**Scientific writing**

Clinical Relevance

Epigenetic dysregulation is implicated in a wide range of diseases:

- **Cancer:** Aberrant DNA methylation leading to oncogene activation or tumor suppressor silencing
- **Metabolic disorders:** Altered gene expression affecting insulin signaling and lipid metabolism
- **Neurodegenerative diseases:** Epigenetic changes affecting neuronal survival and function

Understanding the interplay between genome and epigenome provides insights into disease mechanisms and potential therapeutic targets.

Key Takeaways

- DNA stores genetic information in a stable, sequence-based format
- The epigenome regulates gene expression dynamically
- Aging is associated with epigenetic alterations
- Environmental and nutritional factors influence epigenetic mechanisms
- The genome–epigenome interaction is central to health and disease

📚 Scientific References

1. López-Otín C, Blasco MA, Partridge L, Serrano M, Kroemer G. The hallmarks of aging. *Cell*. 2013;153(6):1194–1217.
2. Bird A. Perceptions of epigenetics. *Nature*. 2007;447(7143):396–398.
3. Goldberg AD, Allis CD, Bernstein E. Epigenetics: a landscape takes shape. *Cell*. 2007;128(4):635–638.
4. Jones PA. Functions of DNA methylation. *Nat Rev Genet*. 2012;13(7):484–492.
5. Bannister AJ, Kouzarides T. Regulation of chromatin by histone modifications. *Cell Res*. 2011;21(3):381–395.
6. Horvath S. DNA methylation age of human tissues and cell types. *Genome Biol*. 2013;14(10):R115.
7. Sen P, Shah PP, Nativio R, Berger SL. Epigenetic mechanisms of longevity and aging. *Cell*. 2016;166(4):822–839.
8. Feinberg AP. The key role of epigenetics in human disease prevention. *N Engl J Med*. 2018;378(14):1323–1334.
9. Choi SW, Friso S. Epigenetics: a new bridge between nutrition and health. *Adv Nutr*. 2010;1(1):8–16.
10. Jaenisch R, Bird A. Epigenetic regulation of gene expression. *Nat Genet*. 2003;33 Suppl:245–254.

Chapter-10

Dysbiosis - Hallmark of Aging: Role of the Gut Microbiome in Epigenetic Regulation

1. Introduction: Aging Beyond Cells – The Microbial Dimension

Aging is no longer viewed solely as a process driven by intrinsic cellular mechanisms such as genomic instability or mitochondrial dysfunction. Increasing evidence highlights the critical role of the gut microbial ecosystem in modulating the biological aging process.

One of the emerging concepts in modern biomedicine is dysbiosis, a state of imbalance in the microbial community, which contributes significantly to multiple hallmarks of aging, including:

- Chronic inflammation ("inflammaging")
- Altered nutrient sensing
- Epigenetic dysregulation
- Immune system decline

Thus, the gut microbiome acts as a dynamic regulator of host physiology, influencing both health span and lifespan.

2. Microbiota vs Microbiome: Fundamental Distinction

Understanding the difference between these two terms is essential:

Microbiota

Refers to the collection of living microorganisms residing in specific niches of the human body, such as:

- Gastrointestinal tract
- Skin
- Oral cavity

These include:

- Bacteria
- Viruses
- Fungi
- Archaea

👉 In simple terms: *"Who is there?"*

Microbiome

Refers to:

The microbiota plus their genetic material (genomes)

Their functional capabilities and metabolic potential

👉 In simple terms: *"What can they do?"*

3. Dysbiosis: Definition and Biological Impact

What is Dysbiosis?

Dysbiosis is an alteration in the composition, diversity, or function of the microbiota.

Characteristics of Dysbiosis

- Loss of beneficial microbes
- Overgrowth of pathogenic organisms
- Reduced microbial diversity

Consequences of Dysbiosis

Dysbiosis contributes to:

- Chronic inflammation
- Impaired metabolism
- Immune dysfunction
- Increased intestinal permeability ("leaky gut")

These effects directly link dysbiosis to aging and age-related diseases.

4. Epigenetics and the Gut Microbiome: A Bidirectional Relationship

A key concept for PG students is that the interaction between the host and microbiome is bidirectional.

🔁 **Bidirectional Axis**

- Microbiome → modifies host epigenetics
- Host epigenetics → shapes microbiome composition

This interaction forms a microbiome–epigenome axis that regulates:

- Gene expression
- Immune responses
- Metabolic pathways

5. Microbiome → Epigenetic Regulation

The gut microbiota influences host epigenetics primarily through **metabolite production**.

Key Microbial Metabolites

- Short-chain fatty acids (SCFAs), especially **butyrate**
- Folate
- Acetate and propionate

Mechanisms of Action

1. DNA Methylation

- Microbial folate contributes to methyl group availability
- Alters DNA methylation patterns → changes gene expression

2. Histone Modification

- Butyrate acts as a **histone deacetylase (HDAC) inhibitor**
- Leads to:
    - Increased histone acetylation
    - Relaxed chromatin structure
    - Enhanced gene transcription

3. Chromatin Remodeling

- Microbial metabolites influence chromatin accessibility
- Regulate transcriptional activity of host genes

Functional Outcome

These epigenetic modifications regulate:

- Cellular metabolism
- Inflammatory pathways
- Tissue repair mechanisms

6. Microbiome–Immune System–Epigenetic Axis

The gut microbiome plays a central role in shaping the immune system.

Mechanism

- Microbial antigens and metabolites interact with immune cells
- Induce epigenetic changes in:
    - T cells
    - Macrophages
    - Dendritic cells

Impact

- Alters immune cell differentiation
- Modulates cytokine production
- Influences susceptibility to diseases such as:
    - Inflammatory bowel disease
    - Asthma
    - Autoimmune disorders

7. Dysbiosis and Hallmarks of Aging

Dysbiosis contributes to multiple hallmarks of aging:

1. Chronic Inflammation (Inflammaging)

- Dysbiosis → increased endotoxins (e.g., LPS)
- Persistent low-grade inflammation

2. Mitochondrial Dysfunction

- Altered microbial metabolites → impaired energy metabolism
- Increased oxidative stress

3. Epigenetic Alterations

- Disrupted methylation and histone modification patterns
- Abnormal gene expression

4. Immune Dysregulation

- Reduced immune tolerance
- Increased autoimmunity

5. Deregulated Nutrient Sensing

- Altered metabolic signaling (AMPK, mTOR pathways)

8. Clinical Implications of Microbiome–Epigenetic Interaction

The interplay between dysbiosis and epigenetics is implicated in:

- Metabolic syndrome
- Obesity and diabetes
- Neurodegenerative diseases
- Cancer
- Cardiovascular disorders

9. Conceptual Integration

The gut microbiome acts as an **epigenetic modulator of the host genome**, influencing aging at multiple levels:

Dysbiosis

↓

Altered Microbial Metabolites

↓

Epigenetic Changes (DNA methylation, histone modification)

↓

Gene Expression Alteration

↓

Inflammation + Metabolic Dysfunction

↓

Accelerated Aging

10. Conclusion

Dysbiosis represents a critical, yet modifiable, contributor to the aging process. Through its influence on epigenetic mechanisms, the gut microbiome regulates gene expression, immune responses, and metabolic pathways. The disruption of this delicate balance accelerates the progression of age-related diseases and highlights the importance of targeting the microbiome for therapeutic interventions aimed at promoting healthy aging.

Gut–Brain–Endocrine Axis, Dysbiosis, and Aging

The **gut microbiome** plays a central role in maintaining systemic homeostasis and is increasingly recognized as a key regulator of aging biology. Within the framework of the **hallmarks of aging**, **dysbiosis**—an imbalance in gut microbial composition—contributes to chronic inflammation, metabolic dysfunction, and neurodegeneration.

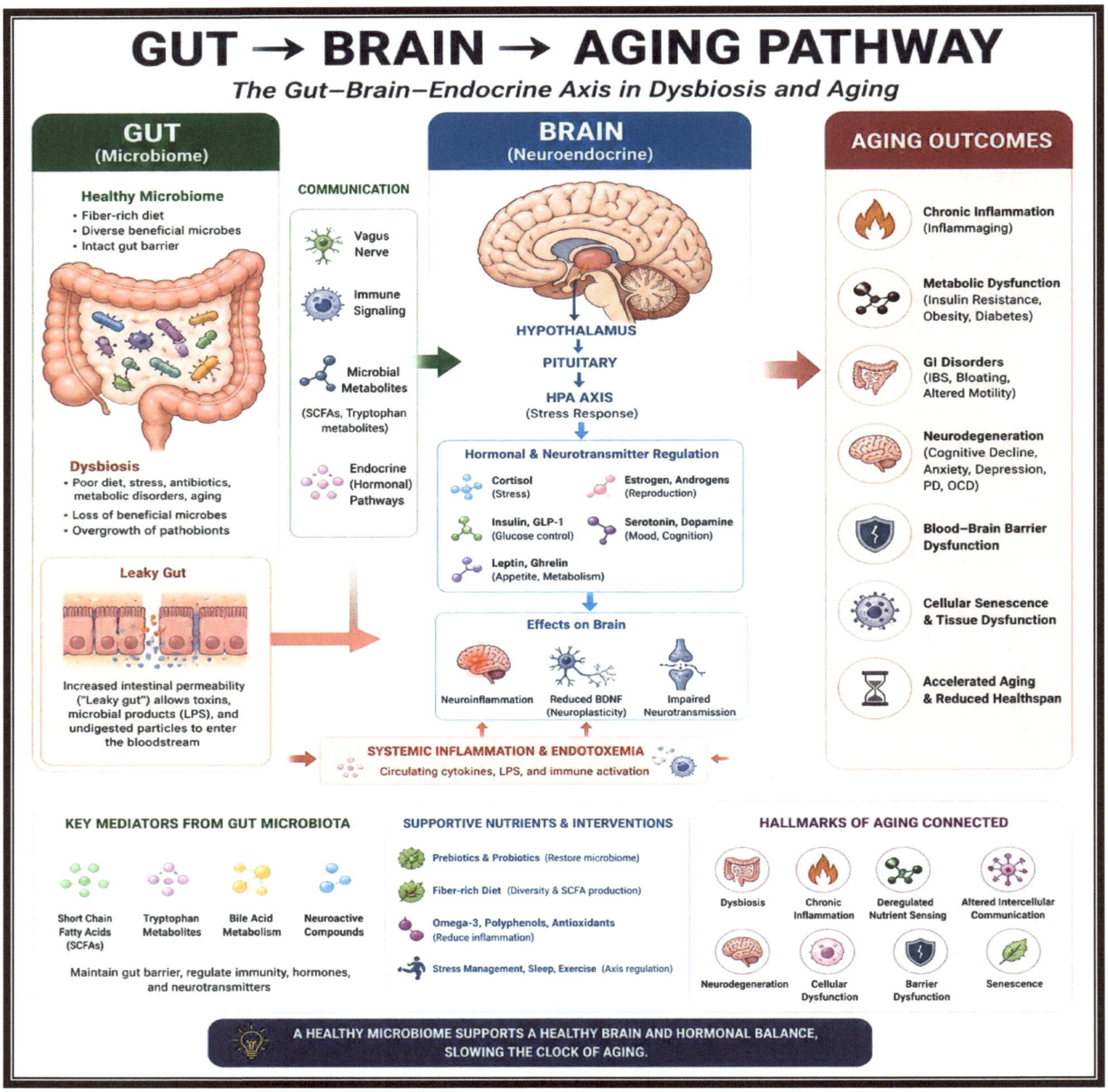

1. The Gut–Brain–Endocrine Axis

The **gut–brain axis** represents a bidirectional communication network linking the gastrointestinal tract and the central nervous system. This communication is mediated through:

- Neural pathways (vagus nerve)
- Immune signaling
- **Endocrine (hormonal) system**, particularly the **hypothalamic–pituitary–adrenal (HPA) axis**

Gut microbiota influences the release of key hormones and signaling molecules, including:

- **Cortisol** (stress response)
- **Insulin and GLP-1** (glucose metabolism)
- **Leptin and ghrelin** (appetite regulation)
- **Serotonin and dopamine** (mood and cognition)

With aging, disruption of this axis contributes to **deregulated nutrient sensing**, **chronic inflammation**, and **metabolic decline**—all core hallmarks of aging.

2. Dysbiosis, Metabolic Dysfunction, and IBS

Dysbiosis is strongly associated with **metabolic syndrome and insulin resistance**, which in turn affect gastrointestinal function.

Key mechanisms include:

- **Hyperinsulinemia and hyperglycaemia** impair enteric nervous system function
- Altered microbiota affect digestion and nutrient absorption
- Increased intestinal fermentation leads to bloating and altered motility

These changes contribute to disorders such as **irritable bowel syndrome (IBS)**, where the gut–brain axis plays a central role in symptoms like abdominal pain and altered bowel habits.

3. Leaky Gut and Blood–Brain Barrier Dysfunction

A critical consequence of dysbiosis is increased intestinal permeability, commonly referred to as **"leaky gut."**

- Disruption of the intestinal barrier allows **toxins, microbial products, and inflammatory molecules** to enter circulation
- This systemic inflammation can impair the **blood–brain barrier (BBB)**
- Increased BBB permeability may contribute to:
    - Neuroinflammation
    - Cognitive decline
    - Neurodegenerative diseases

Thus, dysbiosis links directly to the hallmarks of **altered intercellular communication** and **chronic inflammation**.

4. Neuroendocrine and Mental Health Implications

Gut microbiota influence brain chemistry and behavior through neurotransmitter regulation:

- **Serotonin** (mood, anxiety)
- **Glutamate and GABA** (neural signaling balance)

Emerging evidence suggests that microbial imbalance may contribute to conditions such as:

- Anxiety and depression
- Obsessive–compulsive disorder (OCD)
- Neurodegenerative diseases

Nutritional and metabolic factors (e.g., amino acids, antioxidants, vitamins) may modulate these pathways, although clinical evidence remains evolving.

5. BDNF, Neuroplasticity, and Aging

The gut microbiome also regulates **brain-derived neurotrophic factor (BDNF)**, a key protein involved in:

- **Neurogenesis** (formation of new neurons)
- **Synaptic plasticity**
- **Learning and memory**

Reduced BDNF levels, often observed in dysbiosis and aging, are associated with **cognitive decline and neurodegeneration**, linking gut health to brain aging.

🔷 Integrated Hallmark Perspective

Dysbiosis acts as a central driver connecting multiple hallmarks of aging:

Mechanism	Related Hallmark
Gut microbiome imbalance	Dysbiosis
Chronic inflammation	Inflammaging
Hormonal disruption	Deregulated nutrient sensing
Barrier dysfunction (gut & brain)	Altered intercellular communication
Reduced BDNF	Neurodegeneration/cellular dysfunction

🔷 Conclusion

The gut–brain–endocrine axis represents a critical interface in aging biology. Dysbiosis disrupts this network, leading to metabolic imbalance, inflammation, and impaired neuroplasticity. Understanding and targeting this axis offers promising strategies to improve **health span and resilience against age-related diseases**.

📚 Scientific Reference

- **Hallmarks of Aging (Cell, 2013)**
- https://pubmed.ncbi.nlm.nih.gov/23746838/
- **Gut Microbiota and Brain Interaction**
- https://pubmed.ncbi.nlm.nih.gov/25830558/
- **Gut–Brain Axis and Neuroinflammation**
- https://pubmed.ncbi.nlm.nih.gov/27125916/
- **Microbiome and Aging**
- https://pubmed.ncbi.nlm.nih.gov/30046148/
- **Gut Microbiota and Metabolic Disorders**
- https://pubmed.ncbi.nlm.nih.gov/17167471/
- **Blood–Brain Barrier and Aging**
- https://pubmed.ncbi.nlm.nih.gov/30659149/
- **BDNF and Neuroplasticity**
- https://pubmed.ncbi.nlm.nih.gov/20308767/

🧠 Gut–Brain Axis and Dysbiosis in Aging

🌿 1. Introduction: Gut Microbiome as a Regulator of Aging

The **gut microbiome**—trillions of microorganisms in the digestive tract—plays a central role in human health. It communicates with the brain, immune system, and metabolic pathways through a network known as the **gut–brain axis**.

With aging, disruption of this system (**dysbiosis**) becomes a key contributor to multiple hallmarks of aging, including:

- Chronic inflammation
- Mitochondrial dysfunction

- Immune dysregulation
- Metabolic imbalance

🔄 2. The Gut–Brain Axis: A Bidirectional Communication System

The gut and brain are connected through:

- **Nervous system** (vagus nerve)
- **Endocrine system** (hormones)
- **Immune signaling**
- **Microbial metabolites**

Key Mechanism: Stress Response (HPA Axis)

During stress:

- The hypothalamus activates the **HPA axis**
- Adrenal glands release **cortisol**
- Blood glucose increases to supply energy

👉 Chronic activation leads to:

- Insulin resistance
- Hypertension
- Cognitive dysfunction
- Accelerated aging

⚠️ 3. Dysbiosis and "Leaky Gut"

When gut bacteria become imbalanced:

- The intestinal barrier weakens (**leaky gut**)
- Toxins and bacterial products enter the bloodstream
- The immune system becomes overactive

🚨 Consequences:

- Systemic inflammation
- Autoimmune activation
- Neuroinflammation
- Blood–brain barrier disruption

This contributes to diseases such as:

- Anxiety and depression
- Neurodegeneration
- Metabolic syndrome

🧬 4. Gut–Organ Axes in Aging

Dysbiosis affects multiple organs through interconnected pathways:

❤️ Gut–Heart Axis

- Promotes inflammation and endothelial dysfunction
- Increases risk of cardiovascular disease

🧠 Gut–Brain Axis

- Alters neurotransmitters (serotonin, dopamine)
- Affects mood, cognition, and neuroplasticity

🩺 Gut–Liver Axis

- Leads to fatty liver (NAFLD)
- Promotes metabolic dysfunction

🧂 Gut–Kidney Axis

- Increases inflammatory toxins
- Contributes to chronic kidney disease

🧬 Gut–Endocrine Axis

- Disrupts insulin signaling
- Leads to metabolic syndrome and diabetes

👉 These interconnected pathways explain how **one imbalance (gut dysbiosis)** can accelerate **whole-body aging**.

🧠 5. Dysbiosis, Inflammation, and Neurodegeneration

Dysbiosis promotes:

- Chronic low-grade inflammation
- Oxidative stress
- Reduced neuroprotective factors (like BDNF)

This leads to:

- Cognitive decline
- Neurodegenerative disorders
- Reduced brain adaptability (neuroplasticity)

🌱 6. Anti-Aging Strategies: Restoring Gut Balance

🦠 A. Beneficial Gut Bacteria (Probiotics)

1. *Lactobacillus acidophilus*

- Maintains gut barrier integrity
- Produces neurotransmitters (GABA)
- Reduces inflammation

2. *Bifidobacterium longum*

- Supports immune balance
- Improves digestion and mood
- Produces beneficial metabolites

3. *Akkermansia muciniphila*

- Strengthens gut lining
- Improves insulin sensitivity
- Associated with longevity

4. *Christensenellaceae*

- Linked with lean body composition
- Produces anti-inflammatory metabolites

5. *Clostridium butyricum*

- Produces **butyrate** (key anti-aging molecule)
- Supports mitochondrial health
- Reduces inflammation

🧪 B. Key Nutrients for Gut Repair

🧬 Amino Acids

- **L-Glutamine** → repairs gut lining
- **L-Glycine** → supports tissue repair & anti-inflammation

- **L-Cysteine** → antioxidant and regenerative

🛡️ **Protective Compounds**

- **Zinc L-carnosine** → heals gut mucosa
- **Short-chain fatty acids (SCFAs)** → reduce inflammation

⚡ **C. Microbiome-Derived Anti-Aging Molecule**

🔬 **Urolithin A**

- Produced from foods like pomegranate
- Enhances **mitochondrial function**
- Promotes **mitophagy (cellular cleanup)**
- Linked to improved muscle and cellular health

🥗 7. Lifestyle Recommendations for Healthy Aging

To maintain a healthy gut and slow aging:

✅ **Diet**

- High-fiber foods (vegetables, fruits, whole grains)
- Fermented foods (yogurt, kefir)
- Polyphenol-rich foods (berries, nuts)

🏃 **Lifestyle**

- Regular exercise
- Stress management (reduces cortisol)
- Adequate sleep

❌ **Avoid**

- Excess sugar and processed foods
- Chronic stress
- Unnecessary antibiotics

🧾 8. Conclusion

The **gut microbiome is a central regulator of aging**. Dysbiosis disrupts multiple biological systems—immune, metabolic, neurological—making it a key driver of age-related diseases.

Restoring gut balance through **diet, probiotics, and lifestyle** offers a powerful strategy to:

- Reduce inflammation
- Improve mitochondrial health
- Enhance longevity

📚 Scientific References

- https://pmc.ncbi.nlm.nih.gov/articles/PMC6435494/
- https://pmc.ncbi.nlm.nih.gov/articles/PMC10712442/
- https://www.nature.com/articles/s41580-020-00313-x
- https://pubmed.ncbi.nlm.nih.gov/28899755/
- https://pubmed.ncbi.nlm.nih.gov/27825999/

🧬 Gut–Brain Axis in the NAD⁺–CD38–SIRT Pathway of Aging

🌿 1. Central Concept: Linking Gut Dysbiosis to Cellular Aging

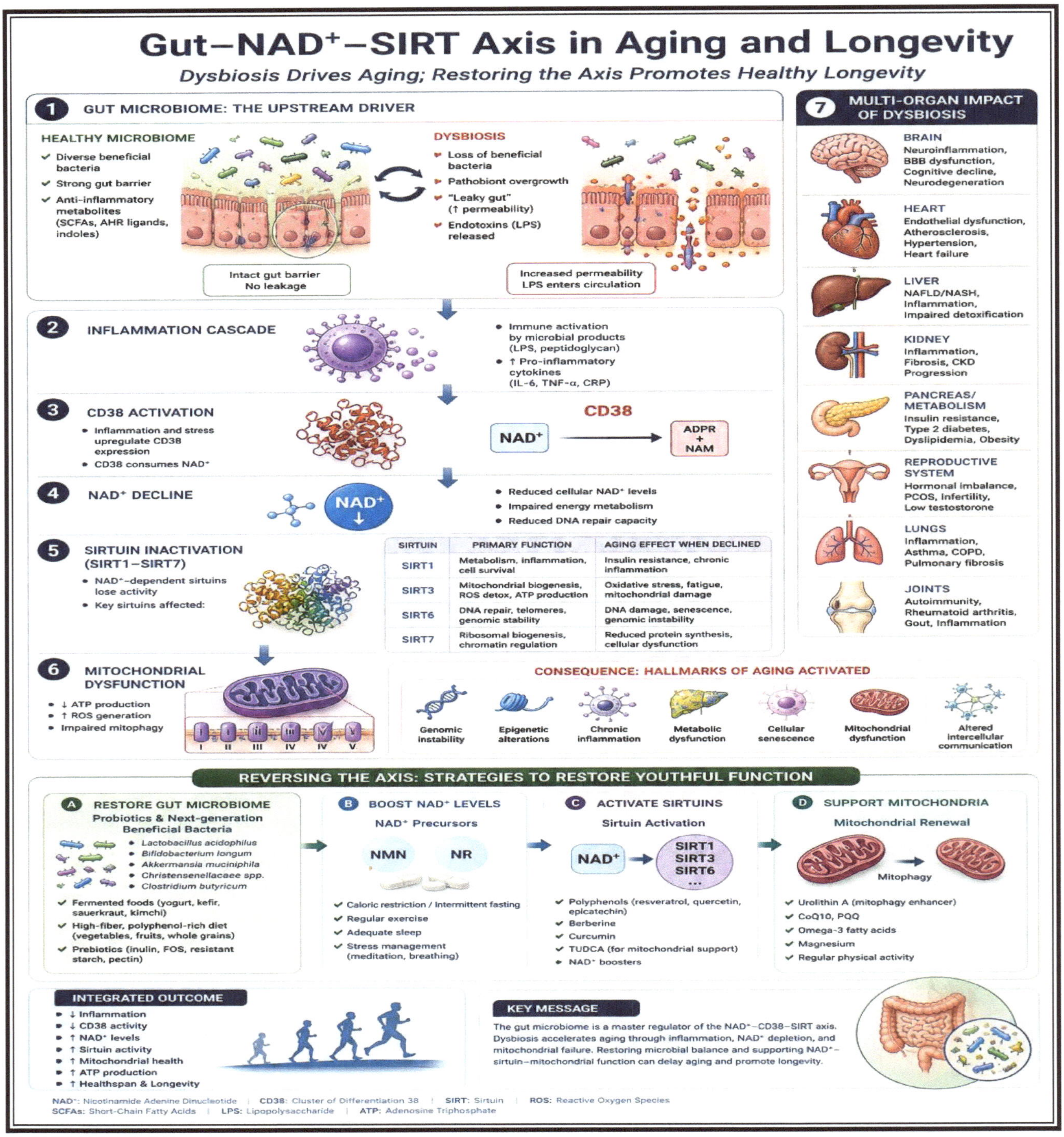

Aging is not only a genetic process but also strongly influenced by metabolic and microbial signals. The **gut microbiome** plays a critical upstream role in regulating:

- **NAD⁺ availability**
- **CD38 activity**
- **Sirtuin (SIRT1–SIRT7) function**
- **Mitochondrial energy (ATP production)**

👉 Dysbiosis acts as a **trigger** that accelerates the decline of this entire pathway.

🔗 2. The Core Aging Axis: NAD^+ → CD38 → Sirtuins → Mitochondria

⚡ NAD^+ (Energy & Longevity Molecule)

- Essential for cellular metabolism and DNA repair
- Required for activation of **sirtuins**

🔥 CD38 (NAD^+ Consumer)

- Enzyme that degrades NAD^+
- Increases with aging and inflammation

🧬 Sirtuins (SIRT1–SIRT7)

- NAD^+-dependent enzymes
- Regulate:
  - DNA repair
  - Inflammation
  - Mitochondrial function

🔋 Mitochondria

- Produce ATP (cellular energy)
- Dysfunction leads to fatigue, disease, and aging

⚠️ 3. How Gut Dysbiosis Disrupts This Pathway

🦠 Step 1: Dysbiosis → Chronic Inflammation

- Harmful bacteria release endotoxins (LPS)
- Activates immune system → chronic inflammation

🔥 Step 2: Inflammation → CD38 Activation

- Inflammatory cytokines increase **CD38 expression**
- Leads to excessive NAD^+ breakdown

⚡ Step 3: NAD^+ Decline

- Reduced NAD^+ availability in cells
- Impairs metabolic and repair processes

🧬 Step 4: Sirtuin Inactivation

- SIRT1, SIRT3, SIRT6 activity decreases
- Results in:
  - Poor DNA repair
  - Increased oxidative stress
  - Epigenetic instability

🔋 Step 5: Mitochondrial Dysfunction

- Reduced ATP production
- Increased ROS (oxidative damage)
- Cellular fatigue and aging

🧠 4. Gut–Brain Axis: Neuroendocrine Amplification

The gut microbiome influences the **HPA axis (stress system)**:

- Stress → ↑ Cortisol
- Cortisol → ↑ blood glucose
- Leads to **insulin resistance**

👉 Insulin resistance further:

- Increases inflammation
- Accelerates NAD^+ depletion
- Worsens mitochondrial dysfunction

This creates a **vicious aging cycle**:

Dysbiosis → Inflammation → CD38 ↑ → NAD^+ ↓ → SIRT ↓ → Mitochondria ↓ → Aging ↑

🧬 5. Blood–Brain Barrier & Neurodegeneration

Dysbiosis contributes to:

- Increased gut permeability (**leaky gut**)
- Disruption of the **blood–brain barrier**

This leads to:

- Neuroinflammation
- Reduced BDNF (brain repair factor)
- Cognitive decline

👉 Linked to:

- Depression
- Parkinson's disease
- Alzheimer's disease

🔄 6. Multi-Organ Impact via NAD^+ Pathway

Gut dysbiosis influences aging across systems:

Axis	Mechanism	NAD^+–SIRT Impact	Outcome
🧠 Brain	Neuroinflammation	↓ SIRT1	Cognitive decline
🧡 Heart	Endothelial dysfunction	↓ SIRT3	CVD
🩺 Liver	Fat accumulation	↓ NAD^+	NAFLD
🧴 Kidney	Toxin accumulation	↓ mitochondrial function	CKD
⚖️ Metabolism	Insulin resistance	↓ SIRT1	Diabetes

🌱 7. Restoring the NAD^+–Gut Axis (Anti-Aging Strategy)

🦠 A. Beneficial Microbiota (Upstream Control)

- **Lactobacillus acidophilus** → reduces inflammation
- **Bifidobacterium longum** → improves metabolic balance
- **Akkermansia muciniphila** → strengthens gut barrier
- **Christensenellaceae** → linked to longevity
- **Clostridium butyricum** → produces butyrate (anti-inflammatory)

👉 Effects:

- ↓ CD38 activity
- ↑ NAD^+ preservation
- ↑ Sirtuin activation

B. NAD^+ Restoration Strategies

- NAD^+ precursors (NMN, NR)
- Caloric restriction
- Exercise

Outcome:

- Reactivation of SIRT1, SIRT3, SIRT6
- Improved mitochondrial ATP production

C. Mitochondrial Support

- **Urolithin A** → enhances mitophagy
- **Short-chain fatty acids (SCFAs)** → improve energy metabolism

D. Gut Barrier Repair

- L-Glutamine → gut lining repair
- Zinc L-carnosine → mucosal healing
- Glycine → anti-inflammatory support

8. Integrated Anti-Aging Model

Unified Pathway:

Healthy Gut Microbiome

↓

Low Inflammation

↓

Low CD38 Activity

↓

High NAD^+ Levels

↓

Active Sirtuins (SIRT1–SIRT7)

↓

Healthy Mitochondria

↓

Efficient ATP Production

↓

Delayed Aging & Longevity

9. Conclusion

The **gut microbiome is a master regulator of the NAD^+–CD38–SIRT pathway**. Dysbiosis accelerates aging by driving inflammation, NAD^+ depletion, and mitochondrial failure.

Conversely, restoring gut health provides a **powerful upstream intervention** to:

- Preserve NAD^+
- Activate sirtuins
- Improve mitochondrial energy
- Slow biological aging

Scientific References

- https://www.nature.com/articles/s41580-020-00313-x
- https://pubmed.ncbi.nlm.nih.gov/28899755/
- https://pubmed.ncbi.nlm.nih.gov/27825999/
- https://pmc.ncbi.nlm.nih.gov/articles/PMC6435494/
- https://pmc.ncbi.nlm.nih.gov/articles/PMC10712442/
- https://pubmed.ncbi.nlm.nih.gov/34509469/

Chapter-11

Loss of Proteostasis as a Hallmark of Aging

Proteostasis (protein homeostasis) means that cells keep their proteins in a healthy balance. This includes:

- making proteins
- folding them into the correct shape
- removing damaged or unnecessary proteins

👉 When this system works properly, cells stay healthy.

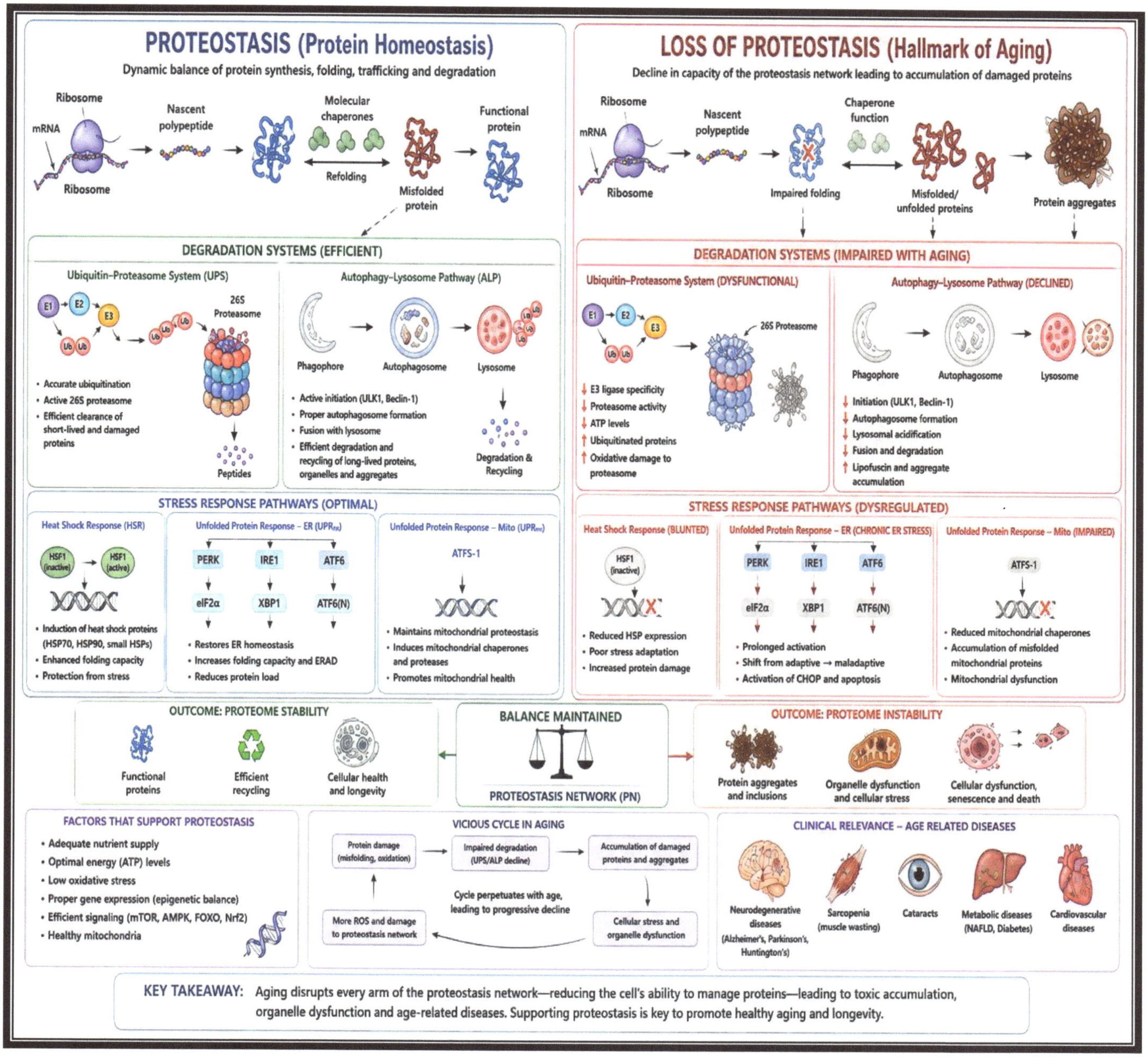

👉 **Protein = machinery (tools), NOT fuel**

👉 **Fuel (glucose/fat) = energy source**

Proteins shown as:

- repair workers 👷
- enzymes ⚙️
- structural parts 🧱
- hormones

🧬 **DNA: The Instruction Manual**

Inside every cell is DNA.

Think of DNA as a CD or blueprint containing instructions:

- how to function
- how to repair
- how to survive

But here's the important part:

👉 **The CD does not change…**
👉 **but how it is played can change.**

🎚️ **Epigenetics: The Control System = Remote Control**

Epigenetics decides:
👉 which genes are ON
👉 which genes are OFF

It is like a remote control for your DNA.

👉 **How your lifestyle becomes faulty when it is controlled through epigenetics remote control:**

- Junk food, stress icons
- Wrong gene activated
- Bad proteins formed:
  - broken tools
  - inefficient workers
- Result:
  - mitochondria weak
  - less ATP

🧱 **Misfolded Proteins = "Wrong Shape Tools"**

Proteins must fold into the correct shape.

👉 If shape is wrong:

- they don't work
- can even become toxic

⚠️ **Damaged Proteins (Oxidative Stress)**

Free radicals damage proteins.

👉 Result:

- weak enzymes
- poor function

🏭 **Poor Quality Control (Loss of Proteostasis)**

Body normally:

- makes proteins
- checks quality
- removes defective ones

When this system fails:
👉 defective proteins accumulate

🧬 **Wrong Protein Expression (Gene Issue)**

Lifestyle can influence:

- which genes are ON

👉 Result:

- less useful proteins
- more harmful pathways (like inflammation)

🧠 **Protein Aggregation (Very Important Clinically)**

Some proteins:
👉 clump together

Seen in:

- Alzheimer's (amyloid plaques)
- Parkinson's

👉 Aging = decline in **protein quality control system**

This is actually one of the real hallmarks: **Loss of proteostasis**

❌ **What is Loss of Proteostasis?**

Loss of proteostasis happens when this balance is disturbed.

- Proteins do not fold properly
- Damaged proteins are not removed efficiently
- Toxic protein clumps (aggregates) build up inside cells

➡️ **This leads to:**

- cell damage
- dysfunction
- aging and diseases

🔍 Key Differences (Very Simple)

✔️ **Proteostasis (Normal State)**

- Balanced protein production and removal
- Proteins function properly
- Cells remain healthy and stress-resistant

❌ **Loss of Proteostasis**

- Protein quality control fails
- Misfolded proteins accumulate
- Cells become stressed and damaged

🧠 **Role in Aging and Disease**

- In young, healthy cells → proteostasis is well maintained
- With aging → this system weakens

➡️ **Leads to diseases like:**

- Alzheimer's (amyloid-β, tau proteins)
- Parkinson's (α-synuclein)

⚙️ Main Components (Proteostasis Network)

1. Chaperones
   - Help proteins fold correctly
2. Degradation systems
   - Proteasome (breaks small proteins)
   - Autophagy (removes large aggregates)
3. Translational control
   - Regulates how many proteins are made

⚠️ What Happens When Proteostasis is Lost?

1. Protein aggregation
   - Misfolded proteins accumulate inside cells
2. Unfolded Protein Response (UPR)
   - Stress response activated when too many misfolded proteins are present
3. Cellular senescence or death
   - Cells stop dividing or die due to damage

🎯 One-Line Summary

Loss of proteostasis is the failure of protein quality control, leading to accumulation of toxic proteins, cellular dysfunction, and aging-related diseases.

Proteostasis (protein homeostasis) refers to the dynamic balance between protein synthesis, folding, trafficking, and degradation. This is maintained by an integrated **proteostasis network (PN)** consisting of molecular chaperones, degradation systems, and stress-response pathways. Aging disrupts this network, leading to accumulation of misfolded, aggregated, or damaged proteins—central to many age-related diseases.

1. Core Concept: Proteostasis Network Collapse

Components of the Proteostasis Network:

- **Protein synthesis machinery** (ribosomes, translation fidelity control)
- **Molecular chaperones** (HSP70, HSP90, small HSPs)
- **Protein degradation systems:**
- **Ubiquitin–proteasome system (UPS)**
- **Autophagy–lysosome pathway (ALP)**
- **Stress response pathways:**
  - Heat shock response (HSR)
  - Unfolded protein responses:
    - **UPR_{ER} (endoplasmic reticulum)**
    - **UPR_{mt} (mitochondria)**

👉 With aging:

- Chaperone efficiency ↓
- Proteasome activity ↓
- Autophagic flux ↓
- Stress responses become blunted

➡️ Result: **Proteome instability + toxic protein accumulation**

2. Molecular Mechanisms Driving Loss of Proteostasis

A. Impaired Protein Folding Capacity

- Reduced expression/activity of **heat shock proteins (HSPs)**
- Decline in **HSF1 (heat shock transcription factor 1)** activation
- Increased burden of unfolded polypeptides

📌 Advanced insight:

- Aging cells show **decoupling between proteotoxic stress and HSF1 activation**
- Epigenetic repression of chaperone genes contributes to failure of adaptive response

B. Dysfunction of the Ubiquitin–Proteasome System (UPS)

- Decreased **E3 ligase specificity**
- Reduced **26S proteasome activity**
- Accumulation of ubiquitinated substrates

📌 Mechanistic detail:

- Oxidative modifications of proteasome subunits impair catalytic function
- Decline in ATP levels affects proteasome assembly

C. Decline in Autophagy–Lysosomal Pathway

- Reduced **macroautophagy initiation (↓ ULK1, Beclin-1)**
- Impaired **lysosomal acidification**
- Accumulation of **lipofuscin** (non-degradable aggregates)

📌 Advanced concept:

- **Selective autophagy failure** (mitophagy, aggrephagy) is critical in aging neurons
- Lysosomal membrane permeabilization contributes to cell death

D. Endoplasmic Reticulum Stress & UPR Dysfunction

- Chronic ER stress due to misfolded proteins
- Dysregulated UPR pathways:
  - PERK–eIF2α
  - IRE1–XBP1
  - ATF6

📌 With aging:

- Adaptive UPR → maladaptive (pro-apoptotic signaling ↑, e.g., CHOP)
- Reduced capacity to restore ER homeostasis

3. Protein Aggregation and Cellular Toxicity

- Misfolded proteins form:
  - **Oligomers (most toxic)**
  - **Amyloid fibrils**
- Aggregates disrupt:
  - Membrane integrity
  - Mitochondrial function
  - Synaptic signaling

📌 Examples:

- Amyloid-β and tau → Alzheimer's
- α-synuclein → Parkinson's
- Huntingtin → Huntington's disease

4. Systems-Level Integration

Interconnection with Other Hallmarks of Aging:

- **Mitochondrial dysfunction** → ROS → protein damage
- **Genomic instability** → defective protein synthesis
- **Epigenetic alterations** → reduced chaperone gene expression
- **Cellular senescence** → impaired proteostasis feedback loops

👉 This creates a **vicious cycle**:

Protein damage → impaired clearance → more damage → cellular dysfunction

5. Quantitative & Biophysical Perspective (Advanced)

- Proteostasis collapse is linked to:
  - **Thermodynamic instability of proteome**
  - Increased **protein misfolding entropy**
- Aging proteome shows:
  - Increased **intrinsically disordered proteins (IDPs)** aggregation tendency
  - Reduced **protein turnover rates**

📌 Emerging concept:

- **Proteostasis boundary model**: cells have a finite buffering capacity against misfolded proteins; aging reduces this threshold

6. Clinical and Translational Relevance

- Loss of proteostasis underlies:
  - Neurodegenerative diseases
  - Sarcopenia
  - Cataracts
  - Metabolic disorders

Therapeutic strategies (research level):

- **Chaperone inducers** (HSP upregulation)
- **Proteasome activators**
- **Autophagy enhancers** (e.g., mTOR inhibition)
- **Chemical chaperones** (stabilize protein folding)

7. High-Yield Summary

- Proteostasis = balance of protein synthesis, folding, and degradation
- Aging → decline in PN efficiency
- Key failures:
  - ↓ chaperones
  - ↓ proteasome
  - ↓ autophagy
  - Dysregulated UPR
- Outcome: protein aggregation → cellular toxicity → disease Top of Form

🔬 Main Causes of Loss of Proteostasis

Think of proteostasis failure as:

👉 **"Too much damaged protein + too little capacity to fix/remove it."**

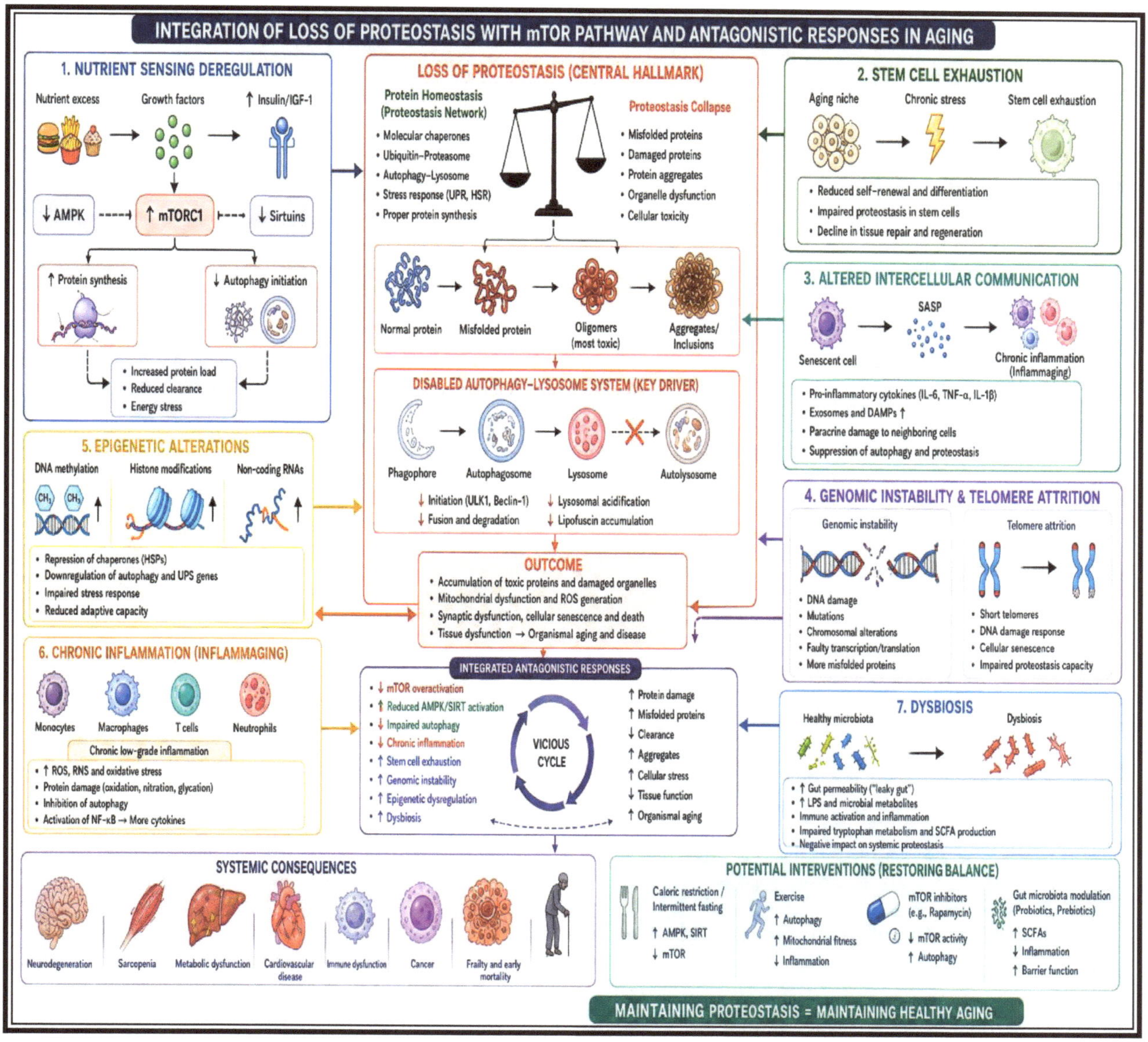

1. Reduced Chaperone Function (Folding Failure)

- Heat shock proteins (HSP70, HSP90) decline with age
- **HSF1 activation becomes weak**

➡️ Result:

- Newly made proteins don't fold properly
- Misfolded proteins accumulate

2. Impaired Protein Degradation

(A) Ubiquitin–Proteasome System (UPS)

- ↓ Proteasome activity
- ↓ ATP → affects degradation
- Oxidative damage to proteasome

➡️ Result: Short-lived and damaged proteins are not cleared

(B) Autophagy–Lysosome Pathway

- ↓ Autophagy initiation (ULK1, Beclin-1)
- ↓ Lysosomal acidity
- Lipofuscin accumulation

➡️ Result: Large aggregates and organelles are not removed

3. Increased Protein Damage

- Reactive oxygen species (**ROS**)
- Glycation (AGEs)
- Oxidation, nitration

➡️ Result:

- Proteins become structurally unstable and misfold

4. Impaired Stress Response Systems

- Heat Shock Response ↓
- ER stress response (UPR) becomes maladaptive

➡️ Result:

- Cells cannot adapt to proteotoxic stress

5. Errors in Protein Synthesis

- Ribosomal fidelity ↓
- Translation errors ↑

➡️ Result:

- More defective proteins are produced

🧠 **Now the MOST IMPORTANT PART (Integration)**

🔗 **Is Loss of Proteostasis Linked to Other Hallmarks of Aging?**

👉 **YES — it is deeply interconnected with ALL major hallmarks**

Let's simplify this like a "chain reaction system" 👇

⚙️ **1. mTOR Pathway (VERY HIGH-YIELD)**

mTOR = **Master regulator of growth & protein synthesis**

With Aging:

- mTOR is **chronically overactive**

Effects:

1. ↑ Protein synthesis → more folding burden
2. ↓ Autophagy → less protein clearance

➡️ Final effect:

👉 **Proteostasis collapse**

📌 Clinical link:

- mTOR inhibition (e.g., rapamycin) → improves proteostasis

2. Nutrient Sensing Deregulation

Includes:

- mTOR ↑
- AMPK ↓
- Sirtuins ↓

Mechanism:

- Nutrient excess → ↑ protein synthesis
- ↓ cellular repair mechanisms

➡ Result:

👉 Increased protein damage + reduced clearance

🧬 **3. Genomic Instability**

- DNA damage → faulty transcription

➡ Result:

- Abnormal proteins are produced
- Increased misfolding load

👉 Proteostasis gets overwhelmed

🧬 **4. Telomere Attrition**

- Short telomeres → cellular stress → senescence

Effect:

- Senescent cells:
    - ↓ autophagy
    - ↓ chaperone activity

➡ Result:

👉 Accumulation of damaged proteins

🧬 **5. Epigenetic Alterations**

- Histone modification changes
- DNA methylation changes

Effect:

- ↓ Expression of:
    - Chaperones (HSPs)
    - Autophagy genes

➡ Result:

👉 Proteostasis machinery itself becomes weak

🧪 **6. Stem Cell Exhaustion**

- Stem cells lose regenerative ability

Effect:

- New cells formed are less efficient
- Reduced repair capacity

➡ Result:

👉 Poor maintenance of proteome

📡 **7. Altered Intercellular Communication**

- Chronic inflammation (**inflammaging**)
- Cytokine imbalance

Effect:

- Inflammatory signals:
  - Increase protein damage (ROS)
  - Suppress autophagy

➡️ Result:

👉 Proteostasis disruption

🔁 **FINAL INTEGRATION**

🔄 **Vicious Cycle:**

1. Protein damage increases
2. Clearance systems fail
3. Aggregates accumulate
4. Cellular stress increases
5. Other hallmarks worsen
6. → More proteostasis failure

🔄 **INTEGRATED FLOW DIAGRAM: Loss of Proteostasis in Aging**

🟢 **STEP 1: Starting Triggers (Root Causes)**

Aging + Lifestyle + Cellular Stress

↓

| Nutrient excess (↑ mTOR) |

| DNA damage (Genomic instability) |

| Telomere shortening |

| Epigenetic changes |

| Stem cell exhaustion |

| Gut dysbiosis |

| Chronic inflammation |

🔵 **STEP 2: Central Control Disruption (mTOR Hub)**

Nutrient excess → ↑ mTOR activation

↓

| ↑ Protein synthesis (load ↑) |

| ↓ Autophagy (clearance ↓) |

↓

Proteostasis burden ↑

👉 Simple meaning:

More protein is made, but less is removed

🟡 **STEP 3: Damage + Repair Imbalance**

Other hallmarks contribute simultaneously:

1. Genomic instability

→ faulty proteins produced

2. Epigenetic alterations

→ ↓ chaperones + ↓ autophagy genes

3. Telomere attrition

→ cellular stress + senescence

4. Stem cell exhaustion

→ poor repair capacity

5. Dysbiosis

→ toxins + inflammation

6. Chronic inflammation

→ ROS ↑ (protein damage ↑)

⬇️ ALL converge into ⬇️

↑ Misfolded proteins + ↑ damaged proteins

🟠 **STEP 4: Failure of Clearance Systems**

Normal systems fail:

❌ Chaperones ↓ (folding fails)

❌ Proteasome ↓ (UPS impaired)

❌ Autophagy ↓ (key event)

❌ Lysosome dysfunction

➡️ Especially important:

mTOR ↑ → Autophagy ↓ → Aggregates ↑

⚫ **STEP 5: Protein Aggregation**

Misfolded proteins

↓

Toxic oligomers

↓

Protein aggregates (amyloid-like)

↓

Cellular toxicity

🔥 **STEP 6: Cellular Consequences**

Aggregates + stress →

| Mitochondrial dysfunction |

| ER stress |

| ROS generation ↑ |

| Inflammation ↑ |

➡️ Feedback loop starts

🔁 STEP 7: Vicious Cycle (MOST IMPORTANT)

Protein damage ↑

↓

Clearance failure

↓

Aggregation ↑

↓

Cell stress ↑

↓

More ROS + inflammation

↓

More protein damage

↓

(repeats)

🧬 FINAL OUTCOME

Loss of proteostasis

↓

Cell dysfunction

↓

Tissue damage

↓

AGING + DISEASE

🧠 Summary

👉 **Loss of proteostasis occurs due to imbalance between protein load and clearance, driven by increased protein damage, reduced chaperone activity, impaired degradation systems, and is strongly amplified by mTOR overactivation and other aging hallmarks.**

👉 **"Aging increases protein damage while reducing the body's ability to fix or remove them — mainly due to mTOR overactivation and failure of autophagy — leading to toxic accumulation and cellular dysfunction."**

📚 Scientific References

- **Carlos López-Otín et al., *Cell (2013)***
- https://doi.org/10.1016/j.cell.2013.05.039
- **Carlos López-Otín et al., *Cell (2023)***
- https://doi.org/10.1016/j.cell.2022.11.001

🔬 Proteostasis & Aging (Core Mechanism Papers)

- ***Cold Spring Harbor Perspectives in Biology***
- **→ Comprehensive review of proteostasis network**
- https://doi.org/10.1101/cshperspect.a033969
- ***Nature Reviews Molecular Cell Biology***
- **→ Proteostasis decline in aging**
- https://doi.org/10.1038/nrm.2016.28
- ***Cell Reports***
- **→ Protein homeostasis and aging mechanisms**
- https://doi.org/10.1016/j.celrep.2021.109771

🧬 **Protein Aggregation & Neurodegenerative Disease**

- **Alzheimer's disease mechanisms (amyloid & tau)**
- https://pmc.ncbi.nlm.nih.gov/articles/PMC10044767/
- **Parkinson's disease (α-synuclein aggregation)**
- https://pmc.ncbi.nlm.nih.gov/articles/PMC3080271/
- **Proteostasis and neurodegeneration**
- https://pmc.ncbi.nlm.nih.gov/articles/PMC3992297/

⚙️ **Proteostasis Network (UPS, Autophagy, Chaperones)**

- **Autophagy and aging**
- https://pmc.ncbi.nlm.nih.gov/articles/PMC8641024/
- **Oxidative stress and protein damage**
- https://pmc.ncbi.nlm.nih.gov/articles/PMC2360465/
- **Proteasome and aging**
- https://doi.org/10.1016/j.arr.2010.10.001

🔥 **Heat Shock Response & HSF1**

- **HSF1 and proteostasis regulation**
- https://doi.org/10.1016/j.tibs.2018.01.006

⚙️ **mTOR, Nutrient Sensing & Proteostasis Link**

- **mTOR and aging**
- https://doi.org/10.1016/j.cell.2016.02.004
- **Nutrient sensing pathways**
- https://doi.org/10.1016/j.cell.2015.02.020

Loss of Proteostasis in Oral Tissues and Dental Regeneration

1. Introduction

Proteostasis (protein homeostasis) refers to the maintenance of protein folding, stability, and degradation. In aging, loss of proteostasis leads to accumulation of misfolded proteins, contributing to cellular dysfunction and impaired regeneration in oral tissues.

2. Proteostasis Mechanisms in Oral Tissues

2.1 Key Systems

- Molecular chaperones (Heat Shock Proteins)
- Ubiquitin–proteasome system
- Autophagy–lysosomal pathway

3. Proteostasis Decline in Aging Oral Tissues

3.1 Misfolded Protein Accumulation

- Impairs:
  - Stem cell function
  - Tissue repair

3.2 Reduced Autophagy

- Leads to:
  - Damaged protein accumulation
  - Cellular senescence

3.3 Oxidative Stress

- ROS damages proteins and enzymes

4. Impact on Dental Stem Cells

- Reduced differentiation capacity
- Impaired regeneration of:
    - Dentin
    - Pulp
    - Periodontal tissues

👉 Dental pulp stem cells rely on proper protein regulation for regeneration

5. Diseases Linked to Proteostasis Loss

- Periodontal disease
- Delayed wound healing
- Pulp degeneration
- Bone resorption

6. Modern Therapeutic Strategies

6.1 Stem Cell Therapy

- Restores:
    - Cellular function
    - Protein balance

👉 **Dental stem cells show strong regenerative potential in tissue repair**

6.2 Proteostasis Modulators

🔹 Heat Shock Protein Activation

- Enhances protein folding

🔹 Autophagy Inducers

- Removes damaged proteins

6.3 Regenerative Endodontics

- Uses:
    - Stem cells
    - Growth factors
- Restores pulp-dentin complex

6.4 Biomaterials & Scaffolds

- Support protein stability
- Enhance cellular repair

7. Future Directions

- Proteostasis-targeting drugs
- Gene therapy
- Exosome-based protein regulation

👉 **Dental stem cells are emerging as a major regenerative tool in modern dentistry**

8. Hallmark Integration

Hallmark	Role
Loss of Proteostasis	Protein misfolding
Stem Cell Exhaustion	Reduced repair
Mitochondrial Dysfunction	ROS production

9. Conclusion

Loss of proteostasis is a critical driver of oral aging. Therapeutic strategies targeting protein quality control systems, combined with stem cell-based regeneration, represent promising approaches for restoring oral tissue health.

📚 Scientific References

- https://pmc.ncbi.nlm.nih.gov/articles/PMC7595477/
- https://pubmed.ncbi.nlm.nih.gov/31271121/
- https://pmc.ncbi.nlm.nih.gov/articles/PMC4367063/

Chapter-12

Antagonistic Responses & Nutrient-Sensing Deregulation - Hallmark of Aging

In the modern framework of aging biology (updated from Carlos LópezOtín and colleagues), **"antagonistic hallmarks"** are processes that are **beneficial early in life but become harmful later**—a concept rooted in the theory of **Antagonistic Pleiotropy**.

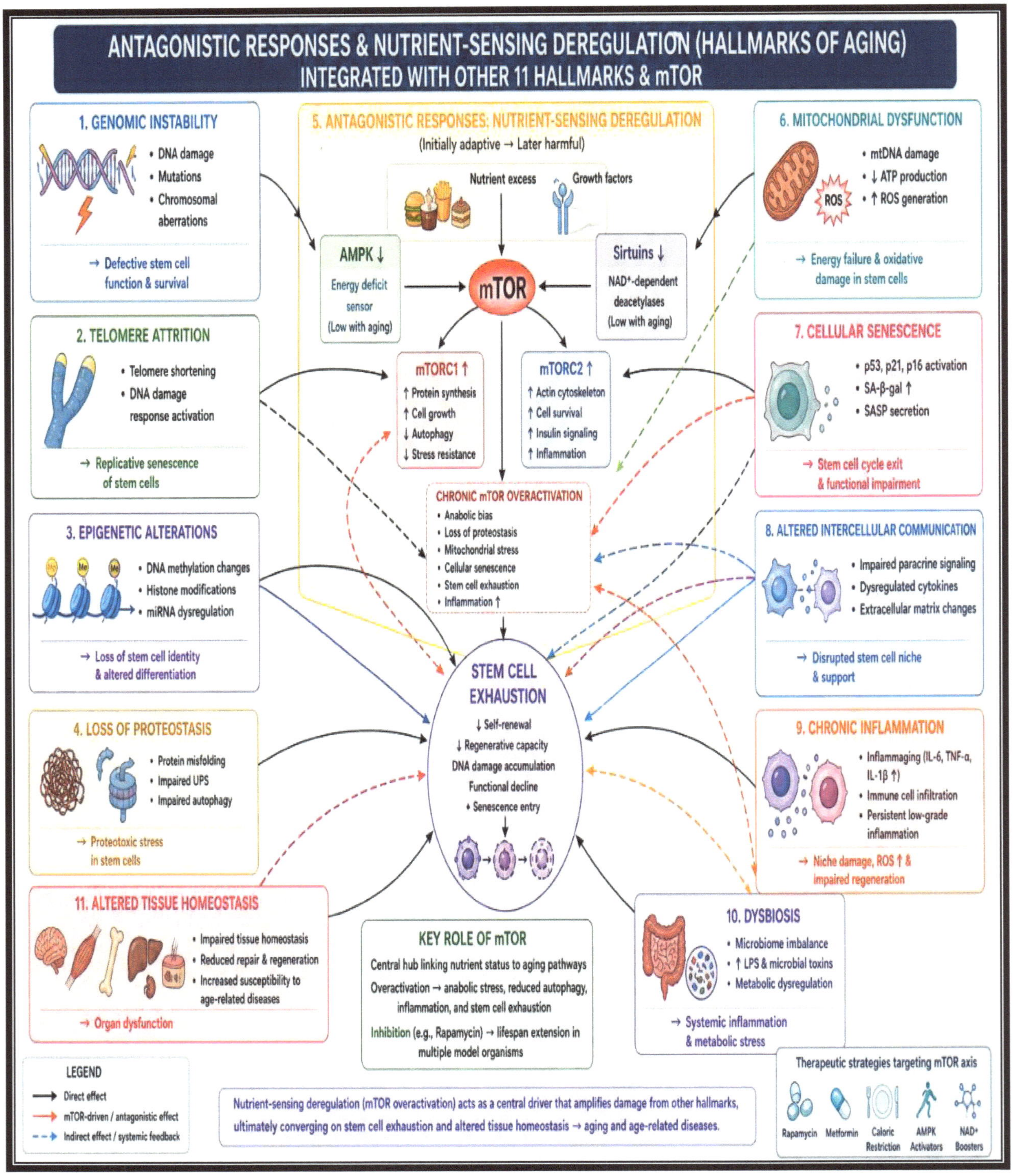

One of the central antagonistic hallmarks is:

🔬 **Deregulated Nutrient Sensing**

🧠 **Core Concept**

Nutrient-sensing pathways evolved to **optimize growth, reproduction, and survival under varying nutrient availability**. However, **chronic activation** of these pathways (common in modern lifestyles with nutrient excess) leads to:

- Cellular hyperfunction
- Impaired stress resistance
- Accumulation of damage

This shift exemplifies antagonistic behavior:

👉 **Pro-growth early in life → Pro-aging later in life**

⚙️ **Major Nutrient-Sensing Pathways**

1. Insulin/IGF-1 Signaling Pathway (IIS)

- Activated by glucose and amino acids
- Promotes:
- Cell growth
- Protein synthesis
- Inhibition of stress resistance genes

📌 With aging:

- Persistent IIS activation → oxidative stress, reduced autophagy
- Downregulates FOXO Transcription Factors (key for stress resistance)

2. mTOR Pathway

- Master regulator of:
  - Protein synthesis
  - Cell growth
  - Anabolism

📌 Chronic activation leads to:

- Reduced autophagy
- Accumulation of damaged proteins/organelles
- Cellular senescence

3. AMP-Activated Protein Kinase (AMPK)

- Activated during low energy (↑ AMP/ATP ratio)
- Promotes:
  - Catabolism
  - Autophagy
  - Mitochondrial biogenesis

📌 Aging:

- AMPK activity declines → reduced metabolic flexibility

4. Sirtuins (SIRT1–7)

- NAD^+-dependent enzymes
- Regulate:
  - DNA repair
  - Mitochondrial function
  - Longevity

📌 Aging:

- NAD$^+$ depletion → decreased sirtuin activity

🔁 Integrated View of Antagonistic Response

Early Life (Adaptive)	Late Life (Maladaptive)
High IIS/mTOR → growth & fertility	Chronic activation → aging, cancer risk
Low AMPK activation	Reduced stress resistance
Balanced metabolism	Metabolic syndrome, insulin resistance

📉 Mechanistic Consequences

1. **Inhibition of Autophagy**
   - Driven by mTOR hyperactivation
   - Leads to **loss of proteostasis**
2. **Mitochondrial Dysfunction**
   - Reduced mitophagy
   - Increased ROS production
3. **Cellular Senescence**
   - mTOR drives SASP (senescence-associated secretory phenotype)
4. **Chronic Inflammation**
   - Nutrient excess → inflammasome activation

📊 Visual Representation (Simplified Flow Diagram)

Nutrient Excess (Glucose, Amino acids)

↓

IIS ↑ & mTOR ↑

↓

↓ Autophagy + ↑ Protein Synthesis

↓

Accumulation of Damaged Proteins

↓

Cellular Senescence + Inflammation

↓

Aging

🖼 Conceptual Diagram

(Text-based since I can't embed actual images directly, but this is how you should visualize it)

Nutrient Availability

/\

Low Nutrients High Nutrients

(Fasting) (Excess)

↓ ↓

AMPK ↑ IIS ↑ + mTOR ↑

↓ ↓

Autophagy ↑ Autophagy ↓

↓ ↓

Cellular Repair Damage Accumulation

↓ ↓

Longevity Aging

🧬 **Clinical & Translational Relevance**

- **Caloric restriction** → ↓ IIS/mTOR, ↑ AMPK & Sirtuins
- Drugs targeting pathways:
    - Rapamycin → inhibits mTOR
    - Metformin → activates AMPK

📌 These interventions mimic **"low nutrient state"**, shifting physiology toward longevity

📚 **Scientific References**

1. Original Hallmarks of Aging Paper

- Authors: Carlos López-Otín et al.
- Journal: *Cell (2013)*

📚 🔬 **Updated/Advanced**

2. Updated Hallmarks (2023 Expansion)

📌 Key points:

- Expanded to **12 hallmarks**
- Includes:
    - deregulated nutrient sensing
    - chronic inflammation
    - dysbiosis

📚 🔬 **Mechanism-Focused Review**

3. Nutrient Sensing Pathways Review

📌 Key points (directly supporting your answer):

- Nutrient sensing = ability of cells to respond to nutrients
- Major pathways:
    - IIS (Insulin/IGF-1)
    - mTOR
    - AMPK
    - Sirtuins

📚 **Scientific References**

- Carlos López-Otín et al., *Cell (2013)*
- → Introduced the **hallmarks of aging**, including deregulated nutrient sensing
- 🔗 https://doi.org/10.1016/j.cell.2013.05.039
- Carlos López-Otín et al., *Cell (2023)*
- → Expanded framework to **12 hallmarks**, reinforcing nutrient sensing role
- 🔗 https://doi.org/10.1016/j.cell.2022.11.001

- Luigi Fontana & Linda Partridge, *Cell (2015)*
- → Reviews **IIS, mTOR, AMPK, sirtuins** in aging and caloric restriction
- 🔗 https://doi.org/10.1016/j.cell.2015.02.020
- Mikhail V. Blagosklonny, *Cell Cycle*
- → Describes **mTOR hyperactivation** as a driver of aging
- 🔗 https://doi.org/10.4161/cc.7.21.6855
- D. Grahame Hardie et al., *Nature Reviews Molecular Cell Biology*
- → Explains **AMPK as an energy sensor** regulating longevity
- 🔗 https://doi.org/10.1038/nrm3311
- Shin-ichiro Imai & Leonard Guarente
- → Covers **sirtuins, NAD⁺, and lifespan control**
- 🔗 https://doi.org/10.1101/cshperspect.a024521
- George C. Williams
- → Origin of **antagonistic pleiotropy theory**
- 🔗 https://doi.org/10.1086/282461

mTOR–AMPK Axis in Aging and Longevity

1. mTOR Signaling: The Growth Switch

The **mechanistic target of rapamycin (mTOR)** is a central cellular signaling pathway that integrates nutrient availability, growth factors, and energy status to regulate cell growth, metabolism, and survival.

When nutrients are abundant—particularly amino acids such as leucine and high insulin levels—mTOR becomes activated and promotes:

- Protein synthesis
- Lipid and nucleotide synthesis
- Cell growth and proliferation
- Suppression of autophagy

mTOR and Autophagy

mTOR acts as a **brake on autophagy**, the cellular recycling process:

- **High nutrients → mTOR ON → Autophagy OFF**
- **Low nutrients/fasting → mTOR OFF → Autophagy ON**

Autophagy is essential for removing damaged proteins and organelles. Chronic suppression of autophagy contributes to:

- Protein aggregation
- Cellular dysfunction
- Accelerated aging

2. mTOR in Aging and Disease

While mTOR is essential for normal physiology, **chronic overactivation** is associated with:

- Cancer (uncontrolled cell growth)
- Type 2 diabetes and insulin resistance
- Cardiovascular disease
- Neurodegeneration
- Chronic inflammation

Persistent mTOR activation reflects a state of **continuous "growth signaling"**, which is beneficial during development but detrimental during aging.

3. AMPK: The Energy Sensor

AMP-activated protein kinase (AMPK) functions as a cellular energy sensor and counterbalances mTOR.

AMPK is activated under conditions of **energy deficit**, such as:

- Fasting
- Caloric restriction
- Exercise

Once activated, AMPK promotes:

- Glucose uptake
- Fatty acid oxidation
- Mitochondrial function
- Autophagy

At the same time, AMPK **inhibits mTOR**, shifting the cell from growth mode to repair mode.

4. AMPK–mTOR Balance: A Longevity Switch

The relationship between AMPK and mTOR represents a fundamental biological trade-off:

State	AMPK	mTOR	Outcome
Fed/High energy	Low	High	Growth, storage
Fasting/Stress	High	Low	Repair, longevity

Healthy aging depends on **dynamic balance**, not complete suppression of either pathway.

5. Integration with NAD⁺–Sirtuin Pathway

The AMPK–mTOR axis is tightly linked with the **NAD^+–SIRT pathway**:

- AMPK activation → increases NAD^+ levels
- NAD^+ activates **sirtuins (SIRT1)**
- Sirtuins promote mitochondrial function and longevity
- Sirtuins and AMPK together suppress mTOR

This creates a **pro-longevity network**:

AMPK → NAD^+ ↑ → SIRT1 ↑ → mTOR ↓ → Autophagy ↑

6. Therapeutic and Lifestyle Modulation

Natural Strategies to Modulate the Axis

To reduce excessive mTOR activation:

- Intermittent fasting
- Caloric restriction
- Reduced excess protein intake (especially constant high leucine intake)

To activate AMPK and longevity pathways:

- Regular physical exercise
- Weight management
- Plant-rich diets (polyphenols)

Key Compounds and Interventions

Intervention	Mechanism
Metformin	Activates AMPK
Rapamycin	Direct mTOR inhibitor
Resveratrol	Activates AMPK and SIRT1
Quercetin	AMPK activation, anti-inflammatory
EGCG (green tea)	AMPK activation
Curcumin	Anti-inflammatory, modulates mTOR
Berberine	Improves insulin sensitivity, activates AMPK

7. Clinical and Aging Implications

Dysregulation of the AMPK–mTOR axis contributes to:

- Metabolic syndrome
- Obesity
- Neurodegenerative disorders
- Cancer progression
- Accelerated biological aging

Targeting this pathway is considered one of the most promising strategies in **geroscience and longevity medicine**.

Key Concept Summary

- **mTOR = Growth, anabolism, aging acceleration (when overactive)**
- **AMPK = Repair, catabolism, longevity promotion**
- Healthy aging requires **periodic activation of AMPK and suppression of mTOR**

Integrated Flowchart: Nutrient Sensing → Aging Axis

DIET/LIFESTYLE INPUTS

(High calories, protein, sugar vs Fasting, exercise, fiber)

↓

GUT MICROBIOME STATUS

(Eubiosis vs Dysbiosis)

↓ ↓

Healthy Microbiome Dysbiosis

(SCFAs, diversity ↑) (Inflammation ↑, LPS ↑)

↓ ↓

Improved Gut Barrier Leaky Gut

↓↓

↓ Inflammation ↑ Systemic Inflammation

↓

NUTRIENT SENSING PATHWAYS

↓↓↓

AMPK ↑ NAD$^+$ ↑ mTOR ↓

(Energy stress) (Sirtuin activation) (Growth suppressed)

↓↓↓

↑ Autophagy ↑ SIRT1/SIRT3 ↓ Protein overdrive

↑ Fat oxidation ↑ Mitochondria ↓ Cellular stress

↑ Insulin sens. ↑ DNA repair ↓ Senescence

↓

CELLULAR HOMEOSTASIS

↓

HEALTHY AGING

🚨 **Opposite Path (Aging Acceleration)**

Overnutrition → Dysbiosis → Inflammation →

↓ AMPK + ↓ NAD$^+$ + ↑ mTOR →

↓ Autophagy + ↑ Insulin Resistance →

Mitochondrial Dysfunction →

CELLULAR SENESCENCE → AGING & DISEASE

📄 **Table: Deregulated Nutrient Sensing (Core Concept)**

Pathway	Trigger	Main Function	Effect on Aging	Key Molecules
mTOR	Nutrients (glucose, amino acids, insulin)	Growth, protein synthesis	↑ Aging when overactive	Leucine, insulin
AMPK	Low energy (fasting, exercise)	Energy balance, repair	↓ Aging (protective)	AMP/ATP ratio

Pathway	Trigger	Main Function	Effect on Aging	Key Molecules
NAD^+–Sirtuins	Calorie restriction, AMPK activation	DNA repair, mitochondrial health	↓ Aging	NAD^+, SIRT1
Gut Microbiome	Diet, antibiotics, lifestyle	Regulates metabolism & inflammation	Dysbiosis → ↑ Aging	SCFAs, LPS

🔄 Functional Comparison Table (mTOR vs AMPK vs NAD^+)

Feature	mTOR	AMPK	NAD^+/Sirtuins
Role	Growth pathway	Energy sensor	Longevity regulator
Activated by	Nutrients, insulin	Fasting, exercise	Calorie restriction
Effect on Autophagy	❌ Inhibits	✅ Activates	✅ Activates
Effect on Aging	Accelerates (if chronic)	Slows aging	Slows aging
Metabolic Effect	Storage, anabolism	Breakdown, catabolism	Mitochondrial efficiency
Interaction	Inhibited by AMPK	Inhibits mTOR	Works with AMPK

🧠 Gut–Brain–Aging Axis Integration

GUT MICROBIOME

▼

Metabolites (SCFAs, serotonin, GABA)

▼

Vagus Nerve + Bloodstream

▼

BRAIN (HPA Axis Activation)

▼

Hormones (Cortisol, Insulin)

▼

Nutrient Sensing Pathways
(AMPK ↔ mTOR ↔ NAD^+)

▼

SYSTEMIC EFFECTS
- Inflammation
- Insulin Resistance
- Mitochondrial Dysfunction

▼

AGING HALLMARKS

⚖️ 5. Simple Clinical Interpretation (For Readers)

Longevity State

- Fasting/exercise
- Healthy gut microbiome
- AMPK ↑ | NAD^+ ↑ | mTOR ↓
- Repair mode ON

Aging State

- Overeating/stress
- Dysbiosis
- AMPK ↓ | NAD^+ ↓ | mTOR ↑
- Damage accumulation

Summary

"Aging is not just the passage of time, but the result of chronic nutrient excess, microbiome imbalance, and persistent activation of growth pathways (mTOR) over repair pathways (AMPK and NAD^+–sirtuins)."

Scientific References

- https://www.ncbi.nlm.nih.gov/pmc/articles/PMC6616936/
- https://pubmed.ncbi.nlm.nih.gov/20303871/
- https://pubmed.ncbi.nlm.nih.gov/19587680/
- https://pubmed.ncbi.nlm.nih.gov/29988155/
- https://www.nature.com/articles/nrm.2016.147
- https://pubmed.ncbi.nlm.nih.gov/25063780/

Chapter-13

Stem Cell Exhaustion as an Integrative Hallmark of Aging

📖 Conceptual Framework

Within the "hallmarks of aging" model proposed by Carlos López-Otín, **stem cell exhaustion** is categorized as an **integrative hallmark**—meaning it is not just an isolated defect but the **final outcome of multiple upstream damages** (genomic instability, proteostasis loss, nutrient deregulation, etc.).

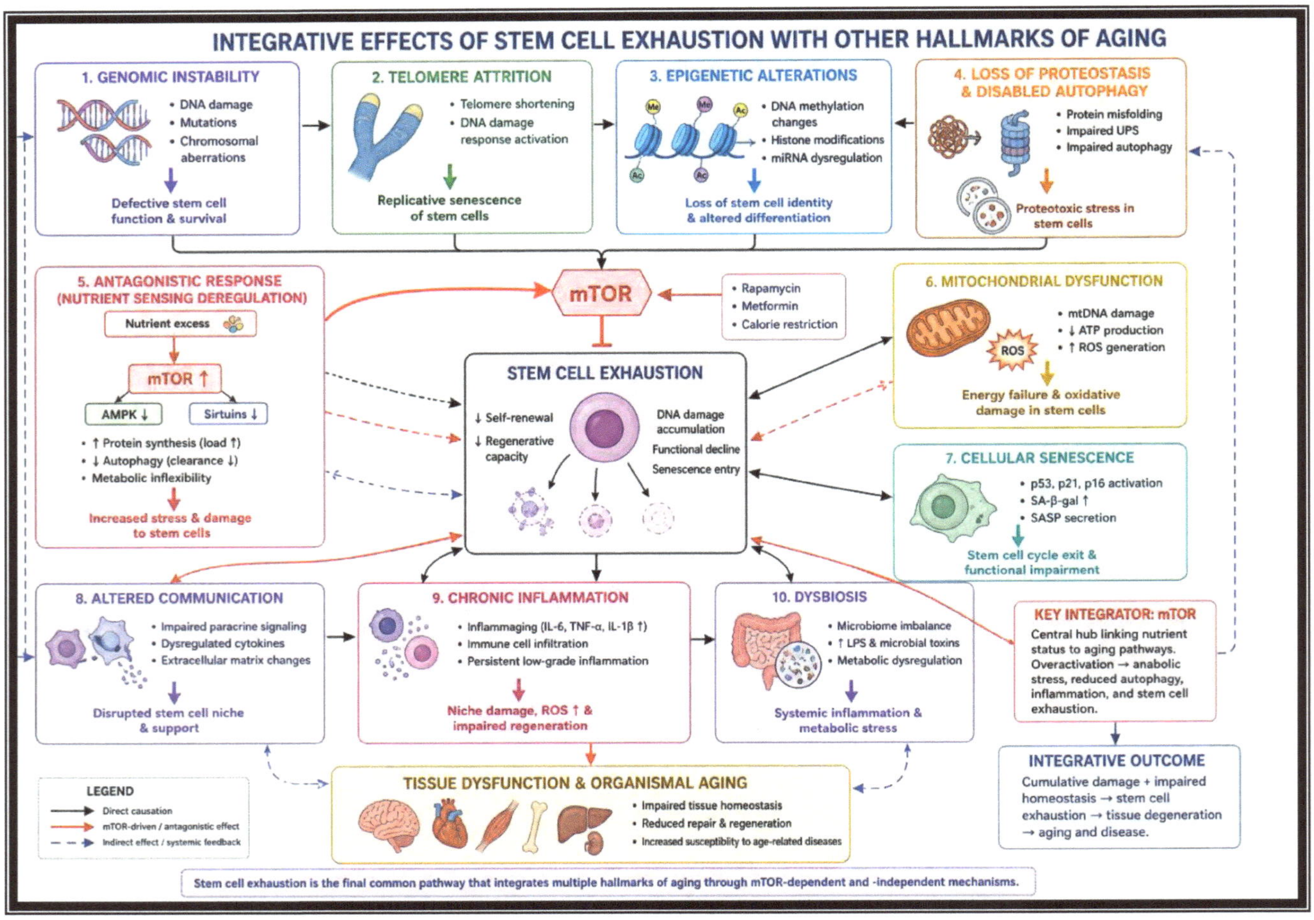

👉 Definition:

Stem cell exhaustion refers to the **progressive decline in the number, self-renewal capacity, and functional potential of tissue-specific stem cells**, leading to impaired tissue homeostasis and regeneration.

🧠 Core Biology

Stem cells maintain tissues through:

- **Self-renewal** (maintaining the stem cell pool)
- **Differentiation** (generating mature cells)

With aging:

- Self-renewal ↓
- Differentiation becomes skewed
- Regenerative capacity declines

➡️ Result: **Tissue degeneration and organismal aging**

🔬 **Types of Stem Cells Affected**

- **Hematopoietic stem cells (HSCs)** → blood system
- **Mesenchymal stem cells (MSCs)** → bone, cartilage
- **Neural stem cells (NSCs)** → brain
- **Epithelial stem cells** → skin, gut

📌 Aging affects each differently, but the underlying mechanisms overlap.

⚙️ **Molecular Mechanisms of Stem Cell Exhaustion**

1. Genomic Damage Accumulation

- DNA damage ↑
- Inefficient repair

📌 Leads to:

- Cell cycle arrest
- Apoptosis

2. Telomere Shortening

- Progressive telomere attrition
- Activation of DNA damage response

📌 Outcome:

- Replicative senescence

3. Epigenetic Drift

- DNA methylation changes
- Histone modification alterations

📌 Result:

- Loss of stem cell identity
- Altered differentiation potential

4. Deregulated Nutrient Sensing

- ↑ mTOR Pathway
- ↓ AMP-Activated Protein Kinase
- ↓ Sirtuins

📌 Effect:

- Increased proliferation stress
- Reduced autophagy → stem cell damage

5. Loss of Proteostasis

- Protein misfolding ↑
- Autophagy ↓

📌 Effect:

- Stem cell functional decline

6. Mitochondrial Dysfunction

- ROS ↑
- ATP ↓

📌 Result:

- Reduced stem cell viability

7. Cellular Senescence

- Activation of p53, p21, p16 pathways
- Entry into irreversible growth arrest

📌 Outcome:

- Stem cells become inactive

🔁 **INTEGRATIVE INTERACTION (VERY IMPORTANT)**

👉 Stem cell exhaustion is **not primary**—it is **secondary to cumulative damage**

🔄 **Vicious Cycle:**

Genomic damage + ROS + mTOR ↑

↓

Stem cell stress ↑

↓

Self-renewal failure

↓

Tissue repair ↓

↓

Accumulation of damage

↓

Further stem cell exhaustion

🖼 **Conceptual Diagram (Easy Visualization)**

Upstream Hallmarks

| Genomic instability |

| Telomere attrition |

| Epigenetic alterations |

| Proteostasis loss |

| Nutrient sensing (mTOR ↑) |

| Mitochondrial dysfunction |

↓

Stem Cell Damage & Stress

↓

↓ Self-Renewal ↓ Differentiation

↓

Stem Cell Exhaustion

↓

Tissue Degeneration

↓

AGING

🔬 Tissue-Level Consequences

Tissue	Effect of Stem Cell Exhaustion
Bone marrow	Anemia, immune decline
Brain	Cognitive decline
Skin	Thinning, delayed wound healing
Muscle	Sarcopenia

📊 Functional Changes in Aged Stem Cells

- Increased quiescence (but dysfunctional)
- Reduced regenerative burst
- Skewed differentiation
  - Example: HSCs → myeloid bias

🧬 Clinical Correlations

- Aging-related diseases:
  - Bone marrow failure
  - Neurodegeneration
  - Osteoporosis
- Reduced recovery after:
  - Injury
  - Infection

💊 Therapeutic Insights (Research Level)

- mTOR inhibition (e.g., Rapamycin)
- NAD^+ boosters → sirtuin activation
- Stem cell niche rejuvenation
- Senolytics (remove senescent cells)

🧬 Stem Cells in the Human Body

🔹 Types of Stem Cells & Their Location

1. **Embryonic Stem Cells (ESCs)**
   - Source: Inner cell mass of blastocyst
   - Potential: Pluripotent (all 3 germ layers)
2. **Adult (Somatic) Stem Cells**
3. Tissue-specific, multipotent:

Type	Location	Function
Hematopoietic Stem Cells (HSCs)	Bone marrow	Blood cell formation
Mesenchymal Stem Cells (MSCs)	Bone marrow, adipose tissue	Tissue repair, immunomodulation
Neural Stem Cells (NSCs)	Brain (SVZ, hippocampus)	Neuron and glial cell formation
Epithelial Stem Cells	Skin, intestine	Barrier regeneration
Muscle Satellite Cells	Skeletal muscle	Muscle repair

4. **Induced Pluripotent Stem Cells (iPSCs)**
    - Somatic cells reprogrammed (e.g., via Shinya Yamanaka factors)

🔄 Endogenous Self-Renewal Mechanisms

Stem cells maintain themselves via:

- **Asymmetric division** → one stem cell + one differentiated cell
- **Niche signaling** (microenvironment):
    - Wnt, Notch, Hedgehog pathways
- **Quiescence regulation** → prevents exhaustion
- **Proteostasis & autophagy** → removes damaged proteins

🧪 Exogenous Regeneration Strategies

Humans can enhance stem cell function via:

- **Stem cell transplantation**
    - Bone marrow transplant (HSCs)
- **MSC therapy**
    - orthopaedics, inflammation
- **iPSC-based regenerative medicine**
- **Growth factors/PRP therapy**
- **Biomaterials & tissue engineering**

⚠️ Causes of Stem Cell Exhaustion (Hallmark of Aging)

Mechanism	Effect
DNA damage	**Genomic instability**
Telomere shortening	**Replicative senescence**
Epigenetic alterations	**Loss of identity**
Mitochondrial dysfunction	**Energy deficit, ROS**
Chronic inflammation	**Tissue damage**
Nutrient sensing dysregulation	**Reduced repair**
Loss of proteostasis	**Protein aggregation**

Aging-Induced Stem Cell Exhaustion

Aging → Cellular Stress → Stem Cell Dysfunction → Reduced Regeneration → Disease

👉 Leads to reduced:

- Self-renewal
- Differentiation capacity

🧬 Diseases Linked to Stem Cell Dysfunction

- Bone marrow failure → anaemia, leukaemia
- Neurodegeneration → Alzheimer's disease, Parkinson's disease
- Muscle wasting → sarcopenia
- Skin aging & poor wound healing
- Osteoarthritis

🩸 Hematopoietic Stem Cells (HSCs)

- Location: Bone marrow niche
- Function:
  - Generate all blood cells (RBCs, WBCs, platelets)
- Aging effects:
  - Myeloid bias
  - Reduced immune function

⚡ Root Causes of Stem Cell Stress

- Reactive oxygen species (ROS)
- Replicative stress
- Protein misfolding
- Environmental toxins
- Metabolic imbalance

🔬 Stem Cells & Proteostasis (YES — Strong Link)

Stem cells rely on **protein homeostasis (proteostasis)**:

- Proper protein folding via chaperones
- Removal of misfolded proteins via:
  - Proteasome
  - Autophagy

👉 When proteostasis fails:

- Misfolded proteins accumulate
- Stem cell function declines
- Leads to aging & disease

🔥 Heat Shock Factor 1 (HSF1)

- Master regulator of stress response
- Activates heat shock proteins (HSPs)

Functions:

- Maintains proteostasis
- Protects stem cells from stress
- Declines with aging → contributes to stem cell exhaustion

💊 Clinical Applications of Stem Cells

1. Orthopedics (Spine/Knee)

- MSC injections → cartilage repair
- Disc regeneration (experimental)

2. Hair Regeneration

- Follicle stem cell activation
- PRP + stem cell therapy

3. Skin/Anti-aging

- MSCs → collagen production
- Wound healing

4. Dentistry

- Dental pulp stem cells → tooth regeneration

5. Cancer

- Bone marrow transplant
- Targeting **Cancer Stem Cells (CSCs)**:
    - Responsible for relapse & resistance

6. Type 1 Diabetes

- Beta-cell regeneration (experimental)
- iPSC-derived insulin-producing cells

🧠 Cancer Stem Cells (CSCs)

- Subpopulation within tumors
- Properties:
    - Self-renewal
    - Drug resistance
- Major cause of:
    - Tumor recurrence
    - Metastasis

🧾 High-Yield PG Summary

👉 Stem cell exhaustion is an **integrative hallmark** because:

- It reflects cumulative damage from other hallmarks
- It leads to failure of tissue regeneration
- It is central to organismal aging

👉 Core mechanism:

"Chronic damage + impaired repair → stem cell dysfunction → tissue degeneration"

📚Scientific References

- Carlos López-Otín et al., *Cell (2013, 2023)*
- → Hallmarks of aging framework, including **stem cell exhaustion**
- https://doi.org/10.1016/j.cell.2013.05.039
- https://doi.org/10.1016/j.cell.2022.11.001
- Shinya Yamanaka
- → Induced pluripotent stem cells (iPSC) and regenerative potential
- https://www.nobelprize.org/prizes/medicine/2012/yamanaka/lecture/
- National Institutes of Health
- → Fundamental concepts of stem cell biology
- https://stemcells.nih.gov/info/basics
- *Nature Reviews Molecular Cell Biology*
- → Molecular regulation of stem cells and aging mechanisms
- https://www.nature.com/articles/nrm.2016.28
- *Cell Stem Cell*
- → Stem cell aging, exhaustion, and regenerative decline
- https://doi.org/10.1016/j.stem.2017.11.010

Additional Supporting Reviews (PMC Articles)

- Stem cell aging and regenerative decline
- https://pmc.ncbi.nlm.nih.gov/articles/PMC10044767/
- Hematopoietic stem cell aging mechanisms
- https://pmc.ncbi.nlm.nih.gov/articles/PMC3080271/
- Stem cells and disease associations
- https://pmc.ncbi.nlm.nih.gov/articles/PMC8641024/
- Proteostasis and stem cell function
- https://pmc.ncbi.nlm.nih.gov/articles/PMC3992297/
- Oxidative stress and stem cell exhaustion
- https://pmc.ncbi.nlm.nih.gov/articles/PMC2360465/

Regenerative Dentistry and Stem Cell-Based Therapies in Aging

Modern Stem Cell–Based Dental Treatments

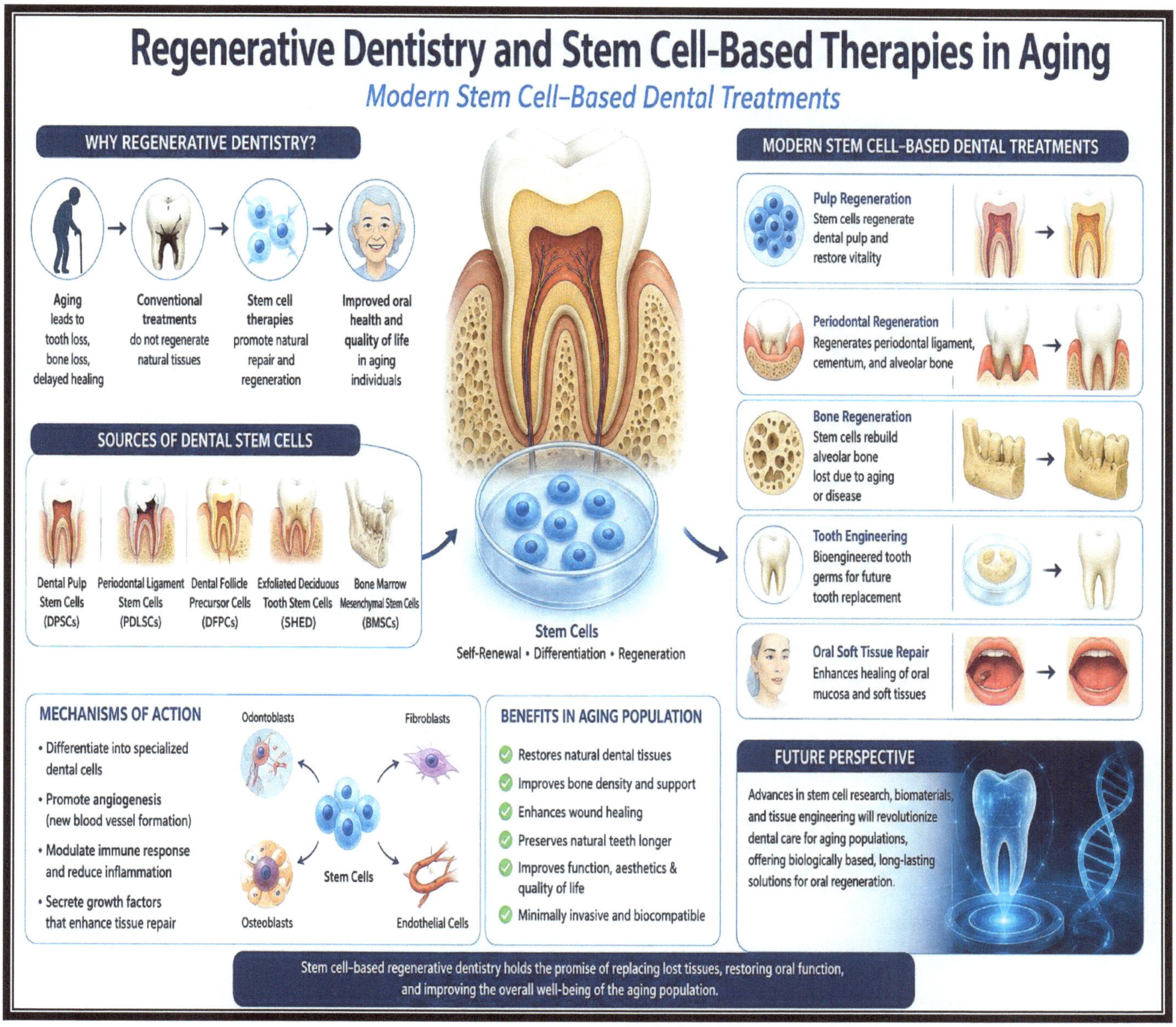

1. Dental Pulp Regeneration

- Uses **Dental Pulp Stem Cells (DPSCs)**
- Can regenerate:
  - Pulp tissue
  - Dentin

📌 Clinical relevance:

- Alternative to root canal (future therapy)

➡️ Regenerative endodontics is emerging but still experimental

2. Periodontal Regeneration

- Uses:
  - Mesenchymal stem cells (MSCs)
  - Periodontal ligament stem cells

📌 Can regenerate:

- Cementum
- Periodontal ligament
- Alveolar bone

➡️ Shows improved healing in periodontal disease

3. Bone Regeneration (Alveolar Bone)

- Stem cells + scaffolds (3D biomaterials)

📌 Used in:

- Dental implants
- Jaw defects

➡️ Scaffold-based regeneration is a key advancement

4. Whole Tooth Regeneration (Future)

- Goal: Grow a **complete natural tooth**
- Based on:
  - Stem cells
  - Developmental signaling pathways

➡️ Still experimental but highly promising

📰 Recent research even explores **natural tooth regrowth using stem cells**

5. Exosome/Secretome Therapy (Newest Trend)

- Stem cells release:
  - Extracellular vesicles (EVs)

📌 Advantages:

- No cell transplantation needed
- Lower immune risk

➡️ Emerging as next-generation therapy

6. Epigenetic Reprogramming of Dental Stem Cells

- Controls differentiation and regeneration
- Influenced by aging and environment

➡️ Key for future precision dentistry

⚠️ Limitations

- Mostly **preclinical or early clinical stage**
- Standardization lacking
- Ethical and regulatory challenges
- Long-term outcomes unclear

➡️ Human trials are still limited despite promising results

🧠 Link to Hallmarks of Aging

Hallmark	Dental Relevance
Stem Cell Exhaustion	Reduced regeneration of pulp, bone
Inflammation	Periodontitis (chronic inflammatory disease)
Loss of Proteostasis	Protein damage in oral tissues
Mitochondrial Dysfunction	Impaired healing
Altered Communication	Disrupted cell signaling in gums

🧾 Summary

Regenerative dentistry represents a translational extension of aging biology, where stem cell exhaustion, chronic inflammation, and impaired proteostasis contribute to oral tissue degeneration. Advances in dental stem cell therapy—including dental pulp regeneration, periodontal repair, and scaffold-based bone regeneration—demonstrate the potential to restore lost structure and function. Although still largely experimental, these approaches illustrate how targeting fundamental hallmarks of aging can enable tissue-specific rejuvenation in the oral cavity.

📚 Scientific References

- https://doi.org/10.1016/j.job.2024.02.006
- https://pmc.ncbi.nlm.nih.gov/articles/PMC10938178/
- https://doi.org/10.3390/cells13121065
- https://doi.org/10.1007/s44337-024-00087-7
- https://doi.org/10.1186/s13287-024-03936-5
- https://doi.org/10.1186/s13072-024-00563-5

Altered Intercellular Communication - Hallmark of Aging

Altered intercellular communication refers to age-associated changes in the way cells signal to each other and to their environment, resulting in impaired coordination between tissues and organs.

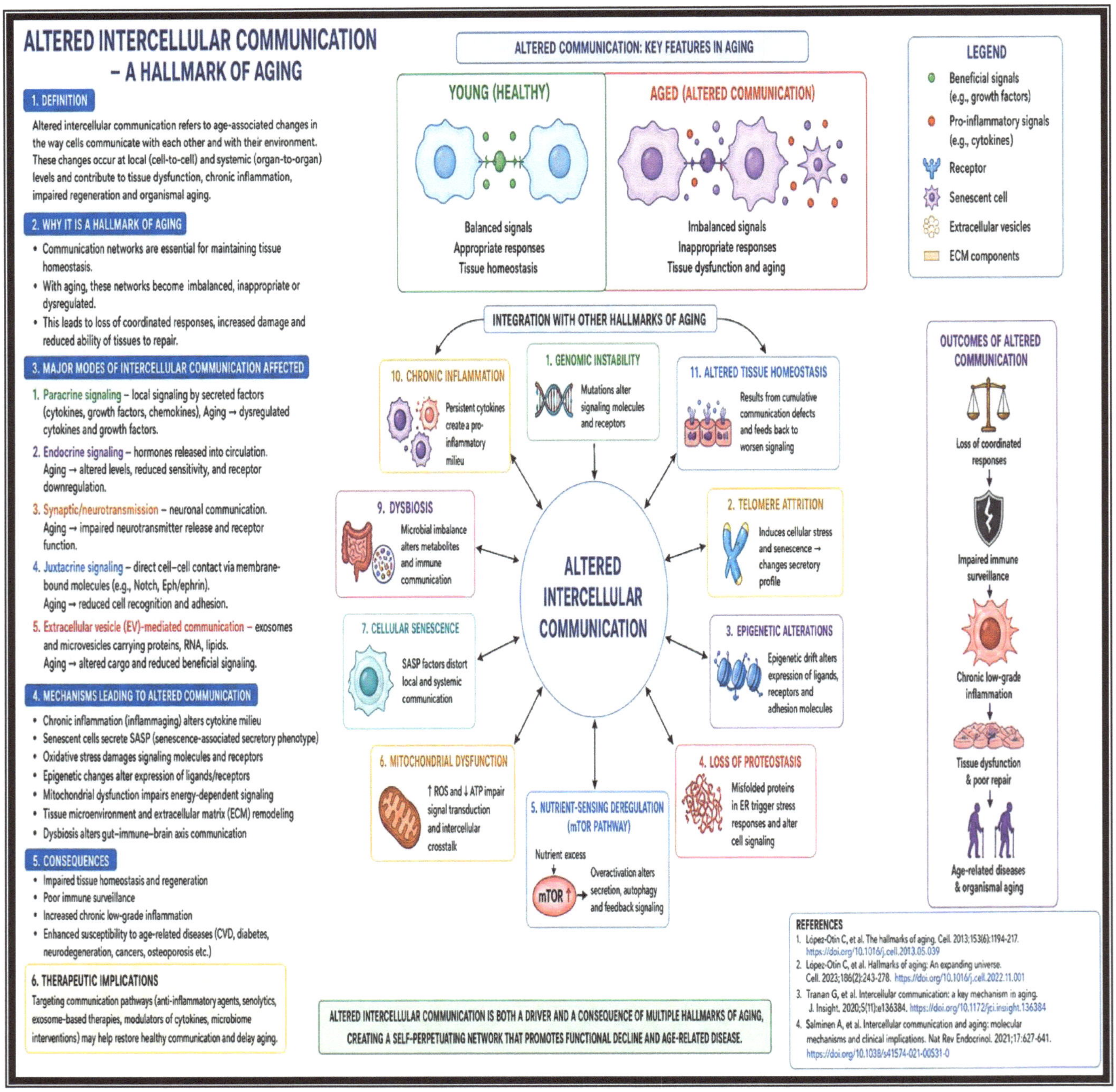

These changes occur at:

- **Local level** (cell-to-cell signaling)
- **Systemic level** (endocrine, immune, neural communication)

👉 The net effect is **loss of tissue homeostasis and increased vulnerability to disease**.

Physiological Importance (Normal State)

In a healthy young organism:

- Cells communicate through **precisely regulated signaling networks**
- These include:
  - growth factors
  - cytokines
  - hormones
  - neurotransmitters

This ensures:

- Proper tissue repair
- Immune surveillance
- Adaptation to stress

❌ What Happens in Aging?

With aging, communication becomes:

- **Dysregulated** (signals are abnormal)
- **Noisy** (inappropriate or excessive signals)
- **Uncoordinated**

➡ Result:

- Cells respond incorrectly to stimuli
- Tissue repair becomes inefficient
- Chronic inflammation develops

Mechanisms of Altered Communication

1. Chronic Low-Grade Inflammation (Inflammaging)

Aging is associated with persistent elevation of:

- IL-6
- TNF-α
- IL-1β

Effects:

- Continuous immune activation
- Tissue damage
- Disruption of signaling balance

2. Cellular Senescence & SASP

Senescent cells release **SASP (Senescence-Associated Secretory Phenotype)**:

- pro-inflammatory cytokines
- growth factors
- proteases

Consequences:

- Alters local microenvironment
- Induces senescence in neighboring cells
- Amplifies inflammation

3. Dysregulation of Paracrine & Endocrine Signaling

- Growth factor signaling becomes abnormal
- Hormonal responsiveness declines

Examples:

- Insulin resistance
- Reduced sensitivity to anabolic signals

4. Impaired Immune Communication

- Decline in immune surveillance
- Altered cytokine signaling

👉 Leads to:

- Increased infections
- Cancer susceptibility

5. Extracellular Vesicle (EV) Changes

- Exosomes carry proteins, RNA, lipids
- With aging:
    - cargo composition changes
    - beneficial signaling decreases

👉 Results in defective intercellular messaging

6. Extracellular Matrix (ECM) Remodeling

- ECM structure changes with age
- Affects:
    - cell adhesion
    - signal transmission

👉 Leads to impaired cell–environment interaction

7. Neuroendocrine Communication Decline

- Reduced hypothalamic regulation
- Altered hormone release

👉 Contributes to systemic aging effects

🔗 **Integration with Other Hallmarks (VERY IMPORTANT)**

Altered communication is both:

👉 **A consequence** of other hallmarks

👉 **A driver** of further aging

Key Interactions:

- **Genomic instability** → abnormal signaling proteins
- **Epigenetic alterations** → altered cytokine/gene expression
- **Loss of proteostasis** → misfolded signaling molecules
- **Mitochondrial dysfunction** → ROS disrupt signaling
- **Nutrient sensing (↑ mTOR)** → pro-inflammatory signaling
- **Cellular senescence** → SASP secretion
- **Dysbiosis** → gut–immune signaling imbalance

👉 This creates a **self-amplifying loop of dysfunction**

🔁 **Vicious Cycle (High-Yield Concept)**

Cellular damage

↓

Abnormal signaling

↓

Chronic inflammation

↓
Tissue dysfunction
↓
More cellular damage
↓
(repeats)

🧬 System-Level Effects

- Impaired tissue repair
- Loss of regenerative coordination
- Increased systemic inflammation
- Reduced stress adaptability

🏥 Clinical Relevance

Altered communication contributes to:

- Cardiovascular disease
- Neurodegeneration
- Metabolic disorders (e.g., diabetes)
- Cancer progression

💊 Therapeutic Perspective (Research Level)

Targets include:

- Anti-inflammatory therapies
- Senolytics (remove senescent cells)
- Cytokine modulation
- Microbiome correction

🧾 High-Yield Summary (Exam Ready)

- Altered intercellular communication = **disruption of signaling networks**
- Driven by:
  - inflammation
  - senescence (SASP)
  - immune dysfunction
- Leads to:
  - tissue dysfunction
  - systemic aging
- Acts as both:
  - **cause and consequence** of other hallmarks

🎯 One-Line Conclusion

Altered intercellular communication represents a breakdown of coordinated cellular signaling, leading to chronic inflammation, impaired tissue function, and progression of aging.

📚 Scientific References

- https://pmc.ncbi.nlm.nih.gov/articles/PMC6449758/
- https://pmc.ncbi.nlm.nih.gov/articles/PMC4036419/
- https://pmc.ncbi.nlm.nih.gov/articles/PMC4166595/
- https://www.cell.com/fulltext/S0092-8674(13)00645-4
- https://www.cell.com/cell/fulltext/S0092-8674(22)01377-0

Altered Intercellular Communication in Aging: with Special Reference to IGF-1 Signaling, Nutrient Sensing, and Protein Intake

1. Aging is not merely a consequence of cellular damage but also a result of progressive dysregulation in communication between cells, tissues, and organ systems.

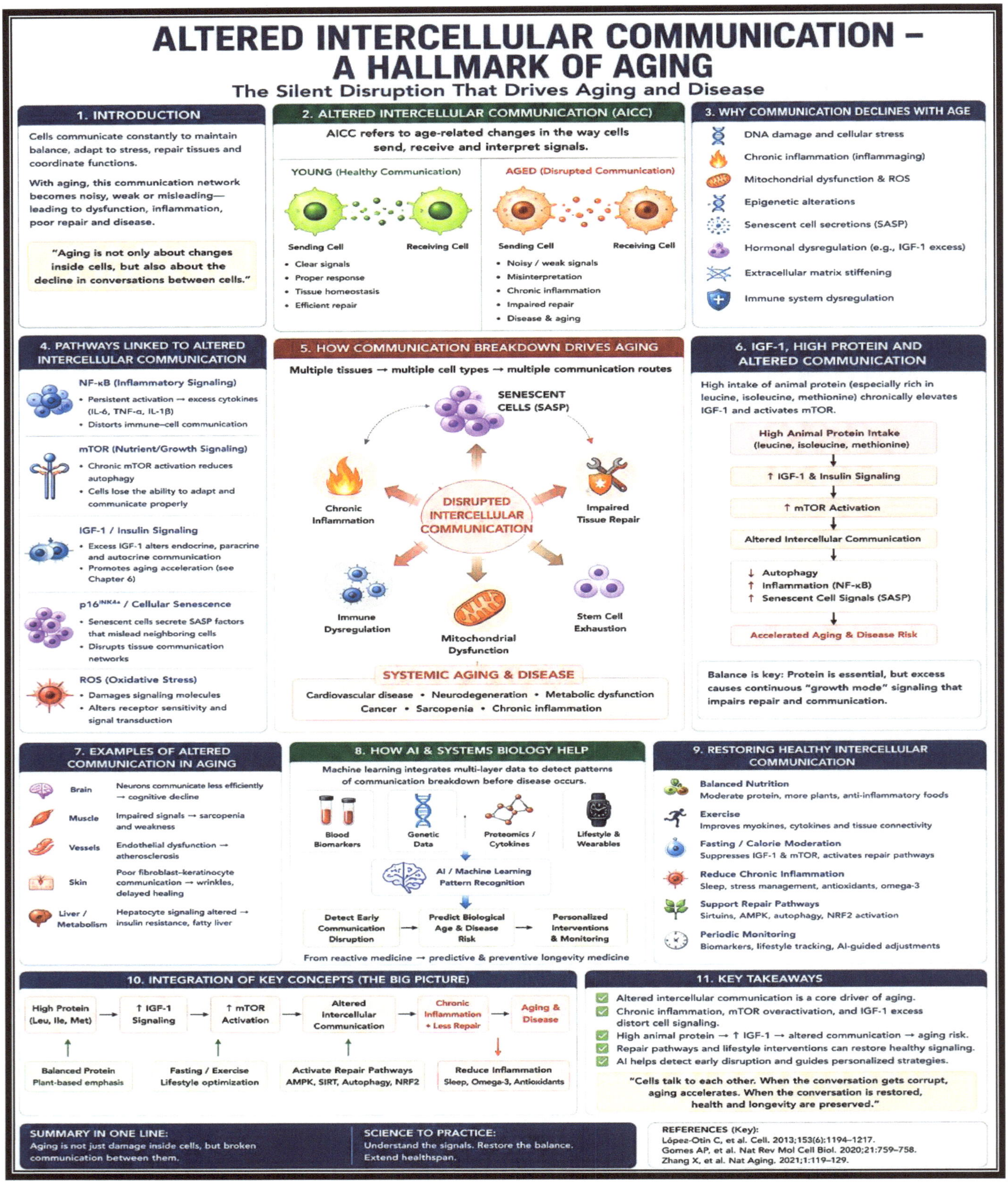

This hallmark—**Altered Intercellular Communication**—represents a critical shift in how biological signals are transmitted, interpreted, and regulated over time.

These signaling changes include:

- Hormonal dysregulation
- Neuroendocrine alterations
- Immune signaling imbalance
- Chronic low-grade inflammation (*inflammaging*)
- Nutrient-sensing pathway disruption (IGF-1, mTOR)

Key Concept:

Aging is not only "cell damage" — it is also "miscommunication between cells."

2. Physiological Basis of Intercellular Communication

Cells communicate through:

A. Endocrine Signaling

- Hormones (e.g., IGF-1, insulin)
- Systemic circulation

B. Paracrine signaling

- Local growth factors
- Cytokines

C. Autocrine signaling

- Self-regulation loops

D. Neural signaling

- Neurotransmitters

E. Immune signaling

- Cytokines (IL-6, TNF-α)

3. IGF-1: Central Regulator of Growth Communication

Definition

Insulin-like Growth Factor 1 (IGF-1) is a peptide hormone primarily produced by the **liver** in response to growth hormone (GH).

Physiological Roles

- Cell proliferation
- Protein synthesis
- Tissue repair
- Metabolic regulation

Conceptual Insight:

IGF-1 is a "growth communication signal" that tells cells: **"Grow, divide, and repair."**

4. The IGF-1 Paradox in Aging

A. Beneficial Role (Short-term/Localized)

- Hair follicle activation
- Wound healing
- Bone regeneration
- Muscle growth

👉 Seen in:

- PRP/GFC therapy
- Dental regeneration
- Fracture healing

B. Harmful Role (Chronic/Systemic Elevation)

- Increased cellular proliferation
- Reduced apoptosis
- Suppressed autophagy
- Increased oxidative stress

👉 Leads to:

- Cancer risk
- Accelerated aging
- Metabolic syndrome
- Cardiovascular disease

💡 **Core Principle:**

IGF-1 is beneficial in **controlled, local signaling**, but harmful when **chronically elevated systemically**.

5. Nutrient Sensing and Protein Intake

A. Role of Dietary Protein

High intake of:

- Animal protein
- Methionine
- Leucine
- Isoleucine

➡️ Activates:

- IGF-1 pathway
- mTOR signaling

B. Molecular Effects

Nutrient	Effect
Leucine	Strong mTOR activation
Methionine	IGF-1 upregulation
Isoleucine	Anabolic signaling

C. Clinical Implication

- Chronic high protein intake → persistent "growth mode"
- Reduced autophagy
- Increased cellular burden

💡 **Important Distinction:**

- Physiological protein intake = beneficial
- Chronic excess = pro-aging

6. Growth vs Longevity Switch

Aging involves a **dynamic balance between two opposing systems**:

A. Growth Pathways (Anabolic)

- IGF-1
- mTOR
- Insulin

👉 Effects:

- Protein synthesis
- Cell proliferation
- Reduced autophagy

B. Longevity Pathways (Catabolic/Repair)

- AMPK
- Sirtuins (SIRT1, SIRT3)
- Autophagy pathways
- FOXO

👉 Effects:

- DNA repair
- Cellular cleanup
- Stress resistance

C. Biological Trade-off

State	Dominant Pathway	Outcome
Growth Mode	IGF-1 ↑ mTOR ↑	Repair ↓ Aging ↑
Longevity Mode	AMPK ↑ Autophagy ↑	Repair ↑ Aging ↓

💡 **Key Insight:**

These systems cannot be maximally active simultaneously.

7. IGF-1 and mTOR Axis in Aging

Mechanism

IGF-1 → IGF-1 receptor → PI3K → AKT → mTORC1

Consequences of Chronic Activation

- Reduced autophagy
- Increased ROS
- Mitochondrial dysfunction
- Cellular senescence

💡 **Clinical Insight:**

Chronic activation of IGF-1/mTOR = "growth without cleanup."

8. IGF-1 and Altered Intercellular Communication

With aging:

A. Dysregulated Hormonal signaling

- Persistent IGF-1 elevation
- Insulin resistance

B. Increased Inflammatory signaling

- NF-κB activation
- Cytokine release

C. Impaired Cellular Feedback

- Reduced sensitivity to signals
- Signal amplification errors

D. Loss of Coordination

- Organs no longer "synchronize"

💡 **Interpretation:**

The body shifts from a **coordinated network → to a noisy, dysregulated system.**

9. Clinical and Research Applications of IGF-1

Localized Therapeutic Uses

- Hair restoration (PRP, GFC)
- Dental regeneration
- Bone healing
- Wound repair
- Muscle recovery

Systemic Considerations

- Growth disorders
- Cachexia
- Metabolic regulation

💡 **Paradox Resolution:**

Local use = controlled signal

Systemic elevation = chronic dysregulation

10. Role of IGF-1 in Major Age-Related Diseases

A. Cancer

- Promotes proliferation
- Inhibits apoptosis

B. Cardiovascular Disease

- Endothelial dysfunction
- Atherosclerosis progression

C. Metabolic Disorders

- Insulin resistance
- Fat accumulation

D. Neurodegeneration

- Mixed effects (context-dependent)

11. Factors That Increase IGF-1 Levels

- High protein diet (especially animal protein)
- Excess calorie intake
- Hyperinsulinemia
- Sedentary lifestyle

- Chronic stress
- Poor sleep

12. Factors That Decrease IGF-1 Activity

- Caloric restriction
- Intermittent fasting
- Plant-based diets
- Exercise (especially aerobic)
- Polyphenols (resveratrol, EGCG)
- Adequate sleep

13. Integration with Hallmarks of Aging

IGF-1 dysregulation contributes to:

- Genomic instability
- Loss of proteostasis
- Disabled autophagy
- Cellular senescence
- Chronic inflammation
- Mitochondrial dysfunction

💡 **System-Level Insight:**

IGF-1 is not isolated—it is a **central connector across multiple hallmarks**.

14. Conceptual Model for PG Students

Three Forces of Aging

1. Growth (IGF-1, mTOR)
2. Repair (Sirtuins, AMPK, Autophagy)
3. Inflammation (NF-κB, Cytokines)

Outcome Equation

👉 Aging = Growth ↑ + Inflammation ↑ + Repair ↓

👉 Longevity = Balanced Growth + Strong Repair + Controlled Inflammation

15. Final Summary

- IGF-1 is essential for growth and survival
- Its effects are **context-dependent**
- Chronic systemic elevation disrupts intercellular communication
- Nutrient signaling (especially protein intake) plays a key regulatory role
- Aging results from **network imbalance**, not a single pathway

📚 Scientific References

🧬 1. IGF-1 and Cancer Risk

Classic Lancet Meta-analysis

Renehan AG, et al.

"Insulin-like growth factor (IGF)-I and cancer risk."

📄 The Lancet (2004)

https://pubmed.ncbi.nlm.nih.gov/15110491/

🔬 Key Finding:

Higher circulating IGF-1 levels were associated with increased risk of:

- prostate cancer
- premenopausal breast cancer

The paper explains that IGF-1 promotes:

- cell proliferation
- survival of damaged cells
- reduced apoptosis

🧬 2. IGF-1 as a Tumor Growth Signal

Nature Reviews Cancer

Pollak M, et al.
"Insulin-like growth factors and neoplasia."

📄 Nature Reviews Cancer

https://www.nature.com/articles/nrc1387?utm_source=chatgpt.com

🔬 Important Concept:

The review explains:

- IGF-1 acts as both a hormone and tissue growth factor
- High-normal IGF-1 may increase cancer susceptibility
- IGF-1 supports survival of genetically damaged cells

🥩 3. Animal Protein → IGF-1 Increase

Nutrition + IGF-1 Review

Kaaks R.
"Nutrition, insulin, IGF-1 metabolism and cancer risk."

https://pubmed.ncbi.nlm.nih.gov/15562834/

🔬 **Key Finding:**
Western diets rich in:

- animal protein
- saturated fats
- excess calories

can increase:

- insulin
- IGF-1 bioactivity

which may promote:

- tumor development
- proliferation
- reduced apoptosis

4. Dairy Protein and IGF-1 Elevation

Human Epidemiology Data

https://pmc.ncbi.nlm.nih.gov/articles/PMC8106105/?utm_source=chatgpt.com

🔬 Key Findings:
Higher dairy and dairy protein intake were associated with:

- higher circulating IGF-1 levels

The paper also discusses:

- whey protein
- casein
- systemic IGF-1 elevation

🥩 5. High Protein Intake and Cancer Mortality

Levine et al. Landmark Study

https://pmc.ncbi.nlm.nih.gov/articles/PMC3988204/?utm_source=chatgpt.com

🔬 Important Findings:
In middle-aged adults:

- high protein intake associated with:
  - higher IGF-1
  - increased cancer mortality
  - increased diabetes mortality

Plant protein showed weaker association than animal protein.

⚖️ Important Scientific Balance

❌ Science does **NOT** say:

"Protein is bad."

✅ Science says:

Chronic overactivation of growth pathways
(IGF-1/mTOR) without adequate repair balance
may accelerate aging and disease risk.

Context matters:

- age
- activity
- muscle mass
- calorie excess
- metabolic health
- protein source
- duration

For example:

- elderly people often need more protein
- athletes differ from sedentary individuals
- localized IGF-1 signaling is therapeutic

🧠 Summary

"IGF-1 and mTOR are essential physiological growth pathways; however, chronic systemic overactivation—particularly in the setting of nutrient excess and persistent anabolic signaling—has been associated with accelerated aging and increased risk of age-related diseases."

Altered Intercellular Communication in Oral Aging and Regenerative Dentistry

1. Introduction

Altered intercellular communication is a key hallmark of aging characterized by disrupted signaling between cells, leading to chronic inflammation, impaired tissue repair, and degeneration. In oral tissues, this manifests prominently in periodontal disease, pulp degeneration, and bone loss.

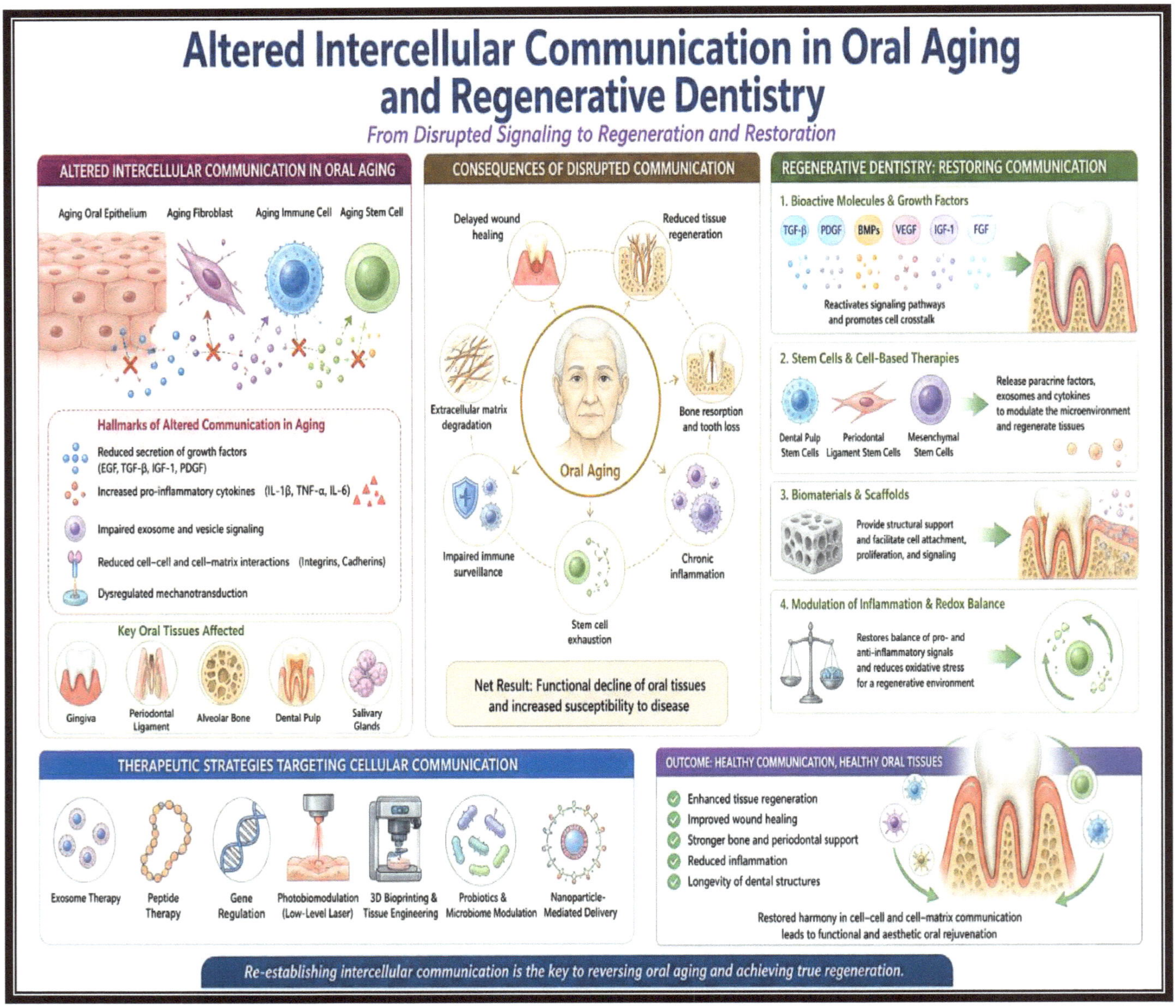

2. Mechanisms of Intercellular Communication in Oral Tissues

2.1 Normal Communication

- Cell–cell signaling via:
  - Cytokines
  - Growth factors
  - Extracellular vesicles (EVs)
- Maintains:
  - Tissue homeostasis
  - Repair and regeneration

2.2 Age-Related Alterations

- **Inflammaging**
  - Chronic low-grade inflammation
  - Increased:
    - IL-6, TNF-α
  - Leads to periodontal destruction
- **Stem Cell Niche Disruption**
  - Altered signaling in dental stem cell microenvironment
  - Impaired regeneration capacity
- **Extracellular Matrix (ECM) Changes**
  - Reduced signaling efficiency
  - Impaired cell adhesion and migration

👉 Dental regeneration is strongly dependent on **microenvironmental signaling and niche regulation**

3. Role in Oral Diseases

- Periodontitis → chronic inflammatory signaling
- Pulp necrosis → disrupted vascular signaling
- Bone loss → impaired osteoblast–osteoclast communication

4. Modern Therapeutic Approaches

4.1 Stem Cell–Mediated Communication

- Mesenchymal stem cells (MSCs):
  - Secrete cytokines and growth factors
  - Enhance regeneration

👉 MSCs improve periodontal and bone regeneration outcomes

4.2 Exosome/Secretome Therapy (Cutting-Edge)

- Cell-free therapy using:
  - Extracellular vesicles
- Benefits:
  - Reduced immune rejection
  - Enhanced signaling restoration

4.3 Growth Factor–Based Regeneration

- Platelet-rich plasma (PRP)
- Bone morphogenetic proteins (BMPs)

4.4 Tissue Engineering & Biomaterials

- Scaffolds mimic natural signaling environment
- Promote:
  - Cell migration
  - Differentiation

5. Clinical Applications

Condition	Therapy
Periodontitis	MSC + scaffold therapy
Bone defects	Growth factors + stem cells
Implantology	Bioactive materials

6. Hallmark Integration

Hallmark	Role in Dentistry
Altered Communication	Chronic inflammation
Stem Cell Exhaustion	Poor regeneration
Inflammation	Periodontal disease

7. Conclusion

Altered intercellular communication is central to oral aging and disease. Emerging therapies targeting signaling pathways—especially stem cell secretome and exosome-based approaches—represent a paradigm shift toward regenerative dentistry.

📚 Scientific References

- https://www.nature.com/articles/s41368-019-0060-3
- https://www.mdpi.com/2673-4095/6/3/65
- https://www.frontiersin.org/articles/10.3389/fphys.2022.1034603/full

Chapter-15

Chronic Inflammation (Inflammaging) - Hallmark of Aging

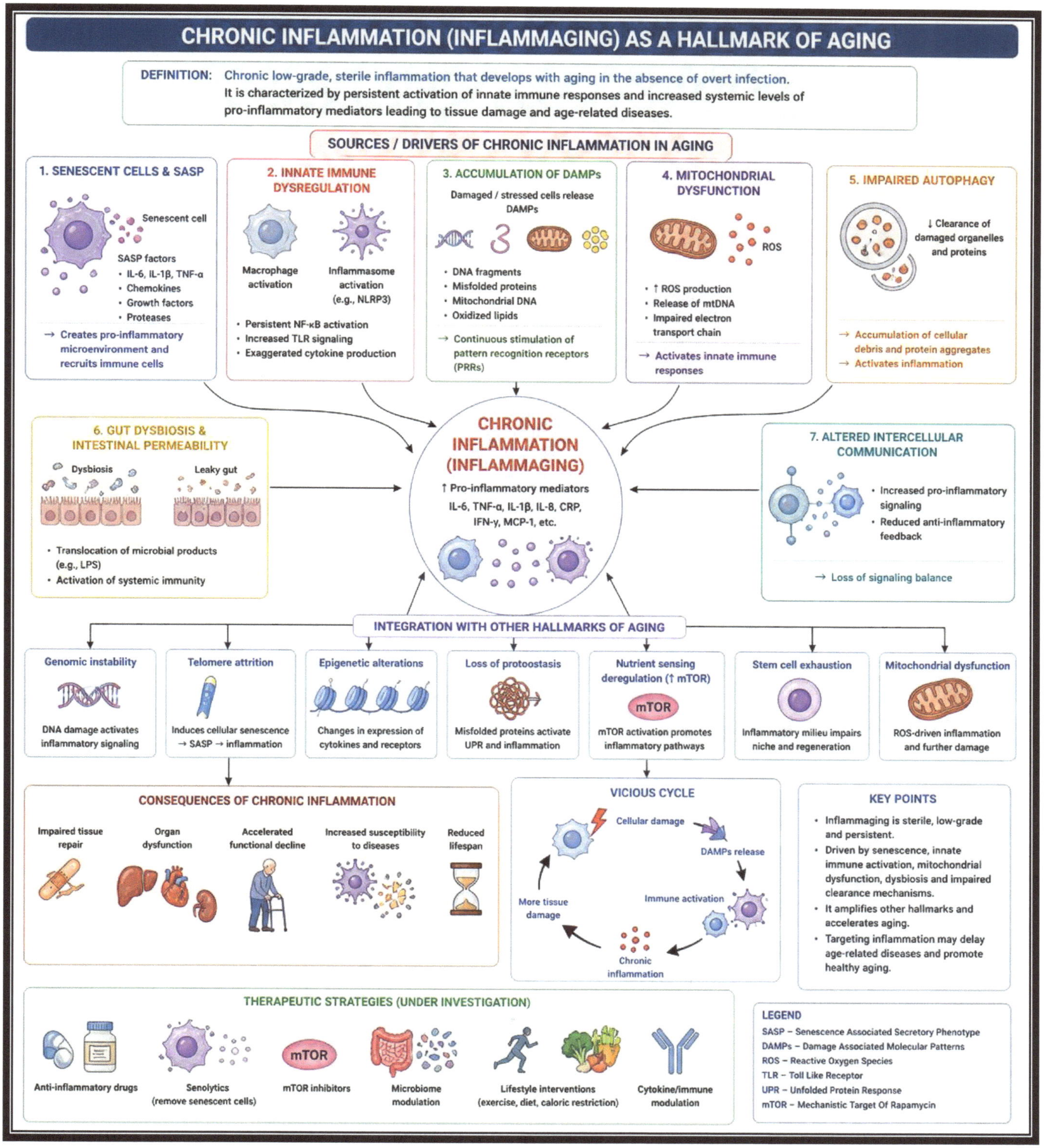

Chronic inflammation, often termed **"inflammaging,"** refers to a **persistent, low-grade, sterile inflammatory state** that develops with advancing age, even in the absence of overt infection.

👉 It is characterized by:

- Mild but sustained elevation of inflammatory mediators
- Continuous activation of innate immune pathways
- Progressive tissue damage over time

🧠 **Physiological Context (Normal vs Aging)**

✔ **In Young Individuals:**

- Inflammation is **acute and tightly regulated**
- Triggered by infection or injury
- Resolves after elimination of the stimulus

❌ **In Aging:**

- Inflammation becomes:
  - **chronic**
  - **systemic**
  - **poorly regulated**

➡️ Result:

- Continuous tissue stress
- Impaired repair and regeneration

⚙️ **Cellular and Molecular Mechanisms**

1. Senescent Cells and SASP

A major driver of chronic inflammation is **cellular senescence**.

Senescent cells secrete:

- Pro-inflammatory cytokines (IL-6, IL-1β, TNF-α)
- Chemokines
- Matrix-degrading enzymes

👉 This is known as **SASP (Senescence-Associated Secretory Phenotype)**

📌 Effects:

- Creates a pro-inflammatory microenvironment
- Spreads inflammation to neighboring cells
- Disrupts tissue structure

2. Innate Immune System Dysregulation

- Aging leads to **hyperactivation of innate immunity**
- Key pathways:
  - NF-κB signaling
  - Inflammasomes (e.g., NLRP3)

👉 Results in:

- Continuous cytokine production
- Increased inflammatory tone

3. Accumulation of Damage Signals (DAMPs)

With aging, damaged cells release:

- DNA fragments
- Misfolded proteins
- Oxidized lipids

👉 These act as **Damage-Associated Molecular Patterns (DAMPs)**

📌 Effect:

- Constant activation of immune receptors
- Sustained inflammation

4. Mitochondrial Dysfunction

- Increased ROS production
- Release of mitochondrial DNA

👉 mtDNA acts as a pro-inflammatory signal

➡️ Amplifies inflammatory pathways

5. Impaired Autophagy

- Reduced clearance of damaged proteins and organelles
- Accumulation of cellular debris

👉 Leads to:

- Activation of inflammatory signaling
- Increased cellular stress

6. Gut Dysbiosis

- Age-related changes in microbiome composition
- Increased intestinal permeability

👉 Leads to:

- Translocation of microbial products (e.g., LPS)
- Systemic immune activation

7. Altered Intercellular Communication

- Increased pro-inflammatory signaling
- Reduced anti-inflammatory feedback

👉 Leads to:

- Loss of signaling balance
- Persistent immune activation

🔗 **Integration with Other Hallmarks**

Chronic inflammation is both:

👉 **A result of other hallmarks**

👉 **A driver of further aging**

Key Links:

- **Genomic instability** → triggers inflammatory signaling
- **Telomere attrition** → induces senescence → SASP

- **Loss of proteostasis** → misfolded proteins → immune activation
- **Mitochondrial dysfunction** → ROS → inflammation
- **Nutrient sensing (↑ mTOR)** → promotes inflammatory pathways
- **Stem cell exhaustion** → impaired tissue repair

👉 This creates a **self-amplifying inflammatory loop**

🔁 Vicious Cycle (High-Yield Concept)

Cellular damage

↓

DAMPs release

↓

Immune activation

↓

Chronic inflammation

↓

Tissue damage

↓

More cellular damage

↓

(repeats)

🧬 Systemic Effects

- Impaired tissue regeneration
- Increased oxidative stress
- Altered metabolic regulation
- Decline in organ function

🏥 Clinical Relevance

Chronic inflammation contributes to:

- Cardiovascular diseases
- Type 2 diabetes
- Neurodegenerative disorders
- Cancer
- Osteoporosis

💊 Therapeutic Implications (Research Level)

Strategies under investigation:

- Anti-inflammatory drugs
- Senolytics (removal of senescent cells)
- mTOR inhibitors
- Microbiome modulation
- Caloric restriction

High-Yield Summary

- Chronic inflammation = **low-grade, persistent inflammation in aging**
- Driven by:
    - senescence (SASP)
    - immune dysregulation
    - mitochondrial dysfunction
- Leads to:
    - tissue damage
    - systemic aging
- Acts as both:
    - cause and consequence of other hallmarks

Conclusion

Chronic inflammation (inflammaging) is a sustained, low-grade inflammatory state driven by cellular damage and immune dysregulation, contributing to tissue dysfunction and progression of aging.

How to combat inflammation in the body

Inflammation can be managed through an anti-inflammatory diet, regular physical activity, adequate hydration, and other lifestyle modifications. Medical treatments are available for chronic cases. Processed foods, added sugars, and trans fats should be avoided, as they are known to increase inflammation.

A diet rich in antioxidants, including those present in fruits, vegetables, nuts, and fatty fish, can help reduce inflammation. Antioxidants neutralize free radicals, thereby mitigating inflammatory processes.

Scientific References

- https://pmc.ncbi.nlm.nih.gov/articles/PMC4166595/
- https://pmc.ncbi.nlm.nih.gov/articles/PMC4717894/
- https://pmc.ncbi.nlm.nih.gov/articles/PMC4036419/
- https://www.cell.com/fulltext/S0092-8674(13)00645-4
- https://www.cell.com/cell/fulltext/S0092-8674(22)01377-0

Adipose Tissue Dysfunction as an Endocrine Driver of Inflammaging

🧬 Hormones Elevated from Adipose Tissue

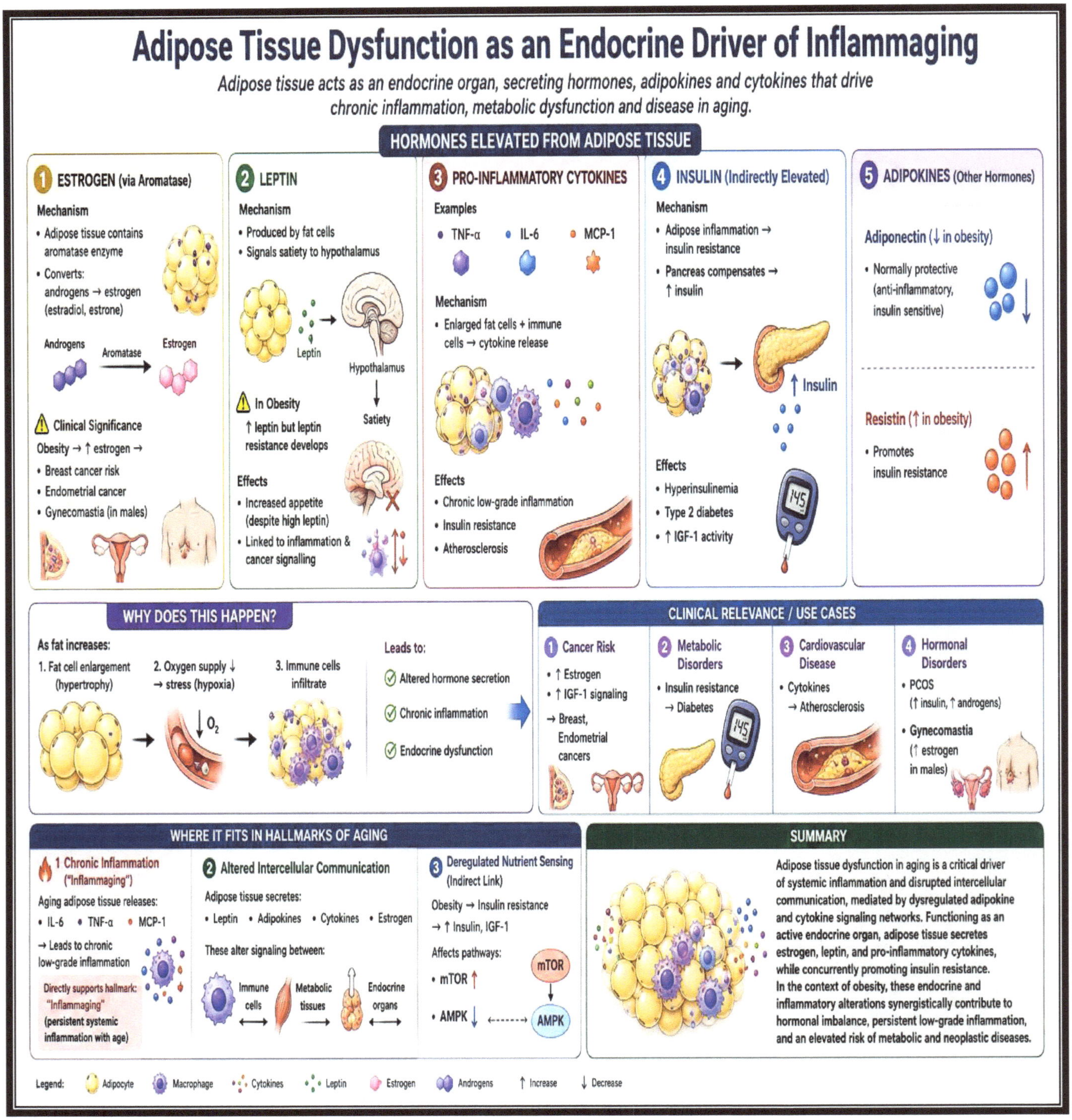

1. Estrogen (via Aromatase)

Mechanism

- Adipose tissue contains **aromatase enzyme**
- Converts:
  - androgens → **estrogen (estradiol, estrone)**

⚠️ Clinical Significance

- Obesity → ↑ estrogen →
  - breast cancer risk
  - endometrial cancer
  - gynecomastia (in males)

🧬 2. Leptin

🔬 Mechanism

- Produced by fat cells
- Signals **satiety** to hypothalamus

⚠️ In Obesity

- ↑ leptin but **leptin resistance** develops

📌 Effects

- increased appetite (despite high leptin)
- linked to inflammation & cancer signaling

🔥 3. Pro-inflammatory Cytokines

Examples

- TNF-α
- IL-6
- MCP-1

🔬 Mechanism

- Enlarged fat cells + immune cells → cytokine release

⚠️ Effects

- chronic low-grade inflammation
- insulin resistance
- atherosclerosis

🍭 4. Insulin (Indirectly Elevated)

🔬 Mechanism

- Adipose inflammation → **insulin resistance**
- Pancreas compensates → ↑ insulin

⚠️ Effects

- hyperinsulinemia
- type 2 diabetes
- ↑ IGF-1 activity

🧬 5. Adipokines (Other Hormones)

🔹 Adiponectin (↓ in obesity)

- Normally **protective** (anti-inflammatory, insulin sensitive)

🔹 Resistin (↑)

- Promotes insulin resistance

❓ Why Does This Happen?

🔬 Core Reason

As fat increases:

- fat cells enlarge (**hypertrophy**)
- oxygen supply ↓ → stress
- immune cells infiltrate

👉 Leads to:

- altered hormone secretion
- chronic inflammation
- endocrine dysfunction

🩺 Use Cases/Clinical Relevance

1. Cancer Risk

- ↑ estrogen + ↑ IGF-1 signaling
  → breast, endometrial cancers

2. Metabolic Disorders

- insulin resistance → diabetes

3. Cardiovascular Disease

- cytokines → atherosclerosis

4. Hormonal Disorders

- PCOS (↑ insulin, ↑ androgens)
- gynecomastia (↑ estrogen in males)

🧬 Where It Fits in *Hallmarks of Aging*

🔥 1. Chronic Inflammation ("Inflammaging")

- Aging adipose tissue releases:
    - **IL-6, TNF-α, MCP-1**
- Leads to **chronic low-grade inflammation**

👉 This directly supports the hallmark:
"Inflammaging" (persistent systemic inflammation with age)

🧪 2. Altered Intercellular Communication

- Adipose tissue secretes:
    - **leptin, adipokines, cytokines, estrogen**
- These alter signaling between:
    - immune cells
    - metabolic tissues
    - endocrine organs

⚙️ 3. Deregulated Nutrient Sensing (Indirect Link)

- Obesity → insulin resistance → ↑ insulin, IGF-1
- Affects pathways:
    - mTOR
    - AMPK

Metabolic Overflow, Chronic Inflammation, and Protein-Driven Oncogenic Pathways in Aging

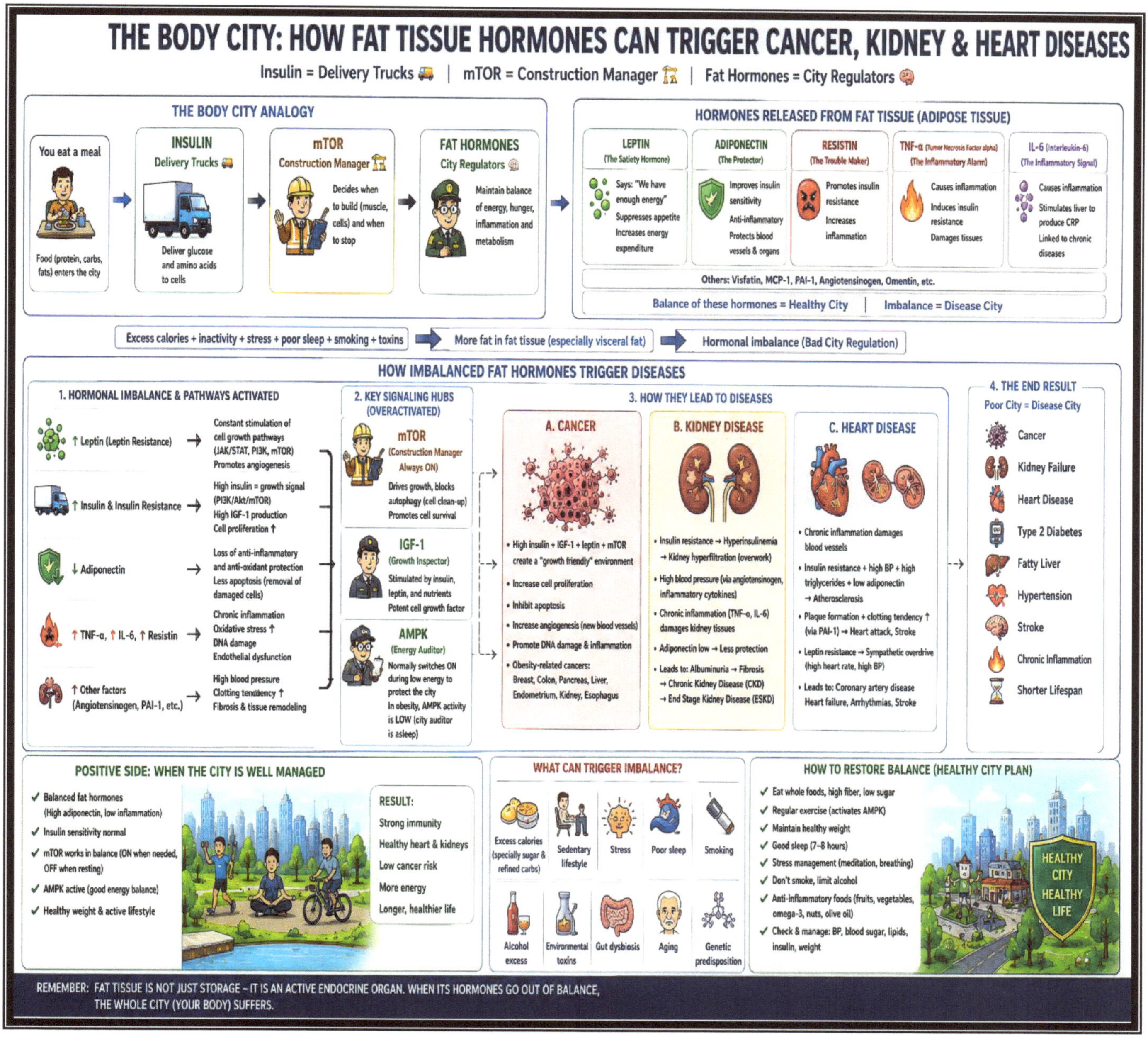

Introduction

Protein is traditionally considered a **non-lipogenic macronutrient**, primarily utilized for structural and functional roles. However, under conditions of **chronic energy excess and metabolic dysregulation**, excess protein contributes indirectly to **lipogenesis, adiposity, and downstream oncogenic pathways**.

Key Concept:

Protein does not directly convert to fat; rather, **metabolic overflow of amino acids under specific conditions leads to fat synthesis and storage**.

Biochemical Basis: Fate of Excess Protein

👉 Excess protein → amino acids → deamination → carbon skeletons → metabolic pathways → fat (only under certain conditions)

🔬 2. Core Biochemical Pathway (When Protein Becomes Fat)

Stepwise:

A. Excess protein intake

B. Amino acids exceed needs for:

- protein synthesis
- enzymes, hormones

C. Liver removes nitrogen (deamination) → urea cycle

D. Remaining carbon skeletons enter:

- pyruvate
- acetyl-CoA
- TCA intermediates

👉 If energy demand is LOW:

TCA cycle is saturated

Citrate exits mitochondria

→ de novo lipogenesis (DNL)

→ fatty acids → triglycerides → adipose storage (especially visceral fat)

Acetyl-CoA

TCA intermediates

⚙️ 3. Key Decision Point (Energy Status)

✅ Lean/Healthy State

High energy demand (exercise, calorie balance)

Amino acids used for:

muscle protein synthesis

repair

immune function

Minimal fat conversion

❌ Pathological State (Important for Exams)

Protein contributes to fat when:

🔺 Conditions:

Caloric surplus (critical)

Sedentary lifestyle

High insulin environment

Chronic mTOR activation

Low metabolic flexibility

🧪 4. Molecular Signaling: Why High Protein Can Promote Fat Storage

A. mTOR Pathway

Triggered strongly by:

Leucine (branched-chain amino acid, BCAA)

High animal protein intake

Leads to:

↑ protein synthesis

↓ autophagy

↑ lipogenesis indirectly (via nutrient abundance signaling)

B. Insulin Response

Protein (especially mixed meals) → insulin secretion

Chronic effects:

Hyperinsulinemia

↓ lipolysis

↑ fat storage

C. IGF-1 Axis

High protein → ↑ **IGF-1**

Effects:

Cell proliferation

Anti-apoptosis

Tumor-promoting environment

D. Hepatic Overload

Excess amino acids → liver metabolism

Leads to:

↑ **acetyl-CoA**

↑ **lipogenesis**

↑ **VLDL secretion**

→ fatty liver → visceral fat

5. Does "Type of Protein" Matter?

Yes—**very important for PG level understanding**:

High-Risk Context (when combined with excess calories)

Red meat (especially processed)

High BCAA load (leucine-rich diets)

High methionine intake

Associated with:

mTOR overactivation

IGF-1 elevation

Insulin resistance

Lower Risk/Protective Context

Plant proteins (lower BCAA density)

Mixed protein with fiber

Calorie-controlled intake

👉 Effects:

Better insulin sensitivity

Less mTOR overdrive

Lower IGF-1 stimulation

🔥 6. Transition: From Fat Storage → Cancer Biology

This is the **critical integration point** from your diagram.

A. Visceral Fat = Endocrine Organ

Produces:

TNF-α

IL-6

Resistin

↓ **Adiponectin**

B. Result: Chronic Low-Grade Inflammation

This leads to:

NF-κB activation

STAT3 signaling

ROS production

👉 Causes:

DNA damage

Epigenetic changes

C. Insulin Resistance + IGF-1 = Growth Signals

Hyperinsulinemia

↑ IGF-1

👉 Activate:

PI3K–AKT–mTOR pathway

Result:

↑ proliferation

↓ apoptosis

↑ angiogenesis

🧬 7. Cancer Link (Mechanistic)

Key Pathways:

1. mTOR Overactivation

Continuous growth signaling

Seen in:

breast cancer

prostate cancer

2. IGF-1 Axis

Promotes:

tumor initiation

tumor progression

3. Chronic Inflammation

TNF-α, IL-6

Drives:

colorectal cancer

liver cancer (NASH → HCC)

4. Oxidative Stress

ROS → DNA mutations

🧠 8. Clinical Integration (Very Important)

Protein → Fat → Cancer happens ONLY when:

✔ Excess calories
✔ Chronic overnutrition
✔ Sedentary Behavior
✔ Visceral fat accumulation
✔ Hormonal dysregulation

🎯 9. High-Yield Summary

Protein is **not inherently lipogenic**

It becomes fat **indirectly via metabolic overflow**

Key switch = **energy surplus + hormonal environment**

Main mediators:

mTOR

Insulin

IGF-1

Cancer risk arises from:

chronic inflammation

insulin resistance

growth signaling pathways

"Protein is like construction material. If the city is growing, it builds muscle. But if the city is already overloaded and inactive, the extra material gets dumped into storage warehouses—fat tissue—which then starts releasing toxic signals that can eventually lead to diseases like cancer."

🎯 Summary

Adipose tissue dysfunction in aging is a critical driver of systemic inflammation and disrupted intercellular communication, mediated by dysregulated adipokine and cytokine signaling networks. Functioning as an active endocrine organ, adipose tissue secretes estrogen, leptin, and pro-inflammatory cytokines, while concurrently promoting insulin resistance. In the context of obesity, these endocrine and inflammatory alterations synergistically contribute to hormonal imbalance, persistent low-grade inflammation, and an elevated risk of metabolic and neoplastic diseases.

Scientific References

1. Hotamisligil GS. Inflammation and metabolic disorders. *Nature.* 2006;444:860–867.
2. Xu H, et al. Chronic inflammation in fat plays a role in obesity-related insulin resistance. *J Clin Invest.* 2003;112(12):1821–1830.
3. Kahn SE, et al. Mechanisms linking obesity to insulin resistance. *Nature.* 2006;444:840–846.
4. Kadowaki T, Yamauchi T. Adiponectin and metabolic syndrome. *Endocr Rev.* 2005;26(3):439–451.
5. Simpson ER, et al. Aromatase expression in human adipose tissue. *Endocr Rev.* 1999;20(3):343–355.
6. Calle EE, Kaaks R. Overweight, obesity and cancer. *Nat Rev Cancer.* 2004;4:579–591.
7. Franceschi C, et al. Inflammaging and its contribution to age-related diseases. *Ann N Y Acad Sci.* 2007;1100:1–10.
8. López-Otín C, et al. The hallmarks of aging. *Cell.* 2013;153(6):1194–1217.

What could be the other probable causes of Hallmarks of aging

Endocrine disruptors

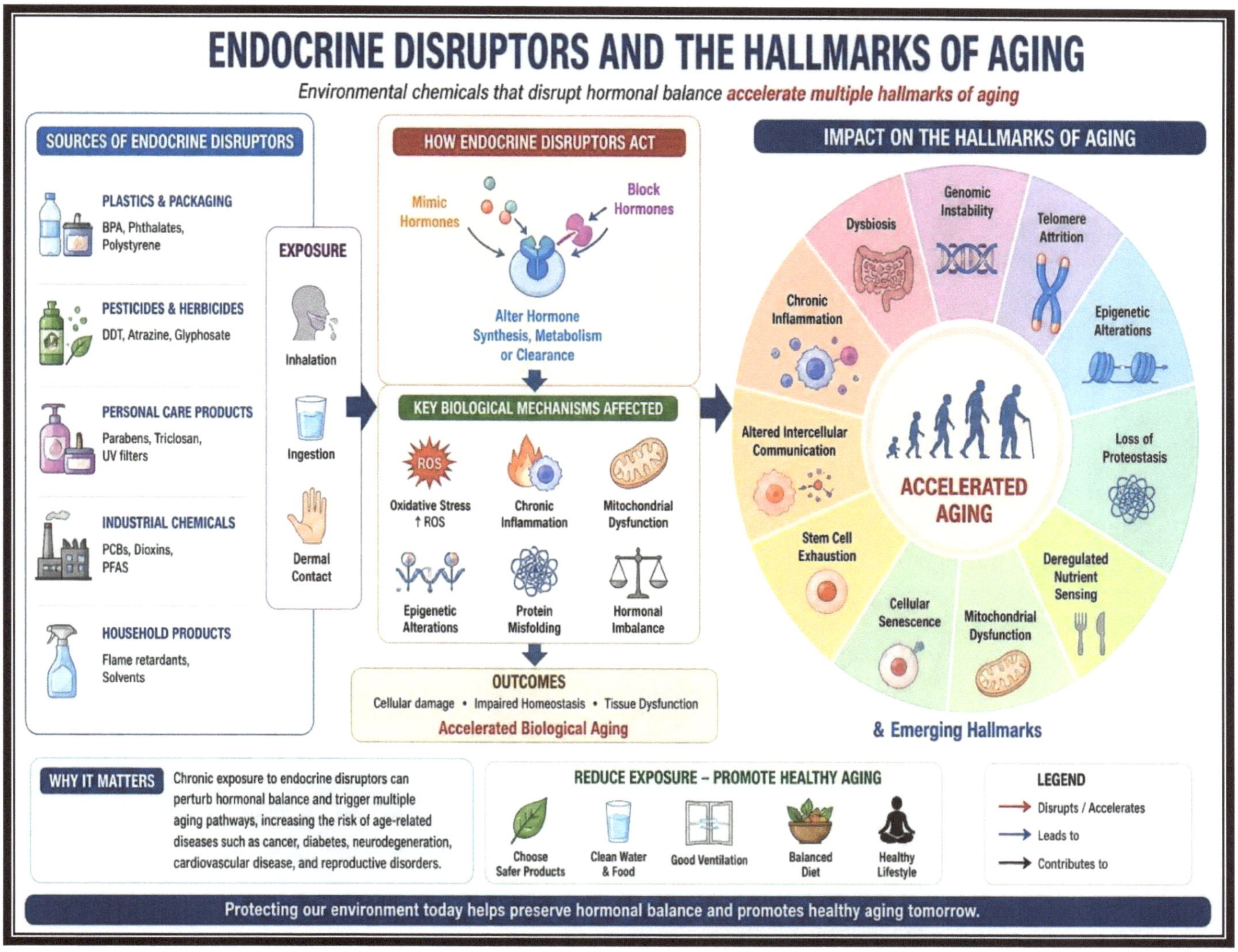

Endocrine disruptors, also known as hormone disruptors, are natural or synthetic chemicals that interfere with the normal functioning of the endocrine system. They can mimic hormones, block their activity, or alter hormone levels, leading to potential adverse effects on growth, metabolism, reproduction, and overall health. These substances are commonly found in everyday products such as plastics, pesticides, cosmetics, and various industrial chemicals. Exposure can occur through ingestion, inhalation, or skin contact, and even low levels of exposure may contribute to developmental, reproductive, neurological, and immune-related disorders.

Common sources of exposure

- Plastics and food packaging:

  Bisphenol A (BPA) and phthalates can leach from food and drink containers.

- Cosmetics and personal care products:

  Everyday items such as makeup, lotions, and sanitizers often hide ingredients like parabens, phthalates, and triclosan.
- Pesticides:

  Organochlorine pesticides, including DDT, are recognized endocrine disruptors.
- Household products:

  Flame retardants found in furniture and electronics, along with some detergents, can also introduce unwanted chemicals into our homes.

Activated charcoal and chelation therapy are both used for detoxification, but each works in its own way and targets different types of toxins.

Activated charcoal is a fine, black powder commonly utilized in emergency medicine to treat specific cases of ingested poisoning or drug overdose.

Chelation therapy relies on special prescription drugs known as chelating agents, named after the Greek word for claw, to latch onto heavy metals and sweep them out of the body.

Chelation therapy is typically administered intravenously. A chelating agent, such as EDTA, is infused directly into a vein, usually in the arm, over a period ranging from 30 minutes to several hours. This approach enables the agent to bind to heavy metals or excess minerals in the bloodstream, facilitating their excretion.

Heavy metals such as mercury and lead are neurotoxins that can substantially impair neurological function, including the regulation of sleep.

- **Mercury Toxicity:** High mercury exposure often brings restless nights, unshakable fatigue, and a fog of sleepiness. In case studies, patients found relief from anxiety, depression, and insomnia, and enjoyed deeper, more restorative sleep after chelation therapy lowered their mercury levels. Mercury tends to build up in the pineal gland, a key player in regulating our sleep cycles.
- **Lead Toxicity:** Patients with lead toxicity have reported improved mood, reduced irritability, and better sleep after chelation therapy lowered their blood lead levels.
- **Iron toxic** chelation therapy uses a medication to bind to and remove excess iron from the body, a condition known as iron overload.

Root Cause (Source of Exposure)

Endocrine-disrupting chemicals (EDCs) are widely present in the environment due to industrialization and modern lifestyle factors. Major sources include:

- Plastic products and food packaging
- Personal care products and cosmetics
- Pesticides and contaminated food/water
- Air pollution and industrial waste

Chronic, low-level exposure over time is particularly concerning, as it can subtly alter hormonal balance without immediate symptoms.

Endocrine disruptors are meaningfully connected to the hallmarks of aging, especially through pathways like hormonal imbalance, inflammation, metabolic dysfunction, and cellular stress.

Chain Reaction in the Context of Aging

Endocrine disruptors can influence multiple **hallmarks of aging** through interconnected biological effects:

1. **Hormonal Imbalance → Cellular Dysregulation**

   Disruption of hormones like estrogen, thyroid hormones, and insulin affects cellular signaling and metabolic balance.

2. **Oxidative Stress and DNA Damage → Genomic Instability**

   Many EDCs increase reactive oxygen species (ROS), contributing to DNA damage—one of the primary hallmarks of aging.

3. **Chronic Inflammation → Altered Intercellular Communication**

   Persistent exposure can promote low-grade inflammation ("inflammaging"), a key driver of age-related diseases.

4. **Metabolic Dysfunction → Deregulated Nutrient Sensing**

   EDCs are linked to insulin resistance and obesity, directly impacting metabolic pathways involved in aging.

5. **Epigenetic Changes → Altered Gene Expression**

   Some disruptors modify DNA methylation and histone activity, influencing how genes related to aging are expressed.

6. **Cellular Senescence**

   Accumulated damage and stress can push cells into a senescent (non-dividing but active) state, contributing to tissue dysfunction.

Summary Insight

Endocrine disruptors do not act through a single pathway. Instead, they create a **multi-layered biological impact**, influencing several hallmarks of aging simultaneously. This makes them an important environmental factor in understanding how external exposures can accelerate or modify the aging process.

Scientific References

- World Health Organization (WHO): Endocrine Disruptors
- https://www.who.int/news-room/fact-sheets/detail/endocrine-disruptors
- Endocrine Society Scientific Statement
- https://www.endocrine.org/topics/edc
- National Institute of Environmental Health Sciences (NIEHS)
- https://www.niehs.nih.gov/health/topics/agents/endocrine
- https://pmc.ncbi.nlm.nih.gov/articles/PMC5118545/
- https://pmc.ncbi.nlm.nih.gov/articles/PMC4448121/
- https://www.ncbi.nlm.nih.gov/books/NBK482294/

Autoimmunity

1. What is Autoimmunity?

Autoimmunity is a pathological state in which the **immune system loses self-tolerance** and mounts an immune response against the body's own cells, tissues, or molecules (autoantigens), leading to **chronic inflammation and tissue damage**.

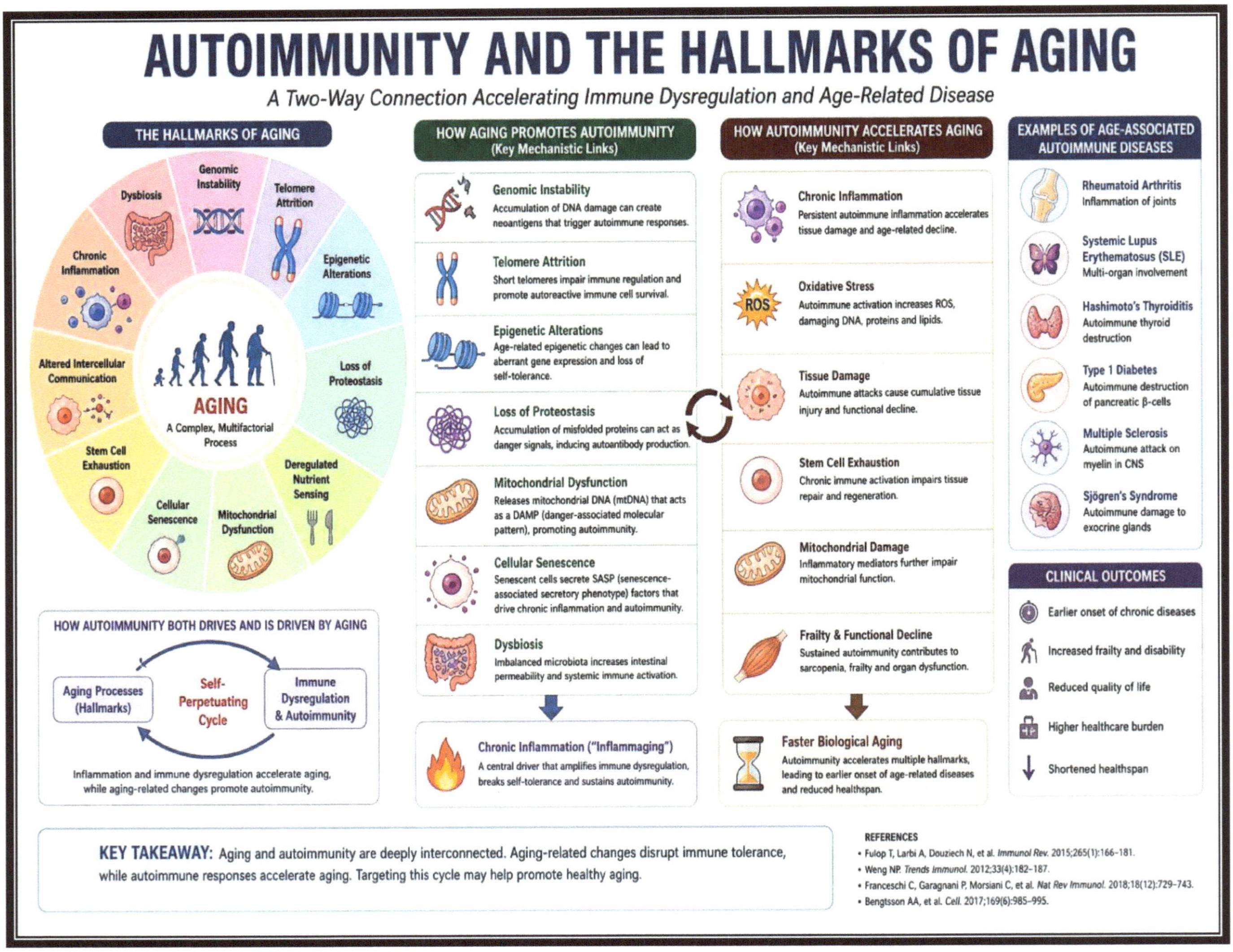

- Normally: immune system distinguishes **self vs non-self**
- In autoimmunity: this discrimination **breaks down**

2. Is Autoimmunity Related to Aging?

Yes. Aging is associated with a process called **"immunosenescence"** (decline in immune function) and **"inflammaging"** (chronic low-grade inflammation).

👉 Together, these create a setting where:

- Self-tolerance weakens
- Damaged molecules accumulate
- Immune system becomes **dysregulated rather than just weak**

➡️ Result: **increased risk of autoimmune diseases with age**

3. Root Cause Concept

Autoimmunity in aging is not due to a single defect but due to a **systems-level breakdown** involving:

- Persistent cellular damage
- Faulty clearance of self-antigens
- Chronic inflammation
- Altered immune signaling

👉 This directly links it to the **Hallmarks of Aging**

4. How Autoimmunity Connects to the 12 Hallmarks of Aging

Below is a **conceptual integration**:

Primary Hallmarks

1. Genomic Instability

- DNA damage → formation of **neoantigens**
- Immune system recognizes altered self as foreign
- 👉 Triggers autoimmune responses

2. Telomere Attrition

- Short telomeres → immune cell dysfunction
- T-cell exhaustion → impaired regulation
- 👉 Loss of immune tolerance

3. Epigenetic Alterations

- Abnormal gene expression in immune cells
- Activation of normally silenced immune pathways
- 👉 Promotes autoantibody production

4. Loss of Proteostasis

- Misfolded proteins accumulate
- These act as **autoantigens**
- 👉 Seen in diseases like lupus

Antagonistic Hallmarks

5. Deregulated Nutrient Sensing

- mTOR overactivation → hyperactive immune cells
- 👉 Promotes inflammation & autoimmunity

6. Mitochondrial Dysfunction

- ↑ ROS → oxidative damage
- Release of mitochondrial DNA (mtDNA)
- 👉 mtDNA acts like a **danger signal (DAMP)** → immune activation

7. Cellular Senescence

- Senescent cells release **SASP (pro-inflammatory cytokines)**
- 👉 Chronic immune activation → autoimmunity

Integrative Hallmarks

8. Stem Cell Exhaustion

- Decline in immune stem cells
- Reduced generation of regulatory immune cells
- 👉 Loss of immune balance

9. Altered Intercellular Communication

- Chronic cytokine signaling (inflammaging)
- 👉 Persistent immune activation

10. Chronic Inflammation (Inflammaging)

- Central driver of autoimmunity
- 👉 Continuous immune stimulation → self-reactivity

11. Dysbiosis (Microbiome Imbalance)

- Gut microbiota changes
- Molecular mimicry (microbes resemble self-antigens)
- 👉 Triggers autoimmune diseases

12. Autophagy Dysfunction

- Failure to clear damaged proteins and organelles
- 👉 Accumulation of autoantigens

5. Chain Reaction (Pathophysiology Flow)

Aging → Hallmark changes → Autoimmunity cascade

1. Cellular damage accumulates
2. Self-antigens increase (damaged DNA, proteins, mtDNA)
3. Clearance mechanisms fail (autophagy ↓)
4. Chronic inflammation (SASP, cytokines)
5. Immune dysregulation (loss of tolerance)
6. Autoantibody formation
7. Tissue-specific or systemic autoimmune disease

6. Real-Life Examples

- Rheumatoid arthritis → immune attack on joints
- Systemic lupus erythematosus → DNA/protein autoantibodies
- Type 1 diabetes → destruction of pancreatic β-cells
- Hashimoto thyroiditis → thyroid autoimmunity

7. Link with Microbiology

Autoimmunity is **deeply connected to microbiology**:

Key Mechanisms:

- **Molecular mimicry** (e.g., bacterial antigens resemble human proteins)
- **Gut microbiome dysbiosis**
- **Chronic infections triggering immune activation**

👉 Example:

- *Streptococcus* infection → rheumatic fever (cross-reactivity)

8. Link with Bioinformatics & AI in Medicine

Why it matters:

- Identification of **autoantigens using omics data**
- Analysis of:
    - Genomics
    - Proteomics
    - Microbiome datasets

AI Applications:

- Predict autoimmune risk
- Pattern recognition in immune responses
- Drug discovery targeting immune pathways

9. Link with Biotechnology

- Development of:
  - Monoclonal antibodies
  - Immunotherapies
  - Vaccines
- Gene editing (CRISPR) for immune disorders
- Biomarker discovery

Key Takeaway

Autoimmunity in aging is:

Not a single disease, but a **systems failure of immune regulation driven by interconnected hallmarks of aging**

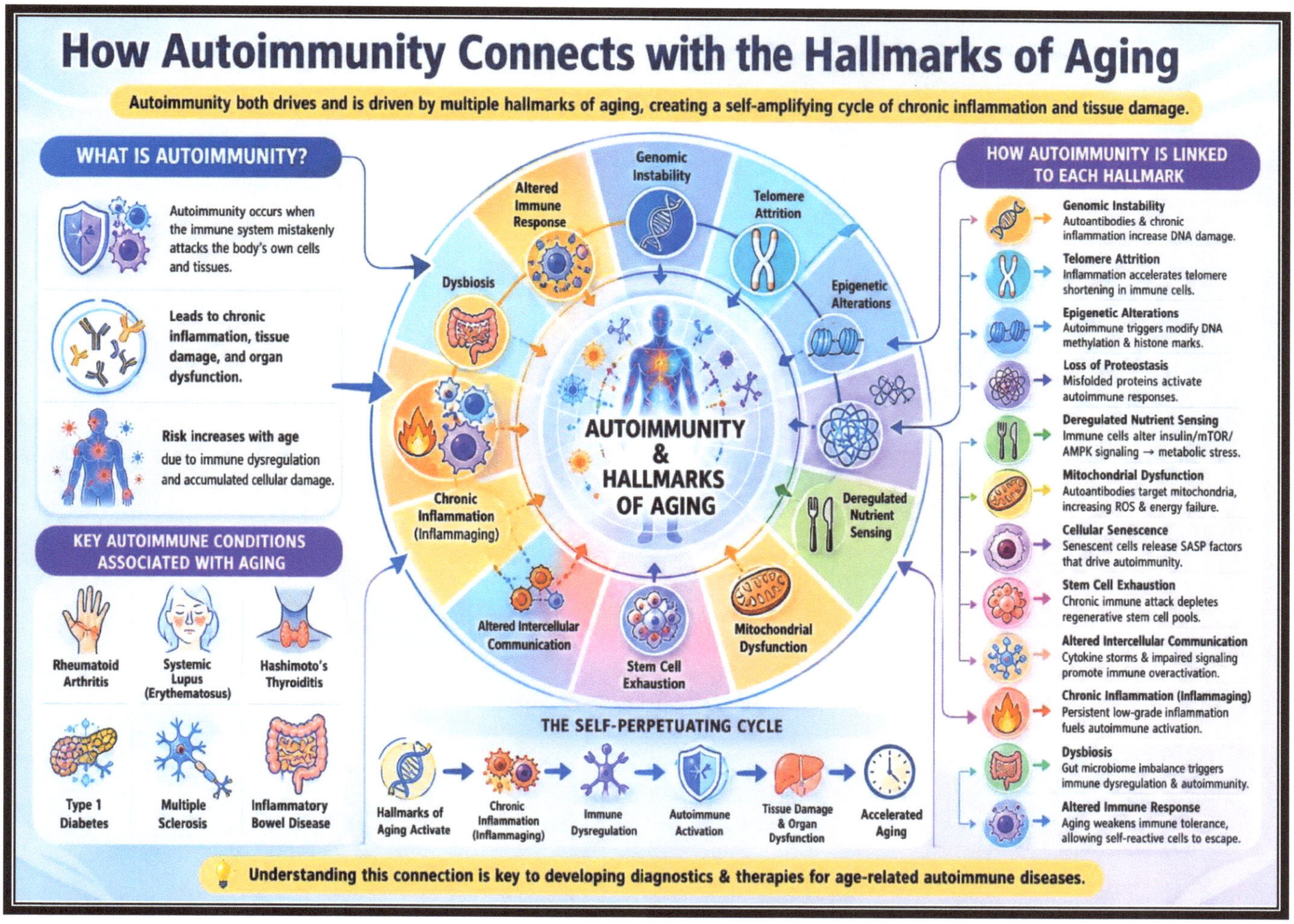

📚 Scientific References

Core Aging Papers

1. **The Hallmarks of Aging**
2. **Hallmarks of Aging: An Expanding Universe**

Autoimmunity & Aging

3. **Immunosenescence and Inflammaging**
4. **Aging and Autoimmunity**

Microbiome & Autoimmunity

5. **Microbiome and Autoimmune Diseases**

Textbooks

- *Robbins Pathologic Basis of Disease*
- *Janeway's Immunobiology*

Ferroptosis

Aging is associated with progressive accumulation of oxidative damage, metabolic imbalance, and cellular dysfunction. Among emerging regulated cell death pathways, **ferroptosis** has gained major attention due to its **iron-dependent lipid peroxidation mechanism** and strong association with age-related diseases.

Unlike apoptosis or necrosis, ferroptosis is uniquely driven by **redox imbalance and iron metabolism**, making it a critical link between metabolism, oxidative stress, and degeneration.

Ferroptosis is an iron-dependent, oxidative form of regulated cell death characterized by lipid peroxidation and depletion of antioxidant defences.

Mechanism:

- Iron (Fe^{2+}) catalyzes ROS formation
- Lipid membranes undergo peroxidation
- Antioxidants like glutathione decline
- Cells undergo irreversible damage

📘 **Is Ferroptosis related to Aging?**

Yes—but **indirectly**, not as a primary hallmark.

Mechanistic links:

Ferroptosis intersects with several hallmarks:

- **Mitochondrial dysfunction** → increases ROS
- **Loss of proteostasis** → lipid damage
- **Deregulated nutrient sensing** → altered iron metabolism
- **Cellular senescence** → promotes oxidative environment

👉 Key idea:

Ferroptosis contributes to age-related tissue damage, not aging itself as a primary driver

Relation to Aging:

Ferroptosis is not a primary hallmark but contributes to aging by:

- Increasing oxidative stress
- Promoting tissue damage
- Enhancing susceptibility to age-related diseases

Key Links to Hallmarks:

- Mitochondrial dysfunction
- Loss of proteostasis
- Cellular senescence
- Altered intercellular communication

Clinical Significance:

- Drives neurodegeneration
- Contributes to cardiovascular aging
- Target for anti-aging therapies

◆ Molecular Mechanisms of Ferroptosis

Iron Metabolism

- Iron (Fe^{2+}) catalyzes **Fenton reaction**
- Generates hydroxyl radicals (•OH)
- Promotes oxidative damage

👉 Iron overload = increased ferroptosis risk

Lipid Peroxidation

- Polyunsaturated fatty acids (PUFAs) in membranes are oxidized
- Leads to:
  - Membrane instability
  - Loss of integrity

Antioxidant System Failure

Key system:

- **Glutathione (GSH)**
- **GPX4 (Glutathione peroxidase 4)**

👉 When GPX4 is inhibited:

- Lipid peroxides accumulate
- Cells undergo ferroptosis

◆ Morphological and Biochemical Features

Morphology:

- Shrunken mitochondria
- Increased membrane density
- Reduced cristae

Biochemical:

- Increased lipid ROS
- Decreased glutathione
- Iron accumulation

◆ Regulation of Ferroptosis

Positive Regulators (Promote Ferroptosis)

- Iron overload
- ROS accumulation
- Lipid peroxidation

Negative Regulators (Inhibit Ferroptosis)

- GPX4
- Glutathione
- Vitamin E
- Ferrostatin-1 (experimental inhibitor)

🔷 Ferroptosis and the Brain (BBB Relevance)

Blood-Brain Barrier (BBB) Connection:

- Brain is highly sensitive to oxidative stress
- Iron accumulation occurs with aging
- Some ferroptosis-targeting drugs must cross BBB

👉 Key concept:

Ferroptosis contributes to neurodegeneration when BBB protection is compromised

🔷 Role in Aging and Age-Related Diseases

Neurodegenerative Diseases

- Alzheimer's disease
- Parkinson's disease

👉 Iron accumulation + oxidative stress

Cardiovascular Diseases

- Atherosclerosis
- Ischemia-reperfusion injury

Cancer

- Dual role:
  - Promotes tumor cell death
  - Can also contribute to resistance

🔷 Therapeutic Implications

Ferroptosis Inhibitors

- Ferrostatin-1
- Liproxstatin-1
- Vitamin E

Ferroptosis Inducers (Cancer Therapy)

- Erastin
- RSL3

Clinical relevance:

- Neuroprotection
- Anti-aging research
- Cancer treatment

📘 Simple Concept Flow

Aging → Iron imbalance ↑ → ROS ↑ → Lipid peroxidation ↑ → Ferroptosis → Tissue damage → Disease

📊 Comparison: Apoptosis vs Ferroptosis vs Necrosis vs Senescence

Feature	Apoptosis	Ferroptosis	Necrosis	Senescence
Definition	Programmed, regulated cell death	Iron-dependent oxidative cell death	Uncontrolled accidental cell death	Permanent cell cycle arrest (cell alive but non-dividing)
Nature	Controlled, physiological	Regulated but metabolic	Uncontrolled, pathological	Non-lethal but dysfunctional

Feature	Apoptosis	Ferroptosis	Necrosis	Senescence
Trigger	DNA damage, stress, development signals	Iron overload, lipid peroxidation, ROS	Injury, toxins, infection	Telomere shortening, DNA damage, stress
Energy Requirement	ATP-dependent	Metabolism-dependent	ATP depletion	Metabolically active
Key Mechanism	Caspase activation	Lipid ROS accumulation, iron catalysis	Cell swelling and rupture	Cell cycle arrest + SASP secretion
Membrane Integrity	Maintained (until late)	Disrupted due to lipid peroxidation	Lost early	Maintained
Inflammation	No (anti-inflammatory)	Yes (moderate)	Yes (highly inflammatory)	Yes (chronic inflammation via SASP)
Cell Morphology	Cell shrinkage, blebbing, apoptotic bodies	Mitochondrial shrinkage, membrane damage	Cell swelling, bursting	Enlarged, flattened cells
DNA Changes	Fragmentation (ladder pattern)	No classic fragmentation	Random degradation	DNA damage persists
Reversibility	Irreversible	Irreversible	Irreversible	Potentially reversible (early stage)
Role in Aging	Removes damaged cells (protective)	Contributes to oxidative damage	Causes tissue injury	Major hallmark of aging
Hallmark of Aging Link	Indirect	Indirect	Indirect	✔ Direct (Cellular Senescence)
Associated Diseases	Cancer (if reduced)	Neurodegeneration, CVD	Acute injury, stroke	Aging, fibrosis, chronic diseases
Therapeutic Target	Cancer therapy (induce apoptosis)	Anti-ferroptotic drugs	Injury management	Senolytics remove these cells

Aging is characterized not only by molecular decline but also by alterations in **cell fate decisions**—whether a cell survives, dies, or becomes dysfunctional. Four major processes govern these outcomes:

- Apoptosis (programmed cell death)
- Ferroptosis (iron-dependent oxidative death)
- Necrosis (uncontrolled cell death)
- Senescence (permanent cell cycle arrest)

Understanding these mechanisms is crucial for linking cellular biology with the **hallmarks of aging**, disease progression, and therapeutic strategies.

📌 **Key Concept:**

Cells respond to stress in four major ways:

- Repair → Survival
- Apoptosis → Controlled removal
- Ferroptosis/Necrosis → Damage-induced death
- Senescence → Survival with dysfunction

Easy Concept Summary

- **Apoptosis** → "Clean cell suicide" (good)
- **Ferroptosis** → "Rusting cell death" (iron + ROS)
- **Necrosis** → "Cell explosion" (damage)
- **Senescence** → "Zombie cells" (alive but harmful)

Conclusion

Ferroptosis represents a critical bridge between **iron metabolism, oxidative stress, and aging-related pathology**. While not a primary hallmark of aging, it significantly contributes to tissue degeneration and disease progression. Targeting ferroptosis offers promising therapeutic potential in extending health span and managing age-associated disorders.

Scientific References

1. Dixon SJ et al. Ferroptosis: an iron-dependent form of cell death (Cell, 2012)
2. Stockwell BR et al. Ferroptosis: mechanisms and disease relevance (Cell, 2017)
3. Tang D et al. Ferroptosis and aging (Cell Research, 2021)
4. Friedmann Angeli JP et al. Ferroptosis in disease (Nature Reviews, 2019)

Stress and Cortisol

Chronic stress is a significant biological factor that influences the aging process. When the body is exposed to prolonged psychological or physical stress, it remains in a sustained "alert" state, leading to continuous release of the hormone cortisol. While cortisol is essential for short-term adaptation, persistently elevated levels can disrupt normal cellular function and accelerate key processes associated with aging.

1. Telomere Shortening

Telomeres are protective structures at the ends of chromosomes that preserve genomic stability. Elevated cortisol levels have been associated with accelerated telomere shortening. Critically shortened telomeres can trigger cellular senescence or programmed cell death (apoptosis), contributing to tissue dysfunction, reduced regenerative capacity, and increased susceptibility to age-related diseases.

2. Oxidative Stress and Inflammation

Chronic stress increases the production of reactive oxygen species (ROS), leading to oxidative damage of DNA, proteins, and lipids. At the same time, it promotes a persistent low-grade inflammatory state, often referred to as "inflammaging." Together, these processes contribute to multiple hallmarks of aging, including genomic instability and altered intercellular communication.

3. Immune System Dysregulation

Sustained elevation of cortisol can impair immune function, reducing the body's ability to respond effectively to infections and cellular damage. Over time, this imbalance contributes to increased vulnerability to chronic diseases and impaired tissue repair.

Stress and Nutritional Imbalance

Stress does not directly "deplete" nutrients, but it significantly alters how the body utilizes, absorbs, and requires them:

- **Increased Metabolic Demand**: Chronic stress raises the body's energy requirements, leading to higher utilization of essential vitamins and minerals involved in energy production and cellular repair.
- **Altered Dietary Patterns**: Stress often influences appetite and food choices, increasing the preference for calorie-dense, nutrient-poor foods while reducing dietary balance.
- **Impaired Digestion and Absorption**: Reduced gastrointestinal blood flow during stress can negatively affect digestion and nutrient absorption, potentially leading to deficiencies despite adequate intake.

Integrated Perspective

Chronic stress creates a compounding effect: it increases the body's nutritional demands while simultaneously impairing nutrient intake and utilization. This imbalance can weaken cellular defence mechanisms, amplify oxidative damage, and disrupt metabolic and immune pathways—thereby accelerating biological aging.

Cortisol sits at the center of the body's **stress response system**, and its long-term imbalance is one of the key biological links between stress and aging.

Cortisol, Stress, and Aging: The Connection

1. What is Cortisol and How is it Linked to Stress?

Cortisol is a hormone released by the adrenal glands as part of the body's stress response, controlled by the **Hypothalamic–Pituitary–Adrenal axis**.

When you experience stress:

1. The brain (hypothalamus) detects stress
2. Signals the pituitary gland
3. Which activates the adrenal glands
4. Leading to the release of cortisol

👉 **Short-term role (beneficial):**

- Increases energy availability
- Enhances alertness
- Helps the body respond to immediate challenges

👉 **Long-term exposure (harmful):**

- Keeps the body in a prolonged "stress mode"
- Disrupts normal physiological balance

2. How Chronic Cortisol Exposure Contributes to Aging

When cortisol remains elevated over time (chronic stress), it affects multiple biological systems and aligns closely with several **hallmarks of aging**:

a. Telomere Shortening (Cellular Aging)

High cortisol levels are associated with faster shortening of telomeres—the protective ends of chromosomes.

👉 Leads to:

- Cellular senescence
- Reduced cell division
- Tissue aging

b. Oxidative Stress and DNA Damage

Chronic cortisol increases the production of reactive oxygen species (ROS).

👉 This causes:

- DNA damage
- Protein and lipid damage
- **Genomic instability** (a key hallmark of aging)

c. Chronic Inflammation ("Inflammaging")

Although cortisol is anti-inflammatory in the short term, long-term imbalance leads to:

- Dysregulated immune signaling
- Persistent low-grade inflammation

👉 Contributes to:

- Age-related diseases
- Altered intercellular communication

d. Immune System Suppression

Prolonged cortisol exposure weakens immune defence:

- Reduced ability to fight infections
- Slower tissue repair
- Increased disease susceptibility

e. Metabolic Dysfunction

Cortisol affects metabolism by:

- Increasing blood glucose
- Promoting fat accumulation (especially visceral fat)
- Contributing to insulin resistance

👉 Linked to:

- **Deregulated nutrient sensing**
- Metabolic aging

f. Epigenetic Changes

Chronic stress and cortisol can alter gene expression without changing DNA sequence.

👉 Leads to:

- Changes in DNA methylation
- Long-term impact on aging pathways

3. Big Picture: Stress → Cortisol → Aging

A simple way to understand:

Chronic Stress → Persistent Cortisol Elevation → Cellular Damage + System Imbalance → Accelerated Aging

4. Key Takeaway

Cortisol is essential for survival in short bursts, but when stress becomes chronic, sustained cortisol exposure disrupts cellular repair, increases oxidative damage, alters immune and metabolic function, and accelerates multiple hallmarks of aging.

📚 **Scientific References**

1. Stress, Cortisol & Telomere Shortening

https://www.sciencedirect.com/science/article/abs/pii/S0306453018309077

👉 This systematic review shows that cortisol response to stress is associated with telomere length, linking stress hormones to cellular aging

2. Stress and Cellular Aging Mechanisms

https://pmc.ncbi.nlm.nih.gov/articles/PMC8920518/

👉 Explains how chronic stress accelerates telomere shortening through cellular mechanisms, including oxidative stress and inflammation

3. Telomere Dysfunction and Aging

https://www.nature.com/articles/s41556-022-00842-x

👉 Confirms that telomere shortening and damage lead to cellular senescence and aging-related dysfunction

4. Psychological Stress and Aging (Meta-analysis)

https://pubmed.ncbi.nlm.nih.gov/26853993/

👉 Demonstrates that psychological stress contributes to disease partly through telomere damage, linking stress to aging and chronic disease.

5. Lifespan Perspective: Stress and Aging Biology

https://pure.psu.edu/en/publications/stress-and-telomere-biology-a-lifespan-perspective/

👉 Shows that stress across life stages is associated with accelerated telomere erosion, reinforcing its role in aging.

Hormesis, Cortisol Dynamics, and the Hallmarks of Aging: Adaptive vs Maladaptive Stress in Human Biology

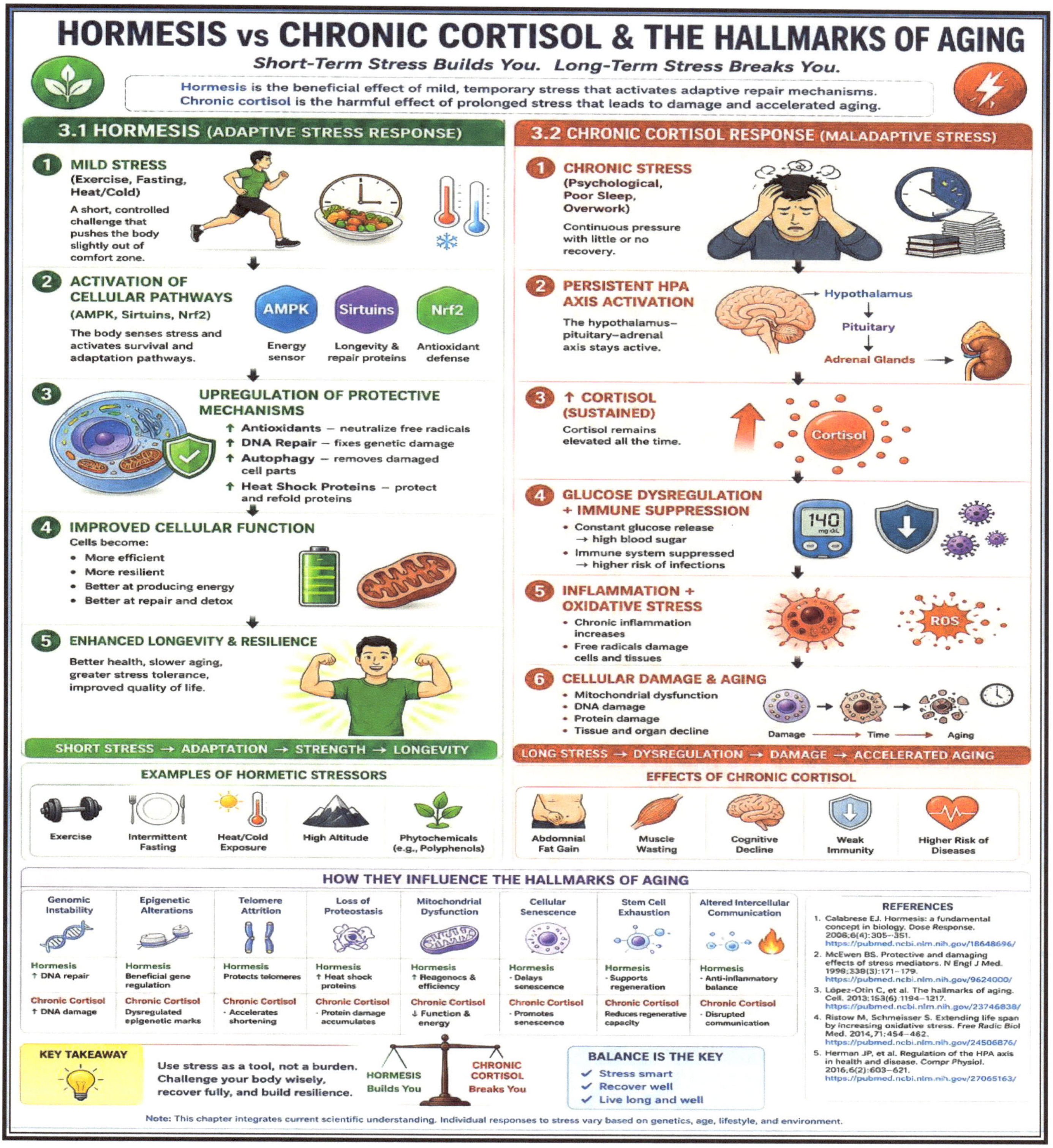

🧠 1. Definition and Core Concept

Hormesis is a biological phenomenon in which **low-dose, transient stressors induce adaptive cellular responses,** enhancing resilience and survival.

Cortisol, the primary glucocorticoid hormone released via the **hypothalamic–pituitary–adrenal (HPA) axis,** mediates the physiological response to stress.

The critical distinction lies in **dose and duration**:

- **Hormesis → adaptive, beneficial stress**
- **Chronic cortisol → maladaptive, harmful stress**

📊 2. Conceptual Framework

👉 Interpretation:

- Low stress → activates repair pathways
- High/prolonged stress → causes cellular damage

🔬 3. Mechanistic Pathways

🔁 3.1 Hormesis (Adaptive Stress Response)

Mild Stress (exercise, fasting, heat/cold)
↓
Activation of Cellular Pathways
(AMPK, Sirtuins, Nrf2)
↓
↑ Antioxidants + ↑ DNA Repair
+ ↑ Autophagy + ↑ Heat Shock Proteins
↓
Improved Cellular Function
↓
Enhanced Longevity & Resilience

👉 **Mild Stress (exercise, fasting, heat/cold)**

This is **controlled, short-term stress**
Examples:

- Exercise
- Skipping a meal (fasting)
- Sauna/cold exposure

👉 Think: *"challenge, not damage"*

👉 **Activation of Cellular Pathways (AMPK, Sirtuins, Nrf2)**

Your body senses:

"Something is stressful—I need to adapt"

So it turns ON special survival systems:

- **AMPK** → energy sensor (boosts energy efficiency)
- **Sirtuins** → longevity & repair proteins
- **Nrf2** → antioxidant defence system

👉 Think: *"emergency repair mode ON"*

👉 **↑ Antioxidants + DNA Repair + Autophagy + Heat Shock Proteins**

Now your body starts **repairing and upgrading itself**:

- **Antioxidants** ↑ → reduce damage
- **DNA repair** ↑ → fix genetic errors
- **Autophagy** ↑ → clean damaged cell parts
- **Heat shock proteins** ↑ → protect proteins

👉 Think:

"Not just repair… but upgrade"

👉 **Improved Cellular Function**

Cells become:

- More efficient
- More resistant to stress
- Better at producing energy

👉 **Enhanced Longevity & Resilience**

Final result:

- Slower aging
- Better health
- Higher stress tolerance

🎯 **Simple Analogy**

Like going to the gym:

- Small stress → muscles break slightly
- Recovery → muscles become stronger

3.2 Chronic Cortisol Response (Maladaptive Stress)

Chronic Stress (psychological, poor sleep)
↓
Persistent HPA Axis Activation
↓
↑ Cortisol (sustained)
↓
Glucose Dysregulation + Immune Suppression
↓
Inflammation + Oxidative Stress
↓
Cellular Damage & Aging

🧠 **Step-by-step meaning**

👉 **Chronic Stress (psychological, poor sleep)**

This is **continuous stress without recovery**

Examples:

- Work pressure
- Anxiety
- Lack of sleep

👉 Think: *"no break, constant pressure"*

👉 **Persistent HPA Axis Activation**

Your brain thinks:

"Danger is still present"

So it keeps activating the stress system:

- Hypothalamus
- Pituitary
- Adrenal glands

👉 This loop = always ON

👉 ↑ **Cortisol (sustained)**

Cortisol is useful in short bursts
BUT here it stays **high all the time**

👉 Think:

"Alarm system stuck ON"

👉 **Glucose Dysregulation + Immune Suppression**

Cortisol does this:

- Releases glucose constantly → high blood sugar
- Suppresses immunity → weak defence

👉 Body is always in "fight mode"

👉 **Inflammation + Oxidative Stress**

Over time:

- Cells get damaged
- Free radicals increase
- Chronic inflammation starts

👉 Silent damage builds up

👉 **Cellular Damage & Aging**

Final result:

- Muscle loss
- Fat gain (especially belly)
- Brain function decline
- Faster aging

🎯 **Simple Analogy**

Like running a car engine at full speed all the time:

- No rest → overheating
- Parts wear out faster

⚖️ **4. Comparative Physiology**

Feature	Hormesis	Chronic Cortisol
Duration	Short, intermittent	Prolonged
Pathways	AMPK, Sirtuins, Nrf2	HPA axis overactivation
Cellular Effect	Repair & adaptation	Damage & inflammation

⚖️ Side-by-Side Simple Understanding

Hormesis (Good Stress)	Chronic Stress (Bad Stress)
Short-term	Long-term
Controlled	Uncontrolled
Builds strength	Causes damage
Repair ↑	Damage ↑
Slows aging	Accelerates aging

🔗 5. Integration with Hallmarks of Aging

Hormesis and chronic cortisol directly influence multiple **hallmarks of aging**:

🔬 5.1 Mitochondrial Dysfunction

- Hormesis → ↑ mitochondrial biogenesis
- Cortisol → ↓ mitochondrial efficiency

🧬 5.2 Epigenetic Alterations

- Hormesis → beneficial gene expression modulation
- Chronic stress → dysregulated epigenetic marks

🔥 5.3 Inflammaging

- Hormesis → anti-inflammatory pathways (Nrf2)
- Cortisol → chronic low-grade inflammation

⚙️ 5.4 Loss of Proteostasis

- Hormesis → ↑ heat shock proteins
- Cortisol → protein damage accumulation

🧠 5.5 Stem Cell Exhaustion

- Chronic stress → ↓ regenerative capacity

🔗 6. Integrated Master Flow (Key Diagram)

Stress Exposure
↓

LOW (Hormesis) HIGH (Chronic Stress)

Adaptive Pathways HPA Axis Overdrive
(AMPK, Sirtuins) ↑ Cortisol
↓ ↓
Cell Repair ↑ Inflammation ↑
Autophagy ↑ Oxidative Stress ↑
↓ ↓
Healthy Aging Accelerated Aging

🧠 7. Clinical and Physiological Outcomes

✅ Hormesis Leads To:

- Improved metabolic flexibility
- Enhanced mitochondrial function

- Better immune resilience
- Increased lifespan (model organisms)

⚠️ Chronic Cortisol Leads To:

- Insulin resistance
- Visceral fat accumulation
- Muscle wasting
- Cognitive decline

🧪 8. Biological Insight

Hormesis represents a **controlled activation of stress-response pathways**, while chronic cortisol reflects **failure of adaptive recovery mechanisms**, leading to systemic dysregulation.

⚠️ 9. Scientific Limitations

- Hormesis threshold varies across individuals
- Excess stress can shift adaptive → harmful
- Chronic cortisol effects depend on genetic and environmental context

🎯 Summary

Hormesis represents a controlled biological challenge that activates repair and resilience pathways, whereas chronic cortisol exposure reflects a failure of recovery, leading to cumulative cellular damage and accelerated aging.

📚 Scientific References

1. Calabrese EJ. *Hormesis: a fundamental concept in biology.* Dose Response. 2008. http://pubmed.ncbi.nlm.nih.gov/18648696/
2. McEwen BS. *Protective and damaging effects of stress mediators.* N Engl J Med. 1998. http://pubmed.ncbi.nlm.nih.gov/9624000/
3. López-Otín C et al. *The hallmarks of aging.* Cell. 2013. http://pubmed.ncbi.nlm.nih.gov/23746838/
4. Ristow M, Schmeisser S. *Mitohormesis.* Cell Metab. 2014. http://pubmed.ncbi.nlm.nih.gov/24506876/
5. Herman JP et al. *Regulation of the HPA axis.* Compr Physiol. 2016. http://pubmed.ncbi.nlm.nih.gov/27065163/

Chapter-17

From Biology to Algorithms: How AI is Transforming the Science of Aging

Aging is a progressive, multifactorial biological process characterized by the gradual decline in cellular, tissue, and systemic function, ultimately increasing vulnerability to disease and death. This process is now systematically understood through the framework of the **"hallmarks of aging,"** which include genomic instability, telomere attrition, epigenetic alterations, loss of proteostasis, mitochondrial dysfunction, deregulated nutrient sensing, cellular senescence, stem cell exhaustion, altered intercellular communication, chronic inflammation, dysbiosis, and impaired autophagy.

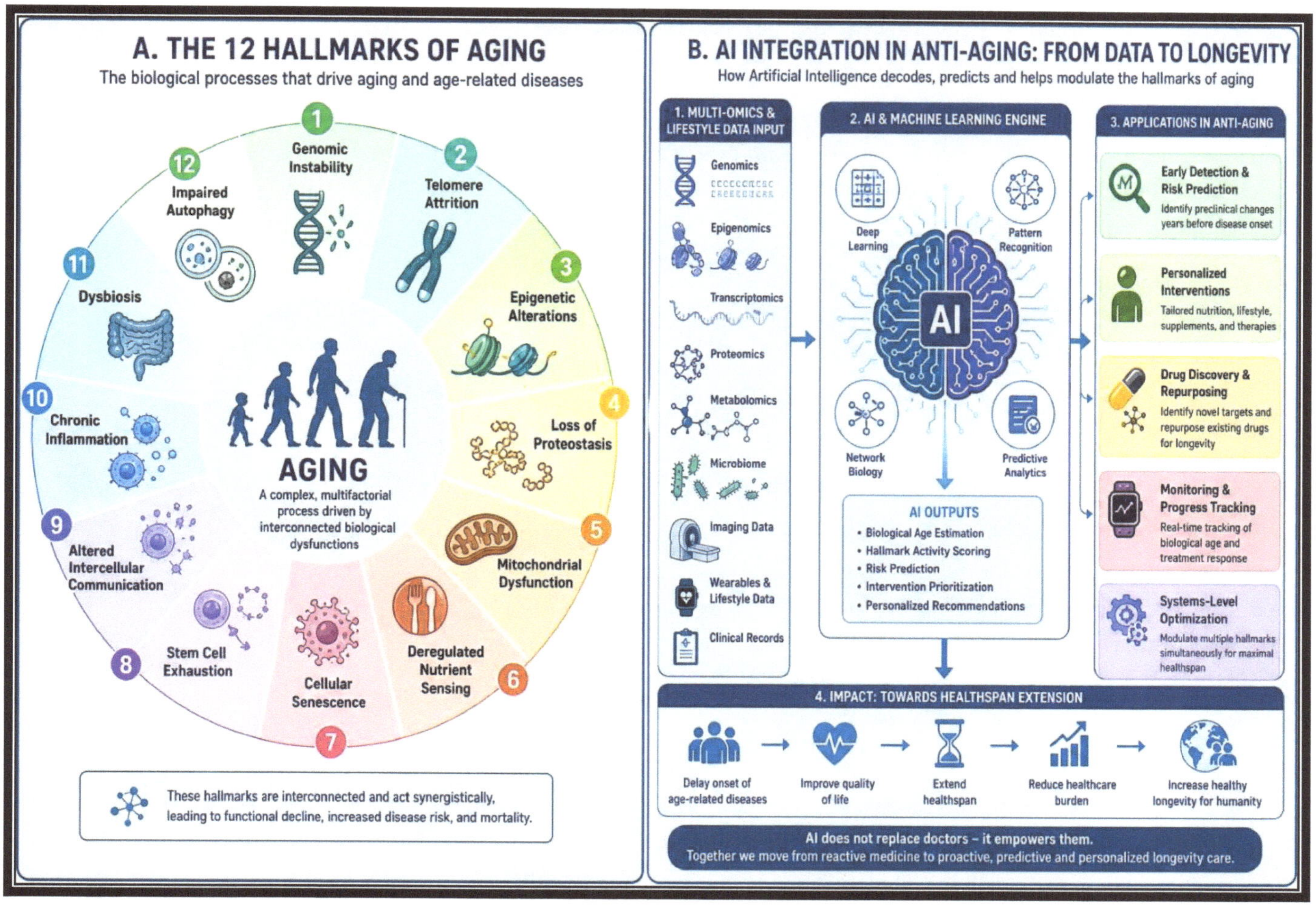

Artificial Intelligence (AI) refers to computational systems capable of learning from complex datasets, identifying patterns, and making predictions or decisions with minimal human intervention. In the context of aging biology, AI is emerging not merely as a tool—but as a transformative force capable of decoding, predicting, and potentially modulating the fundamental processes that drive aging.

For centuries, aging was viewed as an inevitable, irreversible decline. However, the identification of the hallmarks of aging has reframed it as a **biologically regulated and potentially modifiable process**. The challenge lies in the complexity—these hallmarks do not act in isolation but are deeply interconnected, forming a dynamic network of molecular and cellular events.

This is precisely where AI becomes indispensable.

AI systems excel at integrating vast, multidimensional datasets—genomics, proteomics, metabolomics, microbiome profiles, and clinical phenotypes—into coherent, interpretable models. By doing so, AI can:

- Identify early molecular signatures of aging before clinical symptoms appear
- Map interactions between multiple hallmarks simultaneously
- Predict individual aging trajectories
- Suggest targeted interventions tailored to specific biological dysfunctions

In essence, AI shifts medicine from a **reactive model (treat disease)** to a proactive model (predict and prevent aging-related decline).

Future Purpose of This Integration

The integration of AI into aging research serves three major purposes:

1. Precision Longevity

AI enables the transition from generalized anti-aging strategies to personalized longevity medicine, where interventions are tailored based on an individual's biological age, genetic profile, and environmental exposures.

2. Early Disease Prediction

Since most chronic diseases—such as cardiovascular disorders, neurodegeneration, and cancer—are manifestations of underlying aging processes, AI can detect subtle deviations in biological systems years before disease onset.

3. Therapeutic Discovery

AI accelerates drug discovery by:

- Identifying novel molecular targets within aging pathways
- Simulating drug interactions
- Repurposing existing drugs for anti-aging benefits

Genuine Claims vs Hype

It is important to distinguish scientifically validated potential from exaggerated claims.

What AI can genuinely do today:

- Analyze large-scale biological data with high accuracy
- Predict disease risk (e.g., cardiovascular, metabolic disorders)
- Assist in drug discovery and biomarker identification
- Estimate biological age using epigenetic and imaging data

What remains aspirational (but promising):

- Completely reversing aging
- Eliminating all age-related diseases
- Achieving indefinite lifespan extension

AI is not a "cure for aging" yet—but it is significantly accelerating our ability to understand and intervene in aging biology.

Can AI Redefine the Medical Industry?

Yes—but not in a simplistic or immediate way.

AI is poised to redefine medicine across three dimensions:

Decoding Aging with Artificial Intelligence: A New Era in Preventive and Regenerative Medicine

1. Predictive Medicine

AI models can analyze longitudinal health data to forecast disease risk years in advance.

Example:

- Detecting early neurodegenerative changes before clinical symptoms
- Predicting metabolic disorders from subtle biomarker shifts

2. Preventive Medicine

By identifying early dysfunction in aging pathways, interventions can be applied before irreversible damage occurs.

3. Regenerative and Systems Medicine

AI helps in:

- Stem cell therapy optimization
- Tissue regeneration modeling
- Understanding complex system-level interactions across organs

How AI Predicts Diseases in Advance (Mechanistic Explanation)

AI uses multiple approaches:

- Machine Learning Models: Identify patterns in large datasets (e.g., blood markers, imaging)
- Deep Learning: Detect subtle abnormalities in imaging (MRI, CT, histology)
- Network Biology: Map interactions between genes, proteins, and pathways
- Digital Twins: Create virtual models of individuals to simulate disease progression

By integrating these, AI can detect preclinical disease states, sometimes years before symptoms manifest.

Future Outlook: The Next Frontier

The future of AI in anti-aging lies in convergence:

- AI + Genomics → Personalized genetic interventions
- AI + Wearables → Continuous health monitoring
- AI + Regenerative Medicine → Organ repair and replacement
- AI + Microbiome Science → Modulating dysbiosis for longevity

We are moving toward a world where:

- Aging may be slowed, delayed, or partially reversed
- Diseases may be predicted before they occur
- Healthcare may become continuous rather than episodic

AI-Driven Longevity: Targeting the Hallmarks of Aging in the 21st Century

The battle against aging is not a fight against time, but a quest to understand biology at its deepest level. Artificial Intelligence does not replace human insight—it amplifies it. By decoding the intricate language of the hallmarks of aging, AI offers a powerful lens through which we can reimagine health, longevity, and disease.

While immortality remains a philosophical concept, extended health span—free from chronic disease and functional decline—is now an achievable scientific goal.

In this evolving landscape, AI stands not as a distant innovation, but as a central architect in the future of medicine—transforming aging from an inevitability into a manageable, measurable, and potentially modifiable process.

📚 Scientific References

🧬 1. Foundations of Bioinformatics & Systems Biology

- https://www.ncbi.nlm.nih.gov/books/NBK20263/
- https://www.ebi.ac.uk/training/online/courses/bioinformatics-introduction/what-is-bioinformatics/
- https://www.nature.com/scitable/topicpage/systems-biology-a-brief-overview-11878184/

🧬 2. Hallmarks of Aging (Core Framework)

- https://doi.org/10.1016/j.cell.2013.05.039
- https://doi.org/10.1016/j.cell.2023.02.001

🧬 3. Multi-Omics Integration in Aging

- https://www.nature.com/articles/s43587-021-00082-6

- https://www.frontiersin.org/articles/10.3389/fgene.2020.00915/full
- https://www.nature.com/articles/nbt.3935

🧬 4. Bioinformatics Approaches to Hallmarks

Genomic Instability

- https://www.nature.com/articles/nrm2350

Telomere Attrition

- https://www.nature.com/articles/nrg1656

Epigenetic Alterations

- https://genomebiology.biomedcentral.com/articles/10.1186/gb-2013-14-10-r115

Proteostasis

- https://www.nature.com/articles/nrm.2017.36

Mitochondrial Dysfunction

- https://www.cell.com/fulltext/S0092-8674(16)30995-1

Nutrient Sensing (mTOR, AMPK)

- https://www.cell.com/cell-metabolism/fulltext/S1550-4131(13)00444-7

Cellular Senescence

- https://www.nature.com/articles/s41580-018-0063-1

Stem Cell Exhaustion

- https://www.nature.com/articles/nrm.2016.136

Inflammation (Inflammaging)

- https://www.nature.com/articles/s41577-018-0060-3

Dysbiosis (Microbiome)

- https://www.nature.com/articles/s41575-018-0058-8

Autophagy

- https://www.nature.com/articles/nrm.2017.122

🧬 5. Bioinformatics Databases & Tools

- https://www.ncbi.nlm.nih.gov
- https://www.ensembl.org
- https://www.ncbi.nlm.nih.gov/geo/
- https://genomics.senescence.info/genes/
- https://gtexportal.org

🤖 6. AI & Machine Learning in Aging

- https://www.nature.com/articles/s43587-021-00111-4
- https://www.nature.com/articles/s41591-018-0279-9

💊 7. Precision Medicine & Systems Biology

- https://allofus.nih.gov
- https://www.nature.com/articles/nrg2916

⚠️ 8. Challenges & Ethics

- https://www.nature.com/articles/nrg.2016.13
- https://www.nature.com/articles/nrg.2017.104

Chapter-18

Bioinformatics and the Systems-Level Decoding of the Hallmarks of Aging

1.1 Definition

Bioinformatics is an interdisciplinary field that integrates biology, computer science, mathematics, and statistics to collect, store, analyze, and interpret complex biological data.

In the context of aging, bioinformatics enables the **integration of multi-omics datasets**—including genomics, transcriptomics, proteomics, metabolomics, and epigenomics—to uncover molecular signatures, pathways, and networks underlying the hallmarks of aging.

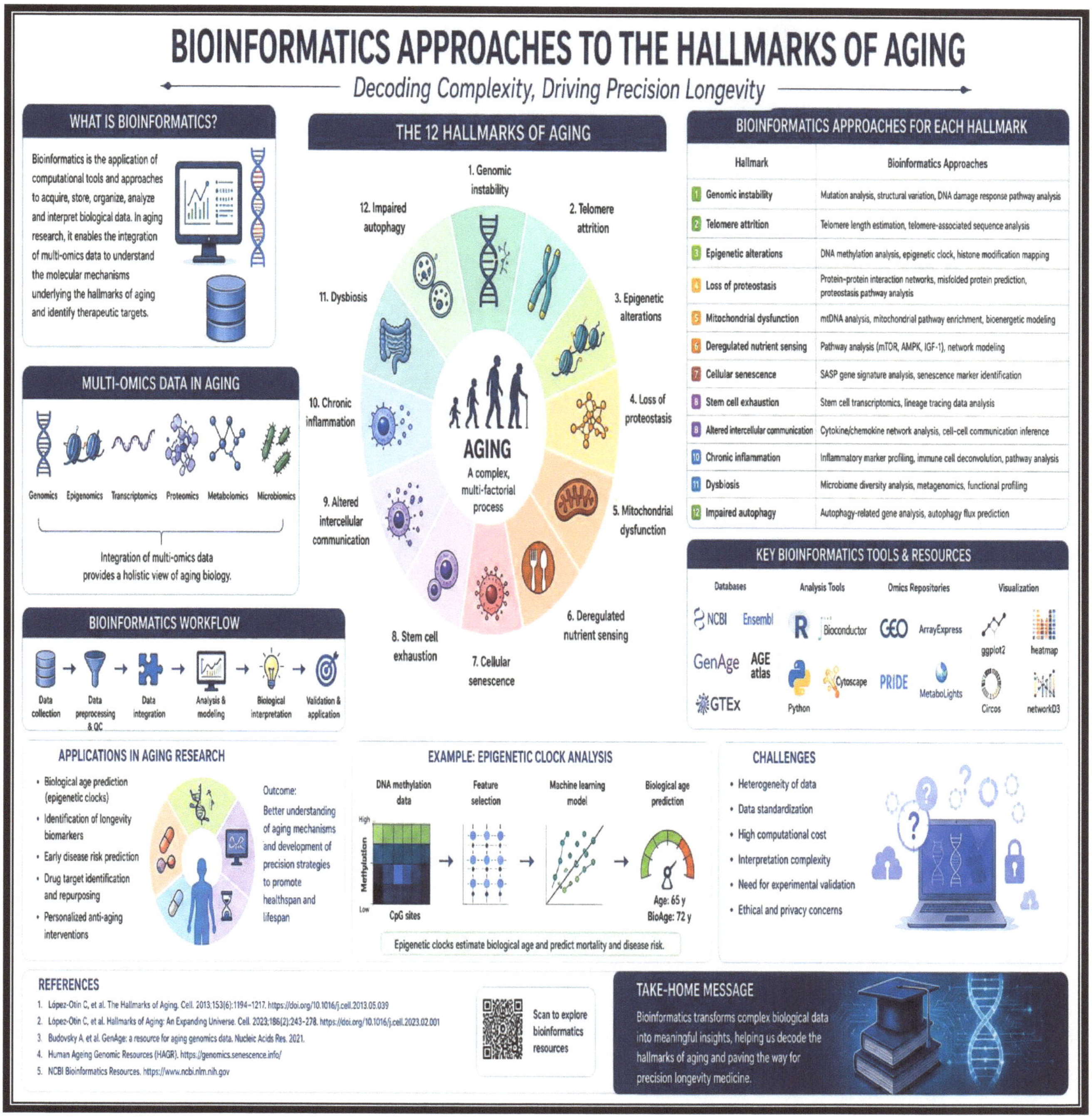

1.2 Introduction: Why Bioinformatics is Central to Aging Research

Aging is a **systems-level biological phenomenon** involving interconnected molecular events rather than isolated mechanisms. Traditional reductionist approaches fail to capture this complexity.

Bioinformatics addresses this gap by:

- Integrating heterogeneous datasets
- Identifying hidden biological patterns
- Modeling interactions between hallmarks
- Predicting disease susceptibility and biological age

1.3 Multi-Omics Integration in Aging

Bioinformatics enables simultaneous analysis of:

- **Genomics** → DNA mutations, genomic instability
- **Epigenomics** → DNA methylation, histone modification (epigenetic alterations)
- **Transcriptomics** → Gene expression changes
- **Proteomics** → Protein folding, aggregation (loss of proteostasis)
- **Metabolomics** → Cellular metabolism (mitochondrial dysfunction)
- **Microbiomics** → Gut flora alterations (dysbiosis)

👉 This integration provides a **holistic view of aging biology**.

1.4 Bioinformatics Approaches to the Hallmarks of Aging

1.4.1 Genomic Instability

- Mutation mapping
- DNA damage response pathway analysis

1.4.2 Telomere Attrition

- Telomere length prediction algorithms
- Sequence-based telomeric analysis

1.4.3 Epigenetic Alterations

- DNA methylation clocks (biological age estimation)
- Histone modification mapping

1.4.4 Loss of Proteostasis

- Protein interaction networks
- Misfolded protein aggregation modeling

1.4.5 Mitochondrial Dysfunction

- Mitochondrial genome analysis
- Bioenergetic modeling

1.4.6 Deregulated Nutrient Sensing

- Pathway analysis (mTOR, AMPK, insulin signaling)

1.4.7 Cellular Senescence

- Senescence-associated secretory phenotype (SASP) profiling

1.4.8 Stem Cell Exhaustion

- Stem cell transcriptomic profiling

1.4.9 Altered Intercellular Communication

- Cytokine network analysis

1.4.10 Chronic Inflammation

- Inflammatory biomarker clustering

1.4.11 Dysbiosis

- Microbiome sequencing and diversity analysis

1.4.12 Impaired Autophagy

- Autophagy-related gene network modeling

1.5 Key Bioinformatics Tools and Technologies

- **Machine Learning & AI Models** → Pattern recognition in aging datasets
- **Network Biology** → Interaction mapping between pathways
- **Molecular Docking** → Drug-target prediction
- **Databases** → Genomic and aging repositories
- **Systems Biology Platforms** → Whole-organism modeling

1.6 Applications in Anti-Aging and Medicine

- Biological age prediction (epigenetic clocks)
- Early disease risk detection
- Drug repurposing for aging-related diseases
- Identification of longevity biomarkers
- Personalized preventive medicine

1.7 Challenges and Limitations

- Data heterogeneity and standardization issues
- Ethical concerns in genetic data usage
- Computational limitations in large-scale modeling
- Need for clinical validation

1.8 Future Perspectives

- Integration with **Artificial Intelligence** for predictive longevity
- Development of **digital twins** for personalized aging simulation
- Real-time health monitoring using wearable-integrated bioinformatics
- Systems-level intervention strategies targeting multiple hallmarks

Scientific References

López-Otín C, et al. The Hallmarks of Aging. Cell, 2013.

https://doi.org/10.1016/j.cell.2013.05.039

López-Otín C, et al. Hallmarks of Aging: An Expanding Universe. Cell, 2023.

https://doi.org/10.1016/j.cell.2023.02.001

Budovsky A, et al. GenAge: Database of Aging Genes.

https://genomics.senescence.info/genes/

National Center for Biotechnology Information (NCBI)

https://www.ncbi.nlm.nih.gov/

Human Ageing Genomic Resources (HAGR)

https://genomics.senescence.info/

Chapter-19

Biotechnology and the Therapeutic Modulation of the Hallmarks of Aging

2.1 Definition

Biotechnology is the application of biological systems, living organisms, or their derivatives to develop products and technologies aimed at improving human health and quality of life.

In aging research, biotechnology focuses on **intervening in biological processes** to delay, prevent, or reverse the hallmarks of aging.

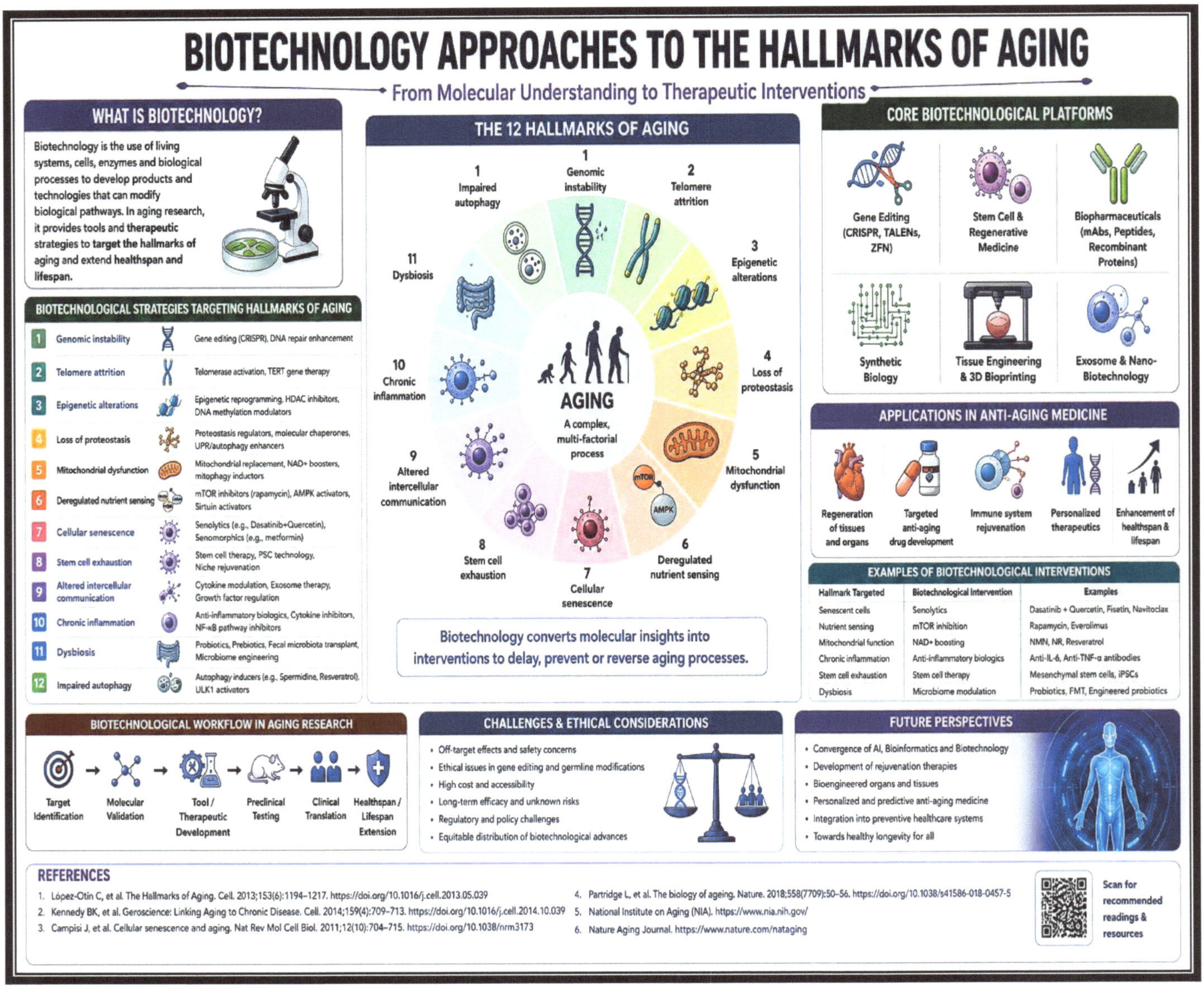

2.2 Introduction: From Understanding to Intervention

While bioinformatics decodes aging, biotechnology **acts upon it**.

It translates molecular insights into **therapeutic strategies** that can modify aging pathways and extend healthspan.

2.3 Biotechnological Strategies Targeting the Hallmarks of Aging

2.3.1 Genomic Instability

- Gene editing (CRISPR-Cas systems)
- DNA repair enhancement

2.3.2 Telomere Attrition

- Telomerase activation therapies

2.3.3 Epigenetic Alterations

- Epigenetic reprogramming
- Histone modification drugs

2.3.4 Loss of Proteostasis

- Proteostasis regulators
- Chaperone-based therapies

2.3.5 Mitochondrial Dysfunction

- Mitochondrial replacement therapy
- NAD^+ boosters

2.3.6 Deregulated Nutrient Sensing

- mTOR inhibitors (e.g., rapamycin analogs)
- AMPK activators

2.3.7 Cellular Senescence

- Senolytics (removal of senescent cells)
- Senomorphics (modulating senescence effects)

2.3.8 Stem Cell Exhaustion

- Stem cell therapy
- Induced pluripotent stem cells (iPSCs)

2.3.9 Altered Intercellular Communication

- Cytokine modulation
- Exosome-based therapies

2.3.10 Chronic Inflammation

- Anti-inflammatory biologics

2.3.11 Dysbiosis

- Microbiome engineering (probiotics, fecal transplant)

2.3.12 Impaired Autophagy

- Autophagy inducers

2.4 Core Biotechnological Platforms

- Gene Editing Technologies (CRISPR, TALENs)
- Stem Cell and Regenerative Medicine
- Biopharmaceuticals (Monoclonal antibodies, peptides)
- Synthetic Biology
- Tissue Engineering and 3D Bioprinting

2.5 Applications in Anti-Aging Medicine

- Regeneration of tissues and organs
- Targeted anti-aging drug development
- Immune system rejuvenation
- Personalized therapeutics
- Enhancement of lifespan and healthspan

2.6 Challenges and Ethical Considerations

- Safety and off-target effects
- Ethical concerns in gene editing
- Accessibility and cost
- Regulatory challenges
- Long-term effects unknown

2.7 Future Outlook

- Convergence of **AI + Biotechnology** for precision longevity
- Development of **whole-body rejuvenation therapies**
- Organoid and lab-grown organ replacement
- Personalized gene therapy
- Preventive biotechnology integrated into routine healthcare

2.8 Conclusion

Biotechnology represents the **interventional arm of aging science**, transforming theoretical understanding into clinical reality. When combined with bioinformatics and AI, it holds the potential to redefine medicine—not merely by treating disease, but by **modulating the biological processes that cause it**.

Scientific References

1. Kennedy BK, et al. *Geroscience: Linking Aging to Chronic Disease*. Cell, 2014.
2. https://doi.org/10.1016/j.cell.2014.10.039
3. Campisi J, et al. *Cellular Senescence and Aging*. Nat Rev Mol Cell Biol.
4. https://doi.org/10.1038/nrm2233
5. Partridge L, et al. *The Biology of Aging*. Nature, 2018.
6. https://doi.org/10.1038/s41586-018-0457-5
7. National Institute on Aging (NIA)
8. https://www.nia.nih.gov/
9. Nature Aging Journal
10. https://www.nature.com/nataging/

CRISPR Technology/Tool

CRISPR (Clustered Regularly Interspaced Short Palindromic Repeats) is a powerful **gene-editing technology** that allows scientists to precisely modify DNA sequences in living organisms.

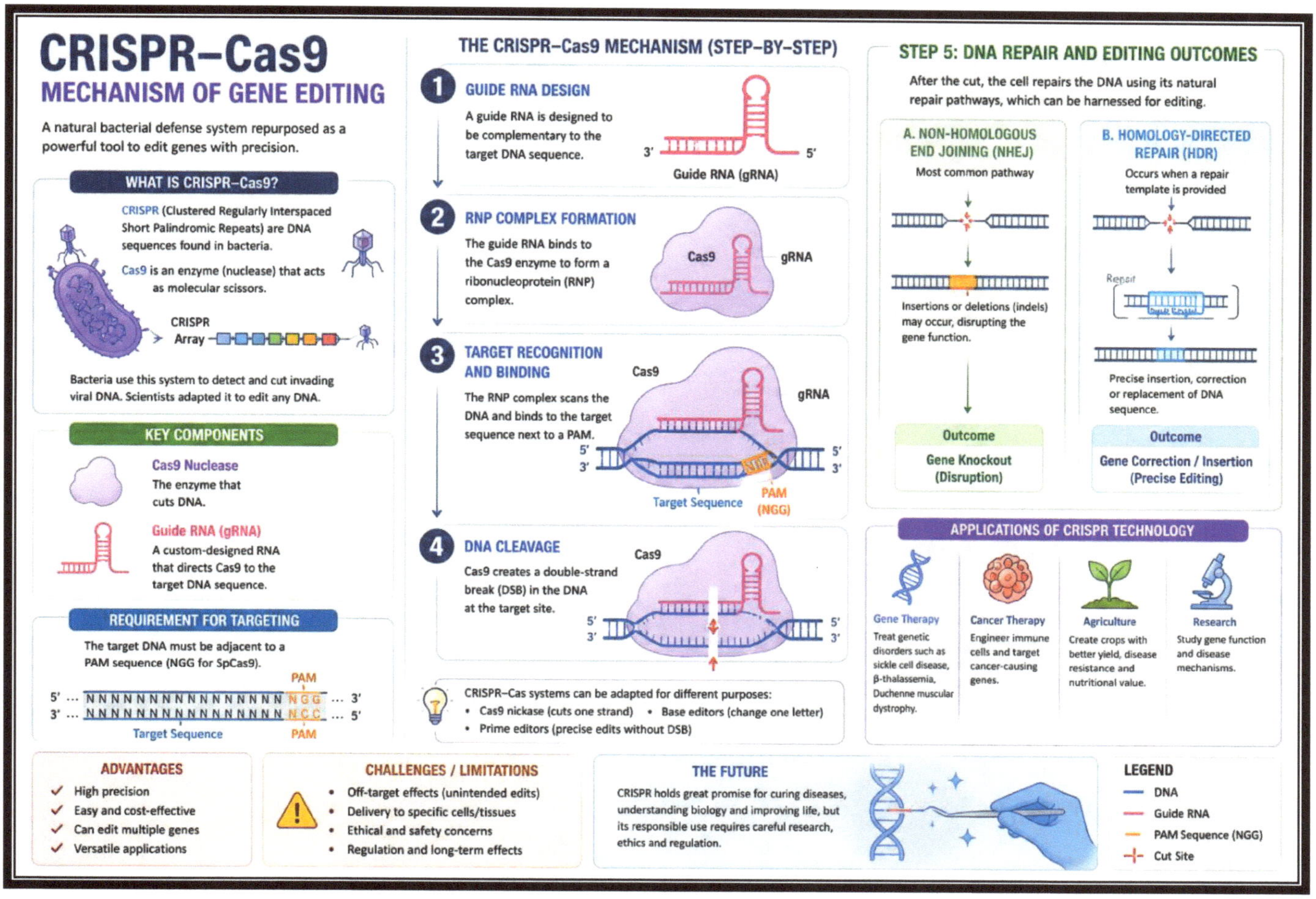

It was developed based on a natural defence system found in bacteria and was widely popularized by scientists like Jennifer Doudna and Emmanuelle Charpentier.

Is CRISPR a Tool or Technology?

CRISPR is **both**:

- **Technology** → because it represents a broader method/platform for gene editing
- **Tool** → specifically, the CRISPR-Cas system (like CRISPR-Cas9) acts as a molecular "scissor" to cut DNA

👉 In simple terms:

CRISPR = technology

Cas9 = tool used within that technology

How CRISPR Works (Step-by-Step)

1. **Guide RNA (gRNA) Design**

   A short RNA sequence is created to match the target DNA.

2. **Target Recognition**

   The guide RNA directs the Cas9 enzyme to the specific DNA location.

3. **DNA Cutting**

   Cas9 cuts the DNA at the targeted site.

4. **DNA Repair/Modification**

   The cell repairs the cut:

   - By disabling a gene, or
   - By inserting or correcting genetic material

👉 This allows precise editing of genes.

Which Field Does CRISPR Belong To?

CRISPR is **interdisciplinary**, similar to your "hallmarks of aging" theme:

- **Biotechnology (Primary field)**

  Used for gene editing, therapeutics, agriculture

- **Molecular Biology & Genetics**

  Core scientific foundation

- **Bioinformatics**

  Used for:

  - Designing guide RNAs
  - Analyzing genetic data
  - Predicting off-target effects

- **Microbiology (Origin)**

  Discovered in bacterial immune systems

👉 **"A key biotechnology tool supported by bioinformatics and rooted in microbiology."**

Is CRISPR Approved in India?

In India:

- CRISPR is **allowed for research purposes**
- Clinical use in humans is **highly regulated**
- Governed by bodies like:
  - Indian Council of Medical Research
  - Department of Biotechnology

👉 Full clinical approval for widespread human gene editing is **still limited and evolving**.

Countries Where CRISPR Has Seen Clinical Progress/Approval

- United States
- United Kingdom
- China

A major milestone:

- First CRISPR-based therapy approved for certain genetic disorders (like sickle cell disease) in the US and UK (recent years).

Future Prospects of CRISPR

CRISPR has **very high potential**, but with careful regulation:

1. Medicine

- Treatment of genetic diseases
- Cancer therapies
- Personalized medicine

2. Aging Research

- Studying genes involved in aging
- Potentially targeting hallmarks like:
    - genomic instability
    - cellular senescence

3. Agriculture

- Disease-resistant crops
- Improved nutritional quality

4. Drug Discovery

- Faster identification of drug targets

Limitations & Ethical Concerns

- Off-target gene edits
- Ethical issues (especially human embryo editing)
- Long-term safety still under study

Gene editing—especially using CRISPR-Cas9—has moved from theory to real clinical breakthroughs. But it's not magic yet: most therapies are still early-stage or limited to specific patients. Here's a clear, **research-grounded overview of where things actually stand (2024–2026)**.

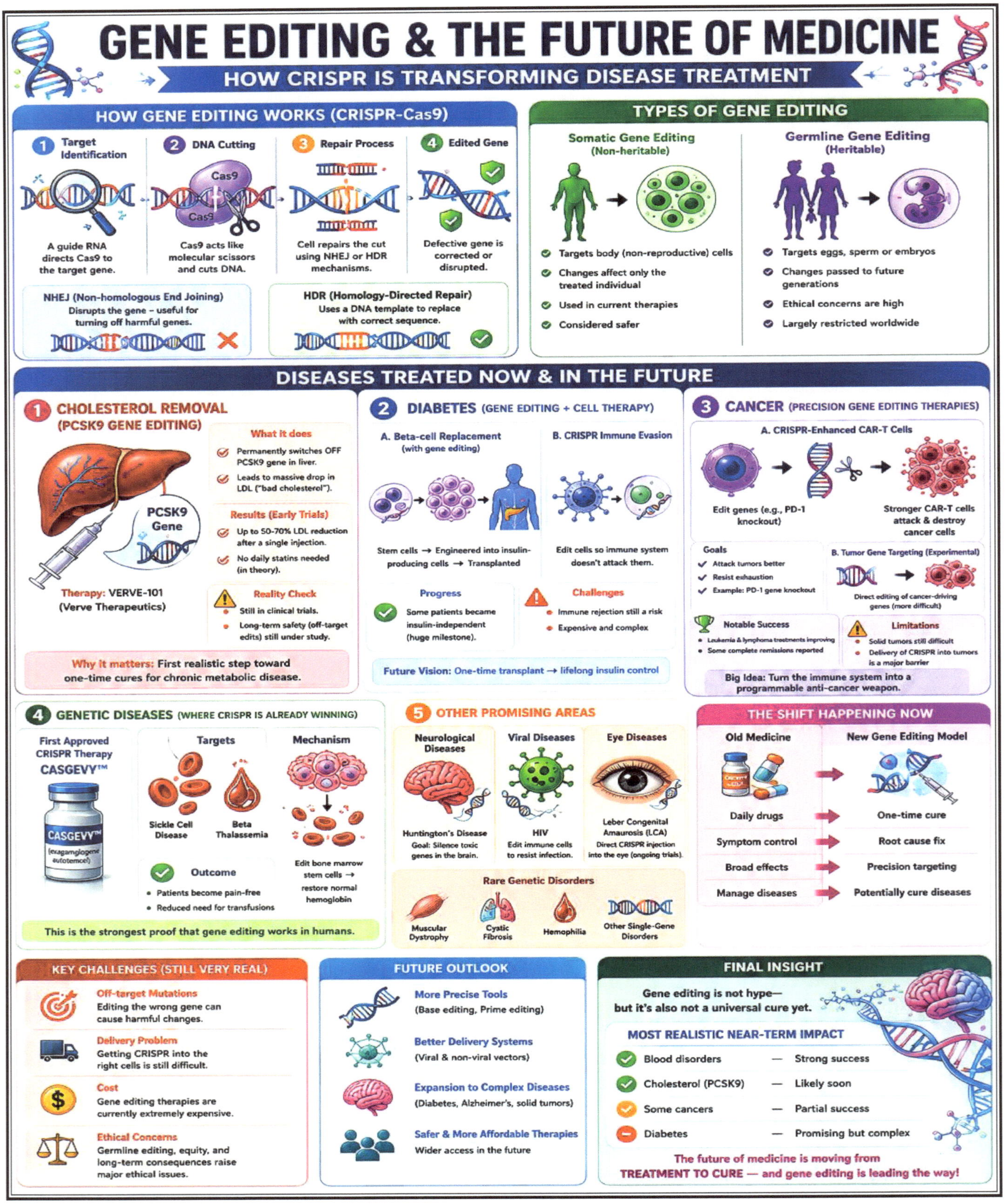

🔬 Breakthrough

Target: **PCSK9 gene** (controls LDL cholesterol levels)

Therapy: VERVE-101 by Verve Therapeutics

💡 **What it does**

Permanently **switches OFF PCSK9 gene in liver**

Leads to **massive drop in LDL ("bad cholesterol")**

📊 **Results (early trials)**

Up to **50–70% LDL reduction** after a *single injection*

No daily statins needed (in theory)

⚠️ **Reality check**

Still in **clinical trials**

Long-term safety (off-target edits) still under study

👉 **Why it matters:** First realistic step toward *one-time cures* for chronic metabolic disease.

🩸 2. Diabetes (Gene Editing + Cell Therapy)

🔬 **Key approaches**

A. Beta-cell replacement (with gene editing)

Companies like Vertex Pharmaceuticals

Therapy: VX-880

👉 Stem cells → engineered into insulin-producing cells → transplanted

B. CRISPR immune evasion

Edit cells so immune system **doesn't attack them**

📊 **Progress**

Some patients became **insulin-independent** (huge milestone)

⚠️ **Challenges**

Immune rejection still a risk

Expensive and complex

👉 **Future vision:** One-time transplant → lifelong insulin control

🧬 3. Cancer (Precision Gene Editing Therapies)

🔬 **Main strategy: Editing immune cells**

A. CRISPR-enhanced CAR-T cells

Modify T-cells to:

Attack tumors better

Resist exhaustion

Example: PD-1 gene knockout

B. Tumor gene targeting (experimental)

Direct editing of cancer-driving genes (harder)

📊 **Notable success**

Leukemia and lymphoma treatments improving

Some **complete remissions** reported

⚠️ **Limitations**

Solid tumors still difficult

Delivery of CRISPR into tumors is a major barrier

👉 **Big idea:** Turn the immune system into a programmable anti-cancer weapon

🧠 4. Genetic Diseases (Where CRISPR is already winning)

🏆 **Major milestone**

First approved CRISPR therapy: Casgevy

Targets:

Sickle Cell Disease

Beta Thalassemia

💡 **Mechanism**

Edit bone marrow stem cells → restore normal hemoglobin

📊 **Outcome**

Patients become **pain-free**

Reduced need for transfusions

👉 **This is the strongest proof that gene editing works in humans.**

🧠 **5. Other Promising Areas**

🧬 **Neurological diseases**

Huntington's Disease

Goal: silence toxic genes in brain

🦠 **Viral diseases**

HIV

Edit immune cells to resist infection

👁️ **Eye diseases**

Leber Congenital Amaurosis

Direct CRISPR injection into eye (ongoing trials)

🎯 **Big Picture (What Medicine is "Banking On")**

🚀 **The shift happening now:**

Old Medicine	New Gene Editing Model
Daily drugs 💊	One-time cure 💉
Symptom control	Root cause fix
Broad effects	Precision targeting

⚠️ **Key Challenges (Still VERY Real)**

Off-target mutations (editing wrong gene)

Delivery problem (getting CRISPR into right cells)

Cost (currently extremely expensive)

Ethical concerns (germline editing)

🧠 Final Insight

Gene editing is not hype—but it's also not a universal cure yet.

👉 The **most realistic near-term impact**:

Blood disorders ✅

Cholesterol ✅ (likely soon)

Some cancers ⚠️ (partial success)

Diabetes ⚠️ (promising but complex)

Summary

CRISPR is a revolutionary gene-editing technology that allows precise modification of DNA. Originating from bacterial immune systems, it is now widely used in biotechnology and supported by bioinformatics for designing and analysing genetic changes. While it holds great promise in medicine, agriculture, and aging research, its clinical use is still carefully regulated in countries like India and continues to evolve globally.

📚 Scientific References

Nature (CRISPR overview):

https://www.nature.com/subjects/crispr-cas-systems

NIH (US National Institutes of Health):

https://www.genome.gov/about-genomics/policy-issues/Genome-Editing

WHO (Human Genome Editing):

https://www.who.int/health-topics/human-genome-editing

ICMR India Guidelines:

https://www.icmr.gov.in

Broad Institute (CRISPR resource):

https://www.broadinstitute.org/what-broad/areas-focus/project-spotlight/crispr

https://pmc.ncbi.nlm.nih.gov/articles/PMC11057861/

https://pmc.ncbi.nlm.nih.gov/articles/PMC7427626/

https://www.cancer.gov/news-events/cancer-currents-blog/2020/crispr-cancer-research-treatment

Broad Institute. CRISPR [Internet]. Available from: https://www.broadinstitute.org/what-broad/areas-focus/project-spotlight/crispr

Doudna JA, Charpentier E. The new frontier of genome engineering with CRISPR-Cas9. Nat Rev Genet. 2014;15(5):317–328.

National Human Genome Research Institute. Genome editing [Internet]. Available from: https://www.genome.gov/about-genomics/policy-issues/Genome-Editing

Verve Therapeutics. Pipeline [Internet]. Available from: https://www.vervetx.com/pipeline/

Musunuru K, et al. In vivo CRISPR base editing of PCSK9 in humans. N Engl J Med. 2023;388:1–12.

ClinicalTrials.gov. Study of VERVE-101 [Internet]. Available from: https://clinicaltrials.gov/ct2/show/NCT05398029

Vertex Pharmaceuticals. Pipeline [Internet]. Available from: https://www.vrtx.com/pipeline/

Shapiro AMJ, et al. Stem-cell–derived beta cells for type 1 diabetes. N Engl J Med. 2021;385:1–10.

ClinicalTrials.gov. VX-880 trial [Internet]. Available from: https://clinicaltrials.gov/ct2/show/NCT04786262

Stadtmauer EA, et al. CRISPR-engineered T cells in cancer. Nat Med. 2020;26:1–8.

National Cancer Institute. CAR T-cell therapy [Internet]. Available from: https://www.cancer.gov/about-cancer/treatment/research/car-t-cells

June CH, et al. CRISPR-based cancer immunotherapy. Science. 2020;367(6481):1–6.

Vertex Pharmaceuticals. Gene editing [Internet]. Available from: https://www.vrtx.com/what-we-do/our-science/gene-editing/

U.S. FDA. FDA approves first gene editing therapy [Internet]. 2023. Available from: https://www.fda.gov/news-events/press-announcements/fda-approves-first-gene-editing-therapy

NHS England. Gene editing treatment rollout [Internet]. 2023. Available from: https://www.england.nhs.uk/2023/11/nhs-england-first-in-world-to-roll-out-gene-editing-treatment/

NINDS. Huntington's disease [Internet]. Available from: https://www.ninds.nih.gov/health-information/disorders/huntingtons-disease

Dash PK, et al. CRISPR editing for HIV elimination. Nat Commun. 2019;10:1–10.

Editas Medicine. EDIT-101 program [Internet]. Available from: https://www.editasmedicine.com/programs/edit-101/

WHO. Human genome editing: Recommendations [Internet]. 2021. Available from: https://www.who.int/publications/i/item/9789240030381

Fu Y, et al. Off-target effects of CRISPR. Nat Biotechnol. 2013;31(9):822–826.

NHGRI. Ethical issues in genome editing [Internet]. Available from: https://www.genome.gov/about-genomics/policy-issues/Genome-Editing/ethical-issues

Chapter-20

Is Aging a Disease? A Critical Medical Perspective

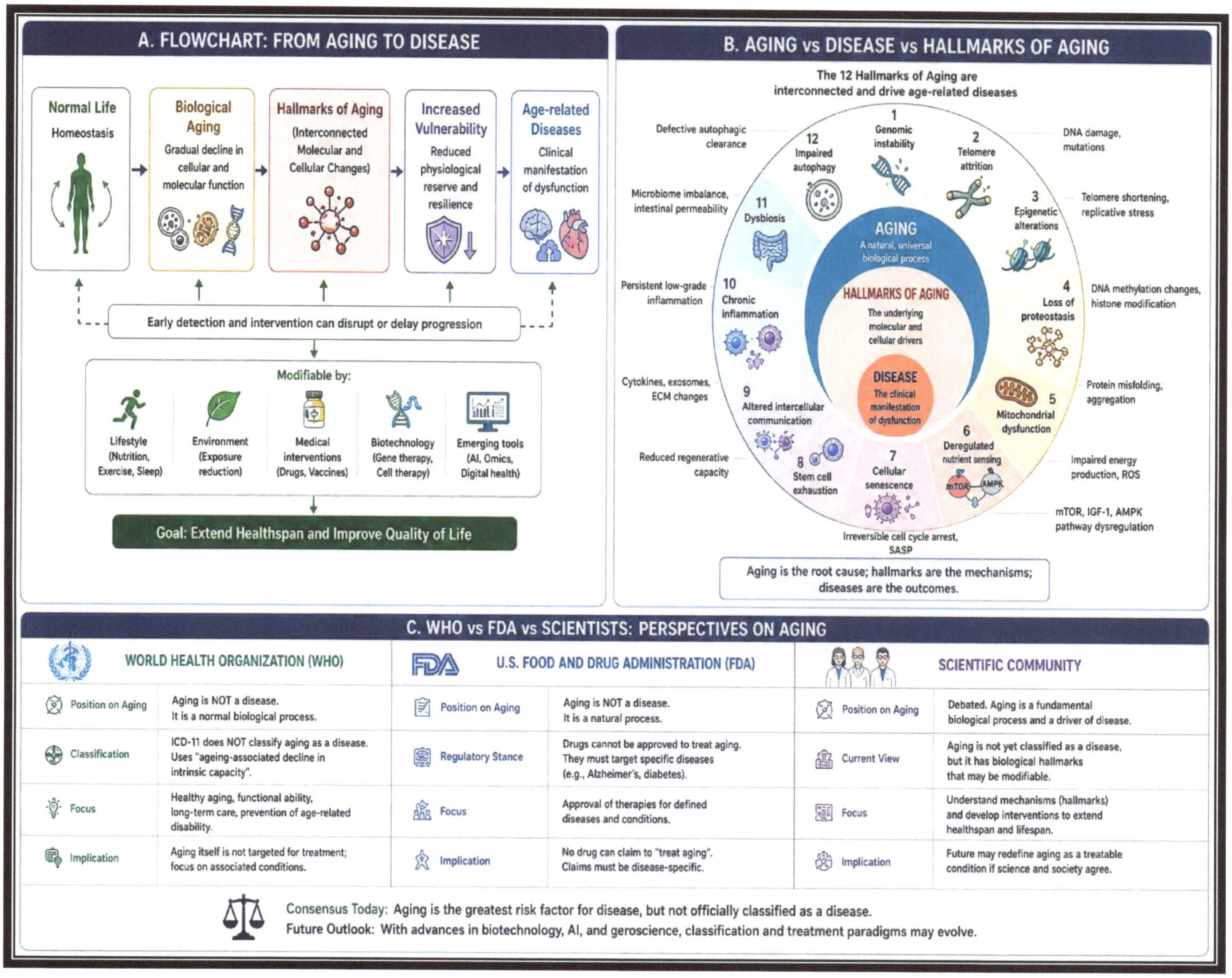

1. Defining the Problem

Aging is traditionally defined as a **progressive decline in physiological function** leading to increased vulnerability to disease and death.

However, the key controversy is:

👉 **Is aging itself a disease, or is it the underlying cause of diseases?**

🧠 2. What Major Medical Bodies Say

2.1 World Health Organization (WHO) Perspective

- WHO **does NOT classify aging as a disease**
- Instead, it uses the concept:
- 👉 **"ageing-associated decline in intrinsic capacity"**

- In ICD-11:
  - Aging is **not a standalone disease**
  - But **"age-related" conditions are coded**

🔑 **WHO Key Idea:**

👉 Aging = **Natural biological process + risk factor for disease**

2.2 U.S. Food and Drug Administration (FDA) Perspective

- FDA clearly states:
- 👉 Aging is **NOT a disease, but a natural process**
- Therefore:
  - Drugs **cannot be approved for "aging"**
  - They must target:
    - Alzheimer's disease
    - Diabetes
    - Cardiovascular disease

🔑 **FDA Key Idea:**

👉 Treat **diseases of aging**, not aging itself

2.3 Indian Perspective (Medical & Policy View)

India does not have a single formal declaration like FDA/WHO, but based on:

- Indian Council of Medical Research
- Ministry of Health and Family Welfare

👉 The approach aligns closely with WHO:

- Aging is treated as:
  - A **natural physiological process**
  - A **public health challenge**
- Focus areas:
  - Geriatric care
  - Non-communicable diseases
  - Healthy aging programs

📌 India emphasizes **"healthy aging"**, not "curing aging"

2.4 Other Global Regulatory Bodies

🇪🇺 **European Medicines Agency**

- Similar to FDA
- Approves drugs for **specific diseases**, not aging

🇯🇵 **Pharmaceuticals and Medical Devices Agency**

- Same stance
- Focus on disease-based approval

⚖️ 3. Why Is There So Much Debate?

This debate exists because **aging sits at the boundary of biology and pathology**.

3.1 Arguments: Aging is NOT a Disease

- It is:
  - Universal
  - Natural
  - Not abnormal
- Scientific argument:
- 👉 Aging = **cause**, diseases = **effects**
- Ethical concern:
  - Labeling aging as disease → **ageism risk**
  - Doctors may ignore treatable conditions

3.2 Arguments: Aging IS a Disease

- Aging has:
  - Defined biological mechanisms (hallmarks)
  - Cellular damage pathways
- Scientific reasoning:
  - If something causes dysfunction → it can be treated
- Benefit:
- 👉 Could accelerate **anti-aging drug development**

🔬 4. Can Aging Be Cured According to These Bodies?

❌ Current Official Position:

- Aging **cannot be cured**
- It is **not classified as a treatable disease**

✅ What CAN be done:

- Delay aging-related diseases
- Improve **health span**
- Target hallmarks indirectly

🔄 Emerging Shift:

- Research shows:
  - Aging processes **can be modified**
- But regulators still require:
- 👉 Disease-specific proof

🚀 5. The Real Scientific Position (Balanced View)

👉 Aging is best understood as:

"A modifiable biological process, but not yet a clinically defined disease."

✍️ Conclusion

Aging represents a universal, progressive biological process characterized by the accumulation of molecular and cellular damage, ultimately leading to functional decline and increased susceptibility to disease. Despite advances in understanding the hallmarks of aging, major regulatory bodies such as the World Health Organization and U.S. Food and Drug Administration do not currently classify aging as a disease. Instead, aging is viewed as a natural physiological process and a primary risk factor for multiple chronic diseases.

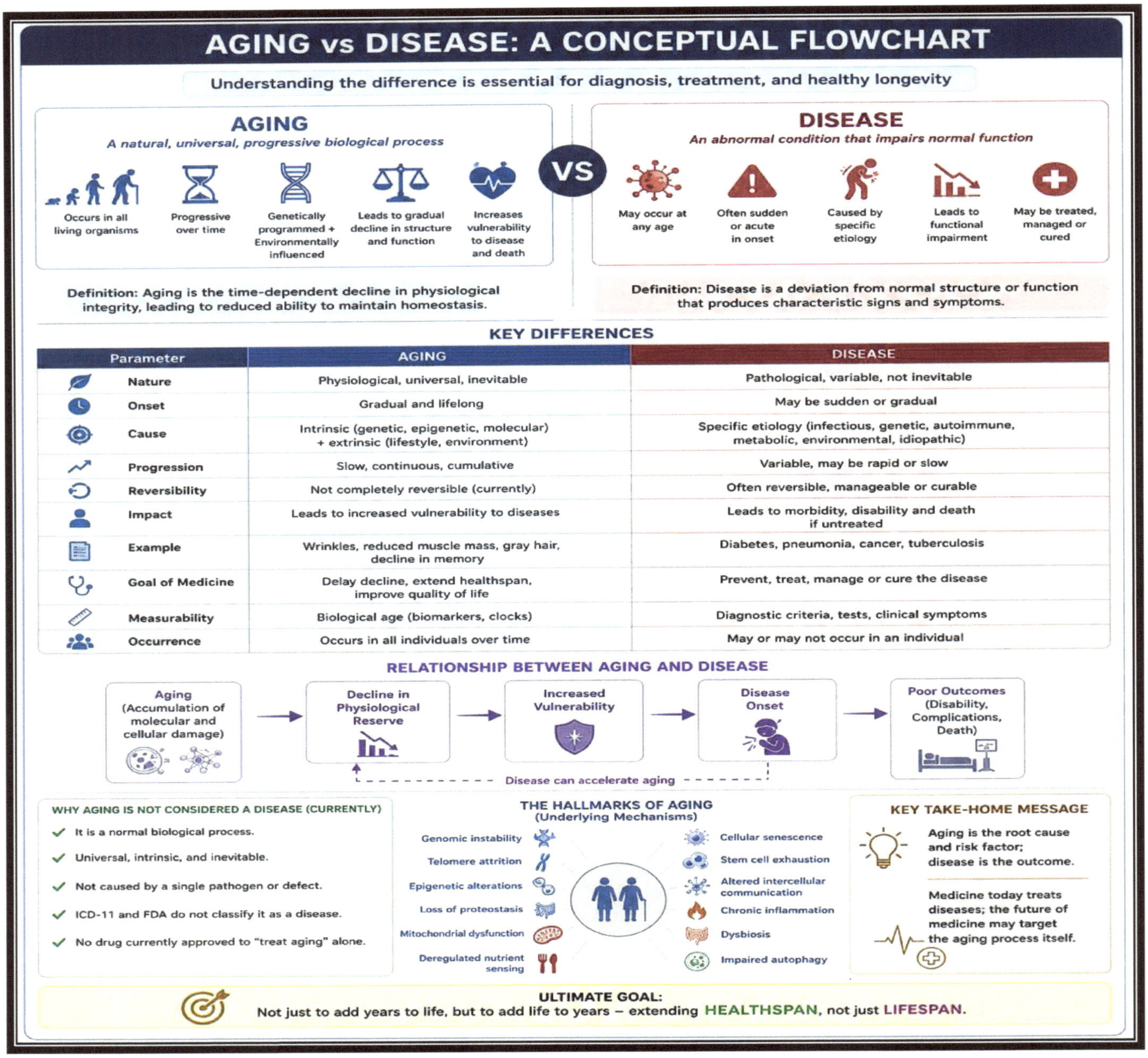

This distinction has significant clinical implications. While diseases associated with aging—such as cardiovascular disorders, neurodegeneration, and metabolic syndromes—are actively targeted for treatment, aging itself remains outside the scope of direct therapeutic approval. However, emerging research in geoscience suggests that aging is biologically modifiable, leading to an ongoing debate regarding its classification.

A balanced perspective recognizes aging as a **central driver of disease rather than a disease entity itself**, while acknowledging that future advancements in biotechnology and artificial intelligence may redefine its clinical status. For medical practitioners, this distinction is critical to avoid both over-medicalization of natural aging and under-treatment of age-related conditions.

🎯 7. What Medical Students Should Understand (Key Takeaway Box)

- Aging ≠ Disease (currently)
- Aging = **Risk factor for most diseases**
- Medicine today = **Treat diseases, not aging itself**
- Future medicine = **May target aging pathways directly**

📚 **Final Conceptual Summary**

👉 *"Aging is not yet a disease—but it is the most important biological process driving disease."*

📚 **Scientific References**

🔬 **1. WHO Position (Aging is NOT a disease)**

- WHO did **not classify aging as a disease in ICD-11** and instead uses functional decline terminology:
- 👉 https://link.springer.com/article/10.1007/s10522-026-10422-3

✔ Key takeaway you can cite:

Aging is considered a **normal biological process**, not a diagnosable disease, and ICD-11 uses "decline in intrinsic capacity" instead.

🔬 **2. ICD-11 & Aging as a Risk Factor (Not a Disease)**

- Aging is recognized as **causally related to diseases**, but not classified as a disease itself:
- 👉 https://journals.sagepub.com/doi/10.1089/rej.2019.2242

✔ Use this line:

Aging is acknowledged as a **causal factor in disease development**, not as a standalone disease.

🔬 **3. Scientific Debate: Should Aging Be Classified as a Disease?**

- Open-access academic discussion:
- 👉 https://www.frontiersin.org/articles/10.3389/fgene.2015.00326/full

✔ Key idea:

Classifying aging as a disease could improve research funding and therapeutic development.

🔬 **4. Ethical Argument Against Calling Aging a Disease**

- Lancet discussion paper:
- 👉 https://www.researchgate.net/publication/354946383_Not_a_disease_a_global_call_for_action_urging_revision_of_the_ICD-11_classification_of_old_age

✔ Key idea:

Labeling aging as a disease may have **negative clinical and social consequences**.

🏛 **5. FDA Position**

- Summary from recent medical reporting:
- 👉 FDA considers aging a **natural process, not a disease**

✔ Key takeaway:

No drug is currently approved by FDA to treat aging itself.

Aging is not currently classified as a disease by major regulatory bodies such as WHO and FDA; rather, it is considered a natural biological process and a major risk factor for disease (WHO ICD-11 framework; FDA position).

📚 **Scientific References**

1. López-Otín et al., *Cell*, 2013 & 2023 (Hallmarks of Aging)
2. WHO ICD-11 Framework on Aging
3. Calimport & Bentley, *Rejuvenation Research*, 2019
4. Zhavoronkov et al., *Frontiers in Genetics*, 2015
5. Banerjee et al., *Lancet Healthy Longevity*, 2021
6. FDA Position on Aging

Chapter-21

An Integrative Biology of Aging

From Molecules to Systems: A Multidisciplinary View of the Hallmarks of Aging

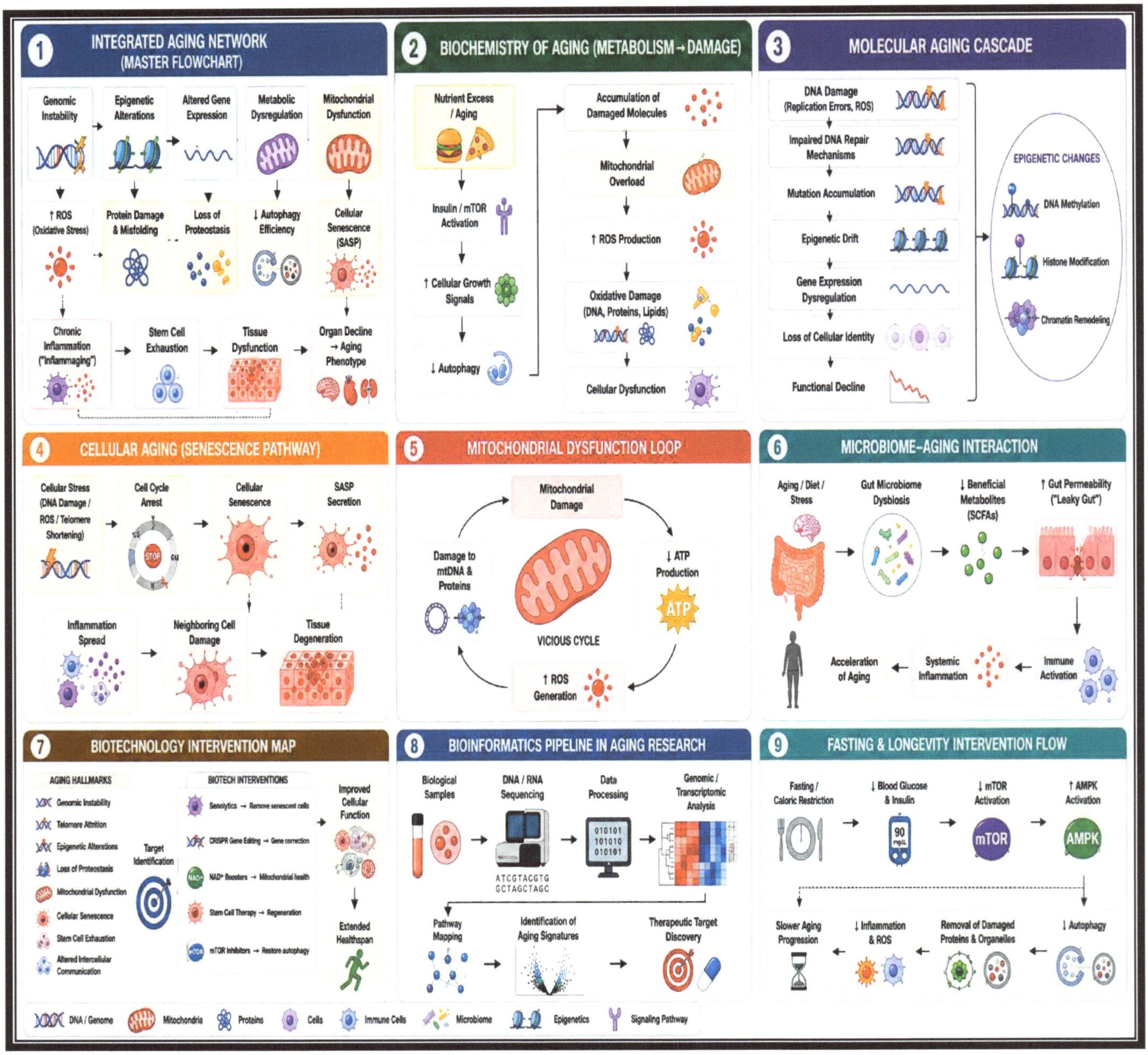

1. Introduction: Aging as a Systems-Level Process

Aging is a complex, multifactorial biological process characterized by the progressive decline in physiological function and increased vulnerability to disease and death. Modern aging research—particularly in **biogerontology**—has established that aging is not driven by a single cause, but rather emerges from interconnected molecular, cellular, and systemic processes.

The framework of the *hallmarks of aging* provides a unifying model that integrates these processes, including genomic instability, loss of proteostasis, mitochondrial dysfunction, cellular senescence, and altered intercellular communication.

Understanding aging requires a **multidisciplinary approach**, combining insights from:

- Biochemistry
- Molecular biology
- Cell biology
- Microbiology
- Biotechnology
- Bioinformatics

This chapter synthesizes these perspectives into a coherent understanding of how aging unfolds and how it may be modulated.

2. Biogerontology: The Foundation of Aging Science

Biogerontology focuses on the biological mechanisms that drive aging and age-related diseases. It seeks to answer key questions:

- Why do organisms age?
- What determines lifespan?
- Can aging be slowed or reversed?

Central to this field is the recognition that aging is **plastic**, meaning it can be influenced by:

- Genetics
- Environment
- Metabolism
- Lifestyle interventions (e.g., fasting, caloric restriction)

Biogerontology connects all downstream disciplines by framing aging as a **modifiable biological program rather than an inevitable decline**.

3. Biochemistry of Aging

3.1 Metabolic Pathways and Aging

Cellular metabolism plays a central role in aging. Key pathways include:

- Glycolysis
- TCA cycle
- Oxidative phosphorylation
- Insulin/IGF-1 signaling
- mTOR pathway

Dysregulation in these pathways leads to:

- Energy imbalance
- Increased production of harmful byproducts
- Reduced cellular repair capacity

3.2 Oxidative Stress

Reactive oxygen species (ROS) are natural byproducts of metabolism. While low levels serve signaling roles, excessive ROS leads to:

- DNA damage
- Protein oxidation
- Lipid peroxidation

This contributes to:

- Mitochondrial dysfunction
- Cellular aging
- Chronic inflammation

3.3 Cellular Energetics

Aging cells show:

- Reduced ATP production
- Impaired mitochondrial efficiency
- Increased metabolic inflexibility

This energy decline affects:

- Repair mechanisms
- Protein turnover
- Stress resistance

🧬 4. Molecular Biology of Aging

4.1 DNA Damage and Genomic Instability

Over time, DNA accumulates damage due to:

- Replication errors
- Environmental stress
- Oxidative damage

This leads to:

- Mutations
- Chromosomal instability
- Impaired cellular function

4.2 Gene Regulation

Aging alters gene expression patterns through:

- Transcriptional dysregulation
- Changes in signaling pathways
- Loss of regulatory precision

This affects:

- Stress responses
- Metabolism
- Cell survival

4.3 Epigenetics

Epigenetic changes include:

- DNA methylation
- Histone modification
- Chromatin remodeling

These changes:

- Alter gene expression without changing DNA sequence
- Serve as biomarkers of biological age
- Are partially reversible

5. Cell Biology of Aging

5.1 Cellular Senescence

Senescent cells are:

- Metabolically active but non-dividing
- Resistant to apoptosis

They secrete inflammatory factors known as:

- SASP (Senescence-Associated Secretory Phenotype)

Consequences:

- Tissue dysfunction
- Chronic inflammation
- Propagation of aging signals

5.2 Stem Cell Exhaustion

With age:

- Stem cell numbers decline
- Regenerative capacity decreases

This leads to:

- Impaired tissue repair
- Organ degeneration

5.3 Signaling Pathways

Key pathways regulating aging include:

- mTOR (growth and metabolism)
- AMPK (energy sensing)
- Sirtuins (stress resistance and longevity)

Imbalance in these pathways accelerates aging.

6. Intersection with Biotechnology

Biotechnology provides tools to both study and intervene in aging.

6.1 Therapeutic Strategies

- Senolytics (removal of senescent cells)
- NAD+ boosters
- mTOR inhibitors (e.g., rapamycin)
- Gene therapy
- Stem cell therapy

6.2 Research Tools

- CRISPR gene editing
- Organoids and tissue models
- High-throughput screening
- Proteomics and metabolomics

These tools enable:

- Mechanistic understanding
- Drug discovery
- Precision medicine approaches

🦠 7. Microbiology: The Microbiome and Aging

The gut microbiome plays a crucial role in aging.

7.1 Microbiome Changes with Age

- Reduced diversity
- Increased pathogenic species
- Altered metabolite production

7.2 Host-Microbiome Interactions

The microbiome influences:

- Immune function
- Metabolism
- Brain function (gut-brain axis)

Dysbiosis contributes to:

- Inflammation
- Metabolic disorders
- Neurodegeneration

💻 8. Bioinformatics and Aging Research

Bioinformatics enables large-scale analysis of aging data.

8.1 Genomics

- Identification of longevity genes
- Mutation analysis
- Population-level studies

8.2 Transcriptomics

- Gene expression profiling
- Aging signatures
- Pathway analysis

8.3 Systems Biology

Integration of multi-omics data helps:

- Map aging networks
- Identify intervention targets
- Predict biological age

🔗 9. Integrated View: How Everything Connects

Aging is not isolated—it is a **networked process**:

- Metabolic dysfunction → increases ROS
- ROS → damages DNA and proteins
- DNA damage → alters gene expression
- Altered expression → drives senescence
- Senescence → increases inflammation
- Inflammation → disrupts microbiome and signaling

This interconnected cascade leads to:

👉 System-wide functional decline

10. Implications for Intervention

Understanding these interactions reveals key intervention points:

- Improve metabolism (fasting, diet)
- Enhance autophagy
- Reduce oxidative stress
- Target senescent cells
- Modulate microbiome
- Use precision biotechnology tools

11. Conclusion

Aging is a **multi-layered biological phenomenon** that emerges from the interplay of biochemical, molecular, cellular, microbial, and computational processes.

The integration of disciplines—from biogerontology to bioinformatics—provides a powerful framework to:

- Understand aging mechanisms
- Identify therapeutic targets
- Extend health span

Future advances will depend on **systems-level thinking**, where aging is treated not as a singular process, but as a dynamic and modifiable biological network.

Master Flowchart

1. Integrated Aging Network

Genomic Instability (DNA Damage)
↓
Epigenetic Alterations
↓
Altered Gene Expression
↓
Metabolic Dysregulation
↓
Mitochondrial Dysfunction
↓
↑ ROS (Oxidative Stress)
↓
Protein Damage & Misfolding
↓
Loss of Proteostasis
↓
↓ Autophagy Efficiency
↓
Cellular Senescence (SASP)
↓
Chronic Inflammation ("Inflammaging")
↓
Stem Cell Exhaustion
↓
Tissue Dysfunction
↓
Organ Decline → Aging Phenotype

2. Biochemistry of Aging (Metabolism → Damage)

Nutrient Excess/Aging
↓
Insulin/mTOR Activation
↓
↑ Cellular Growth Signals
↓
↓ Autophagy
↓
Accumulation of Damaged Molecules
↓
Mitochondrial Overload
↓
↑ ROS Production
↓
Oxidative Damage (DNA, Proteins, Lipids)
↓
Cellular Dysfunction

3. Molecular Aging Cascade

DNA Damage (Replication Errors, ROS)
↓
Impaired DNA Repair Mechanisms
↓
Mutation Accumulation
↓
Epigenetic Drift
↓
Gene Expression Dysregulation
↓
Loss of Cellular Identity
↓
Functional Decline

4. Cellular Aging (Senescence Pathway)

Cellular Stress (DNA Damage/ROS/Telomere Shortening)
↓
Cell Cycle Arrest
↓
Cellular Senescence
↓
SASP Secretion
↓
Inflammation Spread
↓
Neighboring Cell Damage
↓
Tissue Degeneration

5. Mitochondrial Dysfunction Loop

Mitochondrial Damage
↓
↓ ATP Production
↓
↑ ROS Generation
↓
Damage to mtDNA & Proteins
↓
Further Mitochondrial Dysfunction
↺ (Vicious Cycle)

6. Microbiome–Aging Interaction

Aging/Diet/Stress
↓
Gut Microbiome Dysbiosis
↓
↓ Beneficial Metabolites (SCFAs)
↓
↑ Gut Permeability ("Leaky Gut")
↓
Immune Activation
↓
Systemic Inflammation
↓
Acceleration of Aging

7. Biotechnology Intervention Map

Aging Hallmarks
↓
Target Identification
↓
Biotech Interventions
├─ Senolytics → Remove senescent cells
├─ CRISPR → Gene correction
├─ NAD+ Boosters → Mitochondrial health
├─ Stem Cell Therapy → Regeneration
└─ mTOR Inhibitors → Restore autophagy
↓
Improved Cellular Function
↓
Extended Health span

💻 8. Bioinformatics Pipeline in Aging Research

Biological Samples
↓
DNA/RNA Sequencing
↓
Data Processing
↓
Genomic/Transcriptomic Analysis
↓
Pathway Mapping
↓
Identification of Aging Signatures
↓
Therapeutic Target Discovery

🔄 9. Fasting & Longevity Intervention Flow

Fasting/Caloric Restriction
↓
↓ Blood Glucose & Insulin
↓
↓ mTOR Activation
↓
↑ AMPK Activation
↓
↑ Autophagy
↓
Removal of Damaged Proteins & Organelles
↓
Improved Proteostasis
↓
↓ Inflammation & ROS
↓

🌿 The City Inside You - A Storybook Guide to the Hallmarks of Aging

🌱 The Secret Instructions Inside You

Imagine your body is like a huge city made of trillions of tiny houses called *cells*.

Inside every cell, there are **two important things**:

1. The DNA — The Recipe Book 📀

Think of DNA like a big library or a collection of DVDs.

Each DVD is a **gene**.

And each gene contains instructions—like a recipe for making something important in your body.

👉 For example:

- One gene tells your body how to make your hair
- Another helps build your muscles
- Another helps your heart beat

So, DNA is like a **recipe book that never changes much**.

2. The Epigenome — The Reader and Controller 🎛️

Now here's the interesting part.

Just having a recipe book is not enough.

You need someone to decide:

- Which recipe to read
- When to read it
- How much to use

That "someone" is called the **epigenome**.

👉 Think of it like:

- A remote control for your DVDs
- Or a librarian who chooses which book to open
- Or a music DJ who decides which song to play

🎬 **Simple Analogy**

- DNA = DVDs (all the movies you own)
- Epigenome = The person holding the remote

You may own 1,000 movies, but you only watch a few at a time.

⏳ **What Happens as We Age?**

When we are young:

- The "remote control" works perfectly
- The right genes are turned on at the right time

But as we grow older:

- The epigenome gets **confused**
- It starts pressing the wrong buttons
- It plays the wrong "movies" at the wrong time

This is what called:

👉 **"Corrupted biological software"**

💻 **Another Easy Way to Understand**

Think of your body like a computer:

- DNA = Hardware (the machine itself)
- Epigenome = Software (the program running it)

A computer may be perfectly fine…

but if the software gets buggy, things stop working properly.

That's aging.

🌿 **Why This Matters**

The exciting idea is this:

👉 Your DNA doesn't get very damaged

👉 The *instructions are still there*

The problem is:

- The body **forgets how to read them correctly**

And scientists are now asking:

💡 "Can we reset the system?"

💡 "Can we clean the software and make cells young again?"

🧠 One-Line Summary

"DNA is the library of life, but the epigenome is the librarian—and aging happens when the librarian loses track of which book to read."

🌿 The Librarian Who Forgot

A Story About Your Cells, Time, and a Forgetful Helper

Once upon a time, inside your body, there lived a magical city.

This city was not like any city you have seen.

It was made of trillions of tiny houses called **cells**.

Each cell was busy all the time—building, repairing, cleaning, and keeping you alive.

And inside every single cell, there was a very special place…

📚 The Great Library of Life

At the centre of each cell stood a grand library.

This library held the most important collection in the world:

👉 Your DNA

Think of DNA as a giant bookshelf filled with thousands of DVDs or recipe books.

Each DVD (or recipe) is called a **gene**.

Every gene contains instructions:

- How to grow your hair
- How to heal a wound
- How to make your heart beat
- How to think, move, and feel

Everything about you begins here.

And the most amazing part?

This library is almost the same from the day you are born until the day you grow old.

The books don't disappear.

The DVDs don't vanish.

They stay.

🎛️ The Librarian with the Remote

But there was one problem.

The library was too big.

With so many books, how would the cell know:

- Which one to read?
- When to read it?
- How much of it to use?

That's where a very important character comes in.

Meet the **Librarian**.

This librarian is called the **epigenome**.

The librarian's job is simple but powerful:

- Choose the right book
- Open it at the right time
- Close it when it's no longer needed

If DNA is the library…

👉 The epigenome is the one who decides what gets read.

🎬 The Movie Room

Let's imagine it another way.

Inside your cell is also a movie room.

- DNA = a huge collection of movies (genes)
- Epigenome = the person holding the remote

You may own thousands of movies…

But you only watch one at a time.

The remote decides:

- Play
- Pause
- Stop
- Skip

When everything works well, the right movie plays at the right moment.

🌱 When You Are Young

When you are a child, the librarian is sharp and focused.

They:

- Pick the correct books
- Play the right movies
- Turn on the right genes at the right time

Your body works smoothly:

- Cuts heal quickly
- Energy is high
- Skin is fresh
- Organs work perfectly

Everything feels… easy.

⏳ As Time Passes…

But slowly, something begins to change.

The librarian starts getting tired.

Not weak—but confused.

They begin to:

- Misplace books
- Open the wrong pages
- Play the wrong movies

Sometimes they:

- Turn ON genes that should be OFF
- Turn OFF genes that should be ON

It's like:

- Playing a sad movie during a happy moment
- Cooking the wrong recipe for dinner
- Pressing random buttons on a remote

This confusion builds up over time.

💻 The "Corrupted Software"

The scientist explains this beautifully.

They say aging is not just damage.

👉 It is like **corrupted biological software**

Think of your body like a computer:

- DNA = the hardware (the machine)
- Epigenome = the software (the instructions running it)

Your hardware might still be strong…

But if the software gets messy:

- Programs crash
- Things slow down
- Errors appear

That's what aging feels like.

🧩 The Big Surprise

Here's the most exciting part.

The DNA—the library itself—is still mostly intact.

The books are still there.

The recipes are still correct.

👉 The problem is not the instructions…

👉 The problem is how they are being read.

It's as if the body hasn't lost the knowledge—

It has just **forgotten how to use it properly**.

🔄 Can the Librarian Remember Again?

Now imagine this:

What if the librarian could be reminded?

What if:

- The remote could be reset
- The right movies could play again
- The correct books could be opened

Scientists around the world are exploring this idea.

They are asking:

💡 Can we "clean" the epigenome?

💡 Can we restore the instructions?

💡 Can cells remember how to be young again?

And early research suggests…

👉 It might be possible.

🌿 **A Simple Way to Remember**

If this whole story feels big, just remember this:

- DNA is the **library of life**
- Genes are the **books or DVDs**
- The epigenome is the **librarian or remote control**

And aging?

👉 Aging happens when the librarian gets confused.

🧠 **A Thought to Carry with You**

Inside you, right now, is a perfect set of instructions for life.

Not broken.

Not gone.

Just… a little mismanaged.

And the future of science may not be about creating something new—

👉 But about helping your body **remember what it already knows**.

✨ **One-Line Summary**

"We do not age because we lose the instructions for life—we age because our cells forget how to read them."

🌿 The Forgetful Librarian - When the Instructions Go Wrong

The Librarian Who Forgot

(Epigenetic Alterations)

In the great Cell City, every house had a library filled with instructions (DNA).

The Librarian—the epigenome—decided which books to read.

When the city was young, the Librarian was perfect.

But over time, the Librarian grew confused:

- Reading the wrong books
- Ignoring important ones

The city didn't lose its knowledge…

👉 It just forgot how to use it.

The Broken Blueprints

(Genomic Instability)

One day, tiny cracks appeared in the pages of the books.

Letters faded. Words changed.

These books were the DNA.

Every day:

- Sunlight
- Pollution
- Mistakes during copying

…caused small damage.

Workers tried to fix the pages—but not all repairs were perfect.

Over time, the blueprints became harder to trust.

The Fraying Shoelace Tips

(Telomere Attrition)

At the ends of every DNA "string" were little caps—like plastic tips on shoelaces.

These were called telomeres.

Every time a cell copied itself, the caps became shorter.

At first, it didn't matter.

But one day, the caps became too small…

And the cell said:

👉 "I can't divide anymore."

The Trash That Wasn't Taken Out

(Loss of Proteostasis)

Inside Cell City, factories made tiny machines called proteins.

But not all machines were perfect.

Some were broken.

Normally, the city had a cleaning crew that removed the junk.

But as time passed:

- The cleaners slowed down
- Trash began piling up

Broken machines started interfering with everything.

The Power Plants That Dimmed

(Mitochondrial Dysfunction)

Each cell had power plants called mitochondria.

They produced energy—like electricity for the city.

When young:

- Bright
- Efficient
- Strong

But over time:

- They produced less energy
- They leaked harmful "sparks"

The city lights began to dim.

The Noisy Alarm System

(Deregulated Nutrient Sensing)

The city had a control center that sensed food and energy.

When food was available:

👉 "Grow! Build! Expand!"

When food was scarce:

👉 "Repair! Save! Clean!"

But as time passed, the system became confused.

It kept shouting:

👉 "Grow! Grow! Grow!"

Even when the city needed rest and repair.

The Sleeping Workers

(Cellular Senescence)

Some workers in the city stopped working.

They didn't leave.

They didn't help.

They just sat there… taking up space.

Worse, they began spreading complaints:

- Sending negative signals
- Disturbing nearby cells

These were called "senescent cells."

The Exhausted Builders

(Stem Cell Exhaustion)

The city had special builders—stem cells.

They could:

- Repair damage
- Build new structures
- Replace broken parts

But over time:

- They became tired
- Fewer showed up for work

Repairs slowed down.

The city began to wear out.

The Fire That Wouldn't Go Out

(Altered Intercellular Communication/Inflammation)

The cells talked to each other using signals.

When there was danger:

👉 They lit small fires (inflammation) to fix the problem.

But as the city aged:

- The fire alarms kept ringing
- Small fires never stopped burning

Even when there was no danger.

The city was always slightly "on fire."

The Copying Machine That Made Mistakes

(Genomic Copy Errors & Aging Spread)

Every time a cell divided, it copied its instructions.

Like photocopying a page again and again.

At first, copies were clear.

But over time:

- Smudges appeared
- Lines blurred
- Mistakes multiplied

Soon, the copies were no longer perfect.

The City That Remembers

Even after all this…

The city is not lost.

The original instructions are still there.

The library still stands.

The question scientists are now asking:

👉 Can we remind the city how to run correctly again?

Can we:

- Help the Librarian focus?
- Clean the trash?
- Repair the power plants?
- Wake up the builders?

If yes…

Then aging may not just be decline.

👉 It may be something we can **understand, slow, and perhaps one day reset**.

🌟 **Summary**

"Your body is like a city that doesn't break all at once—it slowly forgets how to take care of itself."

🧭 **Overall Structure**

🌿 **The World Inside You**

1. The City Inside You *(Introduction to cells)*
2. The Great Library *(DNA explained)*
3. The Librarian Who Forgot *(Epigenome)*
4. Broken Blueprints (DNA damage)
5. Fraying Shoelace Tips (Telomeres)
6. The Trash Problem (Proteins)

7. Fading Power Plants (Mitochondria)
8. The Confused Control Room (Nutrient sensing)
9. Sleeping Workers (Senescent cells)
10. Tired Builders (Stem cells)
11. The Never-Ending Fire (Inflammation)
12. Mixed-Up Messages (Cell communication)

🏙️ **Main Elements (Label These Clearly)**

- 🏛️ **Library (DNA)**
  → Big central building
  → Shelves/books glowing
- 👩‍🏫 **Librarian (Epigenome)**
  → Holding a remote or checklist
- 🏭 **Factories (Proteins)**
  → Some working, some broken
- ⚡ **Power Plants (Mitochondria)**
  → Bright vs dim
- 🚒 **Fire Stations (Inflammation)**
  → Small vs uncontrolled fires
- 👷 **Construction Workers (Stem Cells)**
  → Busy vs tired
- 🧓 **Idle Workers (Senescent Cells)**
  → Sitting, complaining
- 📡 **Control Tower (Nutrient sensing)**
  → Sending signals
- 🧵 **Shoelace Towers (Telomeres)**
  → With caps shrinking

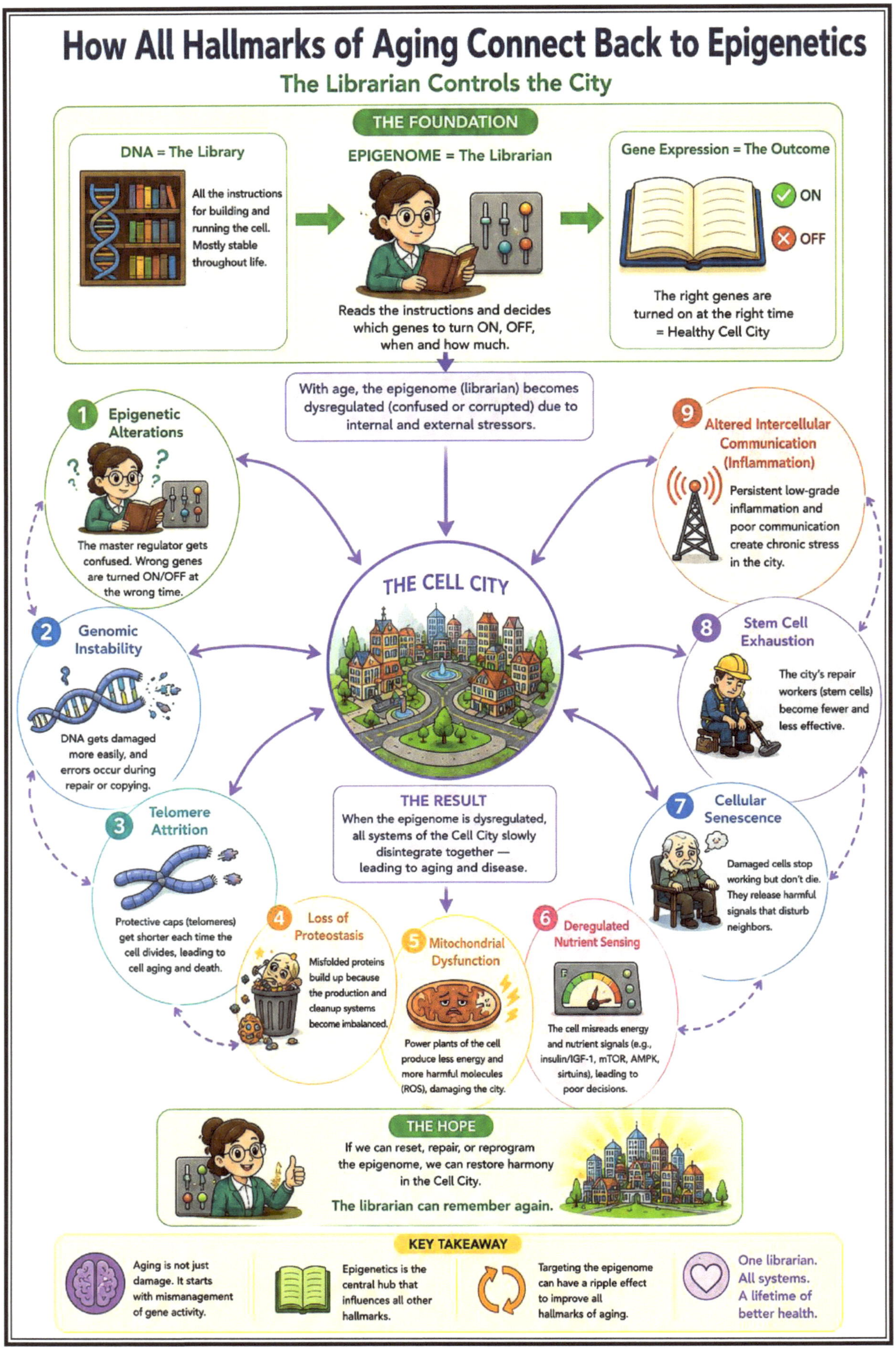
How All Hallmarks of Aging Connect Back to Epigenetics
The Librarian Controls the City
THE FOUNDATION
DNA = The Library
All the instructions for building and running the cell. Mostly stable throughout life.
EPIGENOME = The Librarian
Reads the instructions and decides which genes to turn ON, OFF, when and how much.
Gene Expression = The Outcome
ON
OFF
The right genes are turned on at the right time = Healthy Cell City
With age, the epigenome (librarian) becomes dysregulated (confused or corrupted) due to internal and external stressors.
1 Epigenetic Alterations
The master regulator gets confused. Wrong genes are turned ON/OFF at the wrong time.
2 Genomic Instability
DNA gets damaged more easily, and errors occur during repair or copying.
3 Telomere Attrition
Protective caps (telomeres) get shorter each time the cell divides, leading to cell aging and death.
4 Loss of Proteostasis
Misfolded proteins build up because the production and cleanup systems become imbalanced.
5 Mitochondrial Dysfunction
Power plants of the cell produce less energy and more harmful molecules (ROS), damaging the city.
6 Deregulated Nutrient Sensing
The cell misreads energy and nutrient signals (e.g., insulin/IGF-1, mTOR, AMPK, sirtuins), leading to poor decisions.
7 Cellular Senescence
Damaged cells stop working but don't die. They release harmful signals that disturb neighbors.
8 Stem Cell Exhaustion
The city's repair workers (stem cells) become fewer and less effective.
9 Altered Intercellular Communication (Inflammation)
Persistent low-grade inflammation and poor communication create chronic stress in the city.
THE CELL CITY
THE RESULT
When the epigenome is dysregulated, all systems of the Cell City slowly disintegrate together — leading to aging and disease.
THE HOPE
If we can reset, repair, or reprogram the epigenome, we can restore harmony in the Cell City.
The librarian can remember again.
KEY TAKEAWAY
Aging is not just damage. It starts with mismanagement of gene activity.
Epigenetics is the central hub that influences all other hallmarks.
Targeting the epigenome can have a ripple effect to improve all hallmarks of aging.
One librarian. All systems. A lifetime of better health.

Scientific References

1. **López-Otín C, Blasco MA, Partridge L, Serrano M, Kroemer G. The hallmarks of aging. *Cell.* 2013;153(6):1194–1217. Available from:** https://www.cell.com/fulltext/S0092-8674(13)00645-4
2. **López-Otín C, Blasco MA, Partridge L, Serrano M, Kroemer G. Hallmarks of aging: An expanding universe. *Cell.* 2023;186(2):243–278. Available from:** https://www.cell.com/cell/fulltext/S0092-8674(22)01377-X
3. **Kirkwood TBL. Understanding the odd science of aging. *Cell.* 2005;120(4):437–447. Available from:** https://www.nature.com/articles/35041682
4. **Kitano H. Systems biology: A brief overview. *Science.* 2002;295(5560):1662–1664. Available from:** https://www.nature.com/scitable/topicpage/systems-biology-a-brief-overview-14639358
5. **López-Otín C, Galluzzi L, Freije JMP, Madeo F, Kroemer G. Metabolic control of longevity. *Cell.* 2016;166(4):802–821. Available from:** https://www.cell.com/fulltext/S0092-8674(13)00145-5
6. **Liguori I, Russo G, Curcio F, et al. Oxidative stress, aging, and diseases. *Clin Interv Aging.* 2018;13:757–772. Available from:** https://www.ncbi.nlm.nih.gov/pmc/articles/PMC5927356
7. **Lombard DB, Chua KF, Mostoslavsky R, Franco S, Gostissa M, Alt FW. DNA repair, genome stability, and aging. *Nat Rev Mol Cell Biol.* 2005;6(8):641–654. Available from:** https://www.nature.com/articles/nrm2350
8. **Horvath S. DNA methylation age of human tissues and cell types. *Genome Biol.* 2013;14(10):R115. Available from:** https://genomebiology.biomedcentral.com/articles/10.1186/gb-2013-14-10-r115
9. **Campisi J, d'Adda di Fagagna F. Cellular senescence: When bad things happen to good cells. *Nat Rev Mol Cell Biol.* 2007;8(9):729–740. Available from:** https://www.nature.com/articles/nrm2233
10. **López-Otín C, et al. Stem cell aging. *Nat Rev Mol Cell Biol.* 2013;14(5):306–320. Available from**: https://www.nature.com/articles/nrm3619
11. **O'Toole PW, Jeffery IB. Gut microbiota and aging. *Nat Rev Gastroenterol Hepatol.* 2015;12(6):371–382. Available from:** https://www.nature.com/articles/nrgastro.2017.136
12. **National Center for Biotechnology Information (NCBI). Bioinformatics overview. Available from:** https://www.ncbi.nlm.nih.gov/home/about/
13. **Hasin Y, Seldin M, Lusis A. Multi-omics approaches to disease. *Nat Biotechnol.* 2017;35(9):845–858. Available from:** https://www.nature.com/articles/nbt.3599
14. **Laplante M, Sabatini DM. mTOR signaling in growth control and disease. *Cell Metab.* 2012;23(6):990–1003. Available from:** https://www.cell.com/cell-metabolism/fulltext/S1550-4131(12)00071-3
15. **de Cabo R, Mattson MP. Effects of intermittent fasting on health, aging, and disease. *N Engl J Med.* 2019;381(26):2541–2551. Available from:** https://www.ncbi.nlm.nih.gov/pmc/articles/PMC6520897

"The Messengers of Cell City" - Hormones: Neuroendocrine Control in the Hallmarks of Aging

1. Introduction: Aging Beyond Cells—A Systemic Perspective

Aging is not confined to isolated cellular damage; it is a coordinated, system-wide process involving continuous communication between organs, tissues, and molecular pathways. Among the most important regulators of this communication is the endocrine system.

Hormones function as biochemical messengers that coordinate growth, metabolism, repair, stress responses, and reproduction. Throughout life, these signals maintain physiological balance, or homeostasis. However, with advancing age, hormonal signaling becomes progressively dysregulated.

This endocrine decline does not act independently. Instead, it interacts with and amplifies the established hallmarks of aging—such as genomic instability, mitochondrial dysfunction, cellular senescence, and chronic inflammation—making hormones a central integrative layer in aging biology.

2. The Endocrine System: A Brief Overview

The endocrine system consists of glands that release hormones into the bloodstream, allowing communication across distant organs. Major endocrine organs include:

- Hypothalamus
- Pituitary gland
- Thyroid gland
- Adrenal glands
- Pancreas
- Gonads (testes and ovaries)

These glands regulate critical functions such as:

- Energy metabolism
- Growth and development
- Reproductive function
- Stress adaptation
- Circadian rhythms

Hormonal signaling is tightly regulated through feedback loops. With aging, these feedback mechanisms lose precision, leading to either reduced hormone levels or inappropriate activation.

3. The Neuroendocrine Theory of Aging

The neuroendocrine theory of aging proposes that aging results, in part, from progressive dysfunction of the hypothalamic–pituitary axis, which serves as the master regulator of hormonal balance.

Over time, this system experiences:

- Reduced sensitivity to feedback signals
- Altered hormone secretion patterns
- Disruption of circadian rhythms

This leads to systemic effects including metabolic dysregulation, impaired stress responses, and decreased regenerative capacity.

Thus, aging can be viewed not only as cellular decline but also as a gradual loss of coordinated hormonal regulation.

4. Major Hormonal Changes with Aging

4.1 Growth Hormone and IGF-1 (Somatopause)

Growth hormone (GH) and insulin-like growth factor-1 (IGF-1) decline significantly with age.

Consequences include:

- Reduced protein synthesis
- Decreased muscle mass (sarcopenia)
- Impaired tissue repair
- Reduced stem cell activity

While reduced GH signaling has been associated with increased lifespan in some model organisms, in humans it contributes to functional decline.

4.2 Insulin and Glucose Regulation

Aging is strongly associated with insulin resistance, a condition in which cells respond poorly to insulin.

This leads to:

- Elevated blood glucose levels
- Increased oxidative stress
- Chronic low-grade inflammation

Insulin signaling is a central component of nutrient sensing pathways, directly linking endocrine changes to metabolic hallmarks of aging.

4.3 Sex Hormones: Estrogen and Testosterone

Sex hormones decline with age:

- Estrogen decreases sharply during menopause
- Testosterone gradually declines in men

Effects include:

- Loss of bone density (osteoporosis)
- Reduced muscle mass
- Altered fat distribution
- Increased inflammatory activity

These changes also influence cardiovascular and neurological health.

4.4 Cortisol and Stress Response

Cortisol, the primary stress hormone, often becomes chronically elevated with age due to prolonged stress and dysregulated feedback.

Chronic cortisol elevation contributes to:

- Protein breakdown
- Increased abdominal fat
- Immune suppression
- Impaired cognitive function

Persistent stress signaling accelerates multiple aging processes.

4.5 Melatonin and Circadian Rhythm

Melatonin regulates sleep-wake cycles and has antioxidant properties. Its production declines with age.

Consequences include:

- Sleep disturbances
- Reduced cellular repair
- Increased oxidative stress
- Disruption of circadian gene expression

Circadian dysregulation further amplifies metabolic and inflammatory imbalances.

5. Hormonal Integration of the Hallmarks of Aging

Hormones do not act in isolation. Instead, they influence and connect multiple hallmarks of aging simultaneously.

5.1 Genomic Instability

Hormonal imbalance increases oxidative stress, leading to DNA damage and impaired repair mechanisms.

5.2 Epigenetic Alterations

Hormones regulate gene expression through epigenetic mechanisms such as DNA methylation and histone modification.

5.3 Mitochondrial Dysfunction

Insulin resistance and altered metabolic signaling impair mitochondrial function and energy production.

5.4 Loss of Proteostasis

Hormonal dysregulation reduces protein synthesis and increases accumulation of damaged proteins.

5.5 Cellular Senescence

Chronic stress hormones and metabolic dysfunction promote cellular senescence and the secretion of inflammatory factors.

5.6 Stem Cell Exhaustion

Reduced growth hormone and IGF-1 signaling impair stem cell renewal and tissue regeneration.

5.7 Altered Intercellular Communication

Hormonal imbalance contributes to chronic inflammation ("inflammaging") and disrupted cellular signaling.

5.8 Deregulated Nutrient Sensing

This hallmark is directly mediated by endocrine pathways, including insulin, IGF-1, and mTOR signaling.

6. Circadian Rhythms and Hormonal Aging

Hormone secretion follows daily rhythms controlled by the biological clock. Aging disrupts these rhythms, leading to:

- Irregular cortisol cycles
- Reduced melatonin secretion
- Altered feeding and metabolic patterns

Circadian disruption contributes to metabolic disease, cognitive decline, and reduced physiological resilience.

7. Clinical Implications of Hormonal Aging

Hormonal dysregulation is associated with several age-related conditions:

- Type 2 diabetes
- Obesity and metabolic syndrome
- Sarcopenia (muscle loss)
- Osteoporosis
- Sleep disorders
- Cognitive decline

Understanding endocrine changes is essential for addressing these conditions at a systemic level.

8. Interventions Targeting Hormonal Pathways

While this book focuses on biological understanding rather than treatment, it is important to note that hormonal pathways are modifiable.

Research highlights include:

- Caloric restriction and fasting → improve insulin sensitivity
- Physical activity → supports hormonal balance
- Sleep optimization → restores circadian rhythms
- Pharmacological agents targeting mTOR and AMPK pathways

These approaches aim to restore balance rather than simply increase hormone levels.

9. Integrative Perspective: Hormones as System Coordinators

Hormones function as integrators across biological systems. They:

- Coordinate metabolism with cellular repair
- Link environmental signals with gene expression
- Regulate communication between tissues

Thus, endocrine aging reflects a loss of systemic coordination rather than isolated dysfunction.

10. Conclusion

Aging is a multidimensional process shaped by interconnected biological mechanisms. Hormonal dysregulation plays a central role in this network by influencing metabolism, gene regulation, stress responses, and cellular communication.

Rather than constituting a separate hallmark, endocrine changes act as a unifying layer that connects and amplifies existing hallmarks of aging.

A comprehensive understanding of aging therefore requires integrating endocrine biology with molecular and cellular frameworks.

🌟 **Key Concept**

Hormones are not a separate hallmark of aging—they are the dynamic signals that coordinate and connect all hallmarks across the body.

👉 *"Hormones act as master regulators that connect and amplify all hallmarks of aging through systemic signaling networks."*

🌿 2. STORYBOOK VERSION

"The Messengers of Cell City"

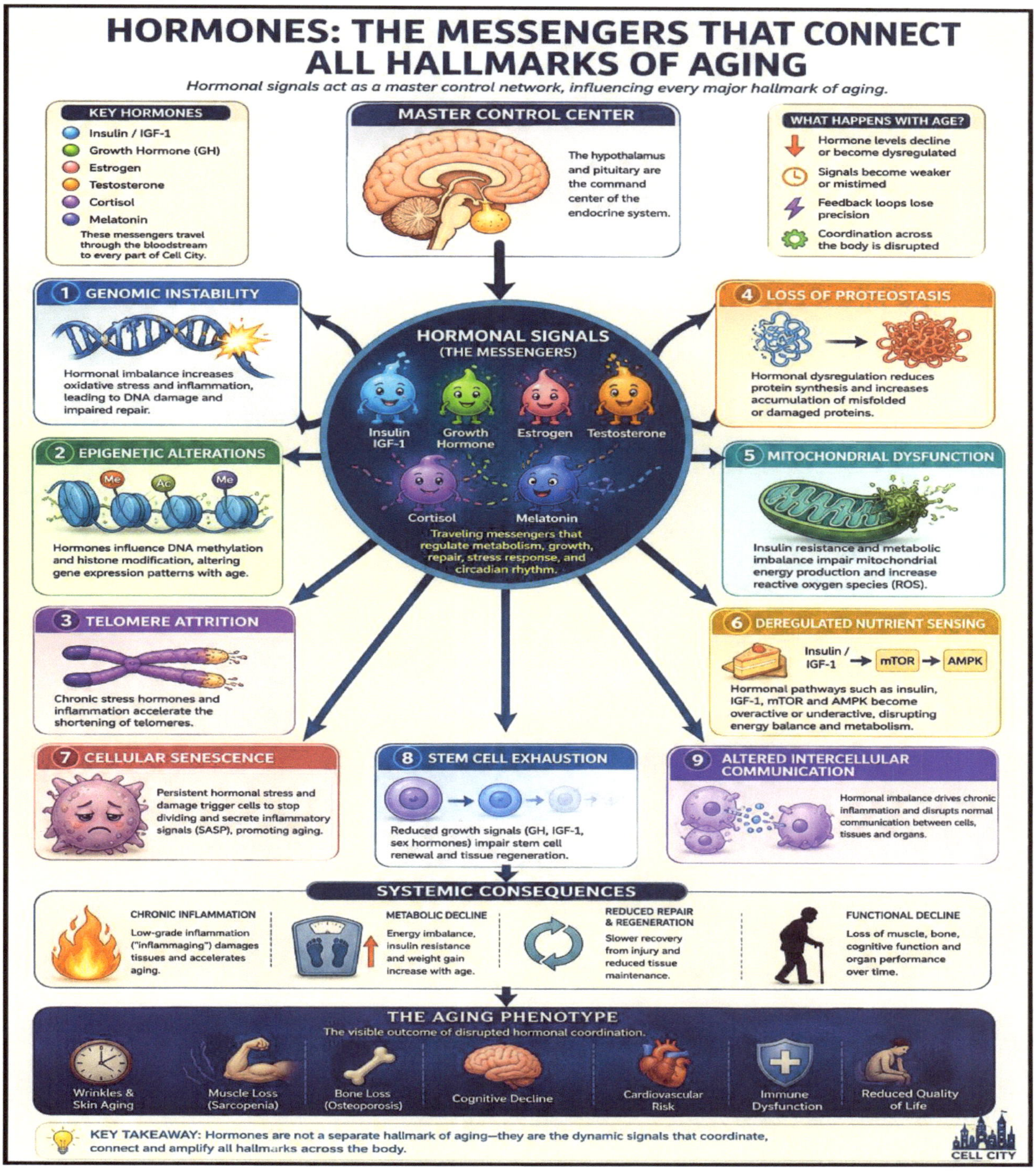

🌆 The City with Invisible Messengers

Inside your body lies a vast and magical place called **Cell City**.

Every building in this city is a cell.
Every cell is busy working—building, repairing, and keeping the city alive.

But something very important keeps everything in order…

👉 **Messages.**

📡 The Messengers of the City

In Cell City, there are special messengers called **hormones**.

They travel everywhere:

- From the brain
- To the muscles
- To the heart
- To every tiny corner of the city

Think of them like:

- Letters 📩
- Phone calls 📞
- Or even WhatsApp messages 📱

They carry instructions like:

- "Grow!"
- "Repair!"
- "Save energy!"
- "Wake up!"
- "Fight danger!"

When the city is young, these messages are:
✅ Clear
✅ Timely
✅ Perfect

Everything runs smoothly.

⏳ What Happens as Time Passes?

As the city ages, something begins to change.

The messengers start making mistakes.

Sometimes:

- Messages arrive late
- Messages are too strong
- Messages are too weak
- Or the wrong message is delivered

It's like:
👉 Getting a "Work!" message when you should be resting
👉 Or a "Grow!" message when repair is needed

This confusion spreads across the city.

🔗 How the Confusion Spreads

Because of wrong messages:

🏛 The Library (DNA) starts getting damaged
→ **Genomic instability**

📚 The Librarian gets confused
→ **Epigenetic alterations**

🧵 The shoelace tips shrink faster
→ **Telomere attrition**

🏭 Factories produce broken machines
→ **Loss of proteostasis**

⚡ Power plants lose energy
→ **Mitochondrial dysfunction**

📡 Control tower keeps shouting "Grow!"
→ **Deregulated nutrient sensing**

👴 Workers stop working
→ **Cellular senescence**

👷 Builders get tired
→ **Stem cell exhaustion**

🔥 Small fires never stop
→ **Chronic inflammation**

🌪 The Big Problem

The problem is not just one mistake.

👉 It's that **all parts of the city are connected**

When messages are wrong:

- Energy drops
- Repairs slow down
- Damage increases

The entire city begins to struggle.

🌟 The Hidden Truth

Here's the most important thing:

👉 The city is not broken.
👉 The instructions are still there.

The real issue is:

The messages are no longer clear.

🔄 A New Hope

Scientists are now asking:

- Can we improve these messages?
- Can we restore balance?
- Can the city communicate properly again?

If yes…

👉 The city may not just age…
👉 It may regain its strength.

🧠 Summary

"Hormones are the messengers of the body—and aging begins when their messages become unclear."

Hormones act as a master communication network linking all hallmarks of aging. Dysregulation of hormonal signals disrupts metabolism, gene regulation, repair systems, and intercellular communication, ultimately driving systemic aging.

In the previous chapter, we saw how the **Control Tower** inside Cell City began sending confusing signals about growth and repair.

But here's something even more important…

👉 The Control Tower does not work alone.

It sends its instructions across the entire city using special messengers.

📡 The Messengers Arrive

These messengers are called **hormones**.

They travel through invisible highways, carrying instructions from one part of the city to another.

They tell cells:

- When to grow
- When to rest
- When to repair
- When to fight danger

When the city is young, these messages are:
✔️ Clear
✔️ Timely
✔️ Perfectly balanced

⏳ When Messages Go Wrong

But as time passes…

The messaging system begins to fail.

- Some messages become too weak
- Some arrive too late
- Some are sent at the wrong time

And slowly…

👉 The entire city begins to lose coordination.

Because:

- Hormones → regulate metabolism → affect mitochondria
- Hormones → influence gene expression → affect epigenetics
- Hormones → control inflammation → affect intercellular communication
- Hormones → regulate stem cells → affect regeneration

👉 So hormones act like a **"master control network"**

This picture shows something very important:

👉 Hormones are not just one part of the system
👉 They connect **every part of the city**

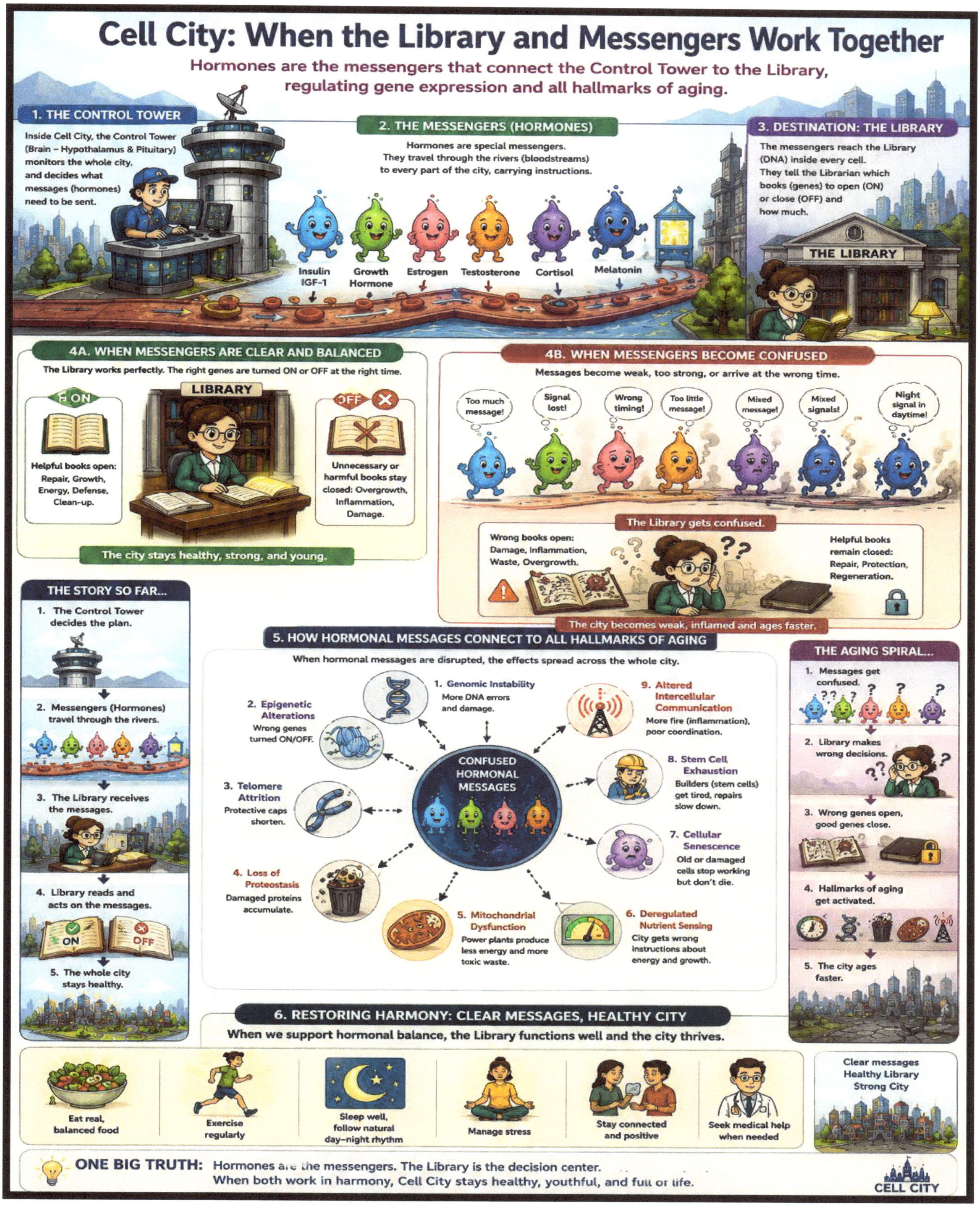
Cell City: When the Library and Messengers Work Together
Hormones are the messengers that connect the Control Tower to the Library, regulating gene expression and all hallmarks of aging.
1. THE CONTROL TOWER
Inside Cell City, the Control Tower (Brain – Hypothalamus & Pituitary) monitors the whole city, and decides what messages (hormones) need to be sent.
2. THE MESSENGERS (HORMONES)
Hormones are special messengers. They travel through the rivers (bloodstreams) to every part of the city, carrying instructions.
Insulin IGF-1
Growth Hormone
Estrogen
Testosterone
Cortisol
Melatonin
3. DESTINATION: THE LIBRARY
The messengers reach the Library (DNA) inside every cell. They tell the Librarian which books (genes) to open (ON) or close (OFF) and how much.
THE LIBRARY
4A. WHEN MESSENGERS ARE CLEAR AND BALANCED
The Library works perfectly. The right genes are turned ON or OFF at the right time.
ON
LIBRARY
OFF
Helpful books open: Repair, Growth, Energy, Defense, Clean-up.
Unnecessary or harmful books stay closed: Overgrowth, Inflammation, Damage.
The city stays healthy, strong, and young.
4B. WHEN MESSENGERS BECOME CONFUSED
Messages become weak, too strong, or arrive at the wrong time.
Too much message!
Signal lost!
Wrong timing!
Too little message!
Mixed message!
Mixed signals!
Night signal in daytime!
The Library gets confused.
Wrong books open: Damage, Inflammation, Waste, Overgrowth.
Helpful books remain closed: Repair, Protection, Regeneration.
The city becomes weak, inflamed and ages faster.
THE STORY SO FAR...
1. The Control Tower decides the plan.
2. Messengers (Hormones) travel through the rivers.
3. The Library receives the messages.
4. Library reads and acts on the messages.
ON
OFF
5. The whole city stays healthy.
5. HOW HORMONAL MESSAGES CONNECT TO ALL HALLMARKS OF AGING
When hormonal messages are disrupted, the effects spread across the whole city.
CONFUSED HORMONAL MESSAGES
1. Genomic Instability
More DNA errors and damage.
2. Epigenetic Alterations
Wrong genes turned ON/OFF.
3. Telomere Attrition
Protective caps shorten.
4. Loss of Proteostasis
Damaged proteins accumulate.
5. Mitochondrial Dysfunction
Power plants produce less energy and more toxic waste.
6. Deregulated Nutrient Sensing
City gets wrong instructions about energy and growth.
7. Cellular Senescence
Old or damaged cells stop working but don't die.
8. Stem Cell Exhaustion
Builders (stem cells) get tired, repairs slow down.
9. Altered Intercellular Communication
More fire (inflammation), poor coordination.
THE AGING SPIRAL...
1. Messages get confused.
2. Library makes wrong decisions.
3. Wrong genes open, good genes close.
4. Hallmarks of aging get activated.
5. The city ages faster.
6. RESTORING HARMONY: CLEAR MESSAGES, HEALTHY CITY
When we support hormonal balance, the Library functions well and the city thrives.
Eat real, balanced food
Exercise regularly
Sleep well, follow natural day–night rhythm
Manage stress
Stay connected and positive
Seek medical help when needed
Clear messages
Healthy Library
Strong City
ONE BIG TRUTH: Hormones are the messengers. The Library is the decision center.
When both work in harmony, Cell City stays healthy, youthful, and full of life.
CELL CITY

When the messengers fail:

- The library gets damaged
- The power plants lose energy
- The factories produce faulty machines
- The workers stop working
- The fires never stop burning

Everything becomes connected in a cycle of decline.

🔗 **The Domino Effect**

Think of it like this:

If one message is wrong…

It doesn't stay in one place.

It spreads.

- A wrong metabolic signal → increases stress
- Stress → damages DNA
- DNA damage → confuses the librarian
- Confusion → creates more problems

👉 **This is how aging spreads through the city.**

🌟 **The Big Insight**

Before this chapter, you may have thought:

👉 **"Each problem happens separately"**

But now you can see:

👉 **Everything is connected through messages**

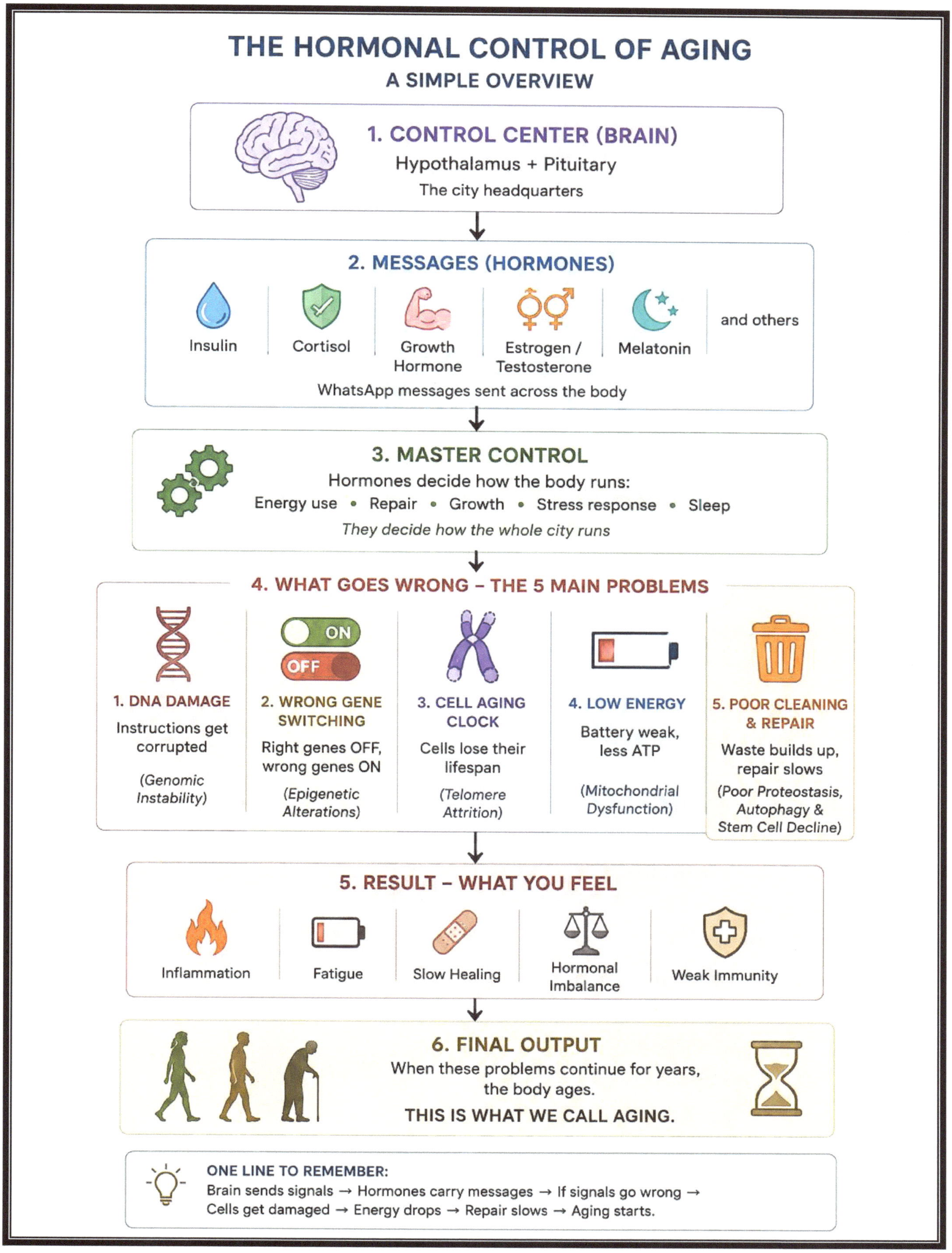
THE HORMONAL CONTROL OF AGING
A SIMPLE OVERVIEW
1. CONTROL CENTER (BRAIN)
Hypothalamus + Pituitary
The city headquarters
2. MESSAGES (HORMONES)
Insulin
Cortisol
Growth Hormone
Estrogen / Testosterone
Melatonin
and others
WhatsApp messages sent across the body
3. MASTER CONTROL
Hormones decide how the body runs:
Energy use • Repair • Growth • Stress response • Sleep
They decide how the whole city runs
4. WHAT GOES WRONG – THE 5 MAIN PROBLEMS
ON
OFF
1. DNA DAMAGE
Instructions get corrupted
(Genomic Instability)
2. WRONG GENE SWITCHING
Right genes OFF, wrong genes ON
(Epigenetic Alterations)
3. CELL AGING CLOCK
Cells lose their lifespan
(Telomere Attrition)
4. LOW ENERGY
Battery weak, less ATP
(Mitochondrial Dysfunction)
5. POOR CLEANING & REPAIR
Waste builds up, repair slows
(Poor Proteostasis, Autophagy & Stem Cell Decline)
5. RESULT – WHAT YOU FEEL
Inflammation
Fatigue
Slow Healing
Hormonal Imbalance
Weak Immunity
6. FINAL OUTPUT
When these problems continue for years, the body ages.
THIS IS WHAT WE CALL AGING.
ONE LINE TO REMEMBER:
Brain sends signals → Hormones carry messages → If signals go wrong →
Cells get damaged → Energy drops → Repair slows → Aging starts.

📚 Scientific References

Hormones and the Hallmarks of Aging

🧬 1. Core Hallmarks of Aging

https://www.cell.com/fulltext/S0092-8674(13)00645-4

https://www.cell.com/cell/fulltext/S0092-8674(23)00181-2

🧠 2. Hormones & Endocrine Aging

https://www.nature.com/articles/nrendo.2016.139

https://academic.oup.com/edrv/article/26/5/610/2355184

https://www.frontiersin.org/articles/10.3389/fendo.2019.00286/full

⚡ 3. Insulin/IGF-1 Pathway

https://www.nature.com/articles/nature05982

https://www.cell.com/cell-metabolism/fulltext/S1550-4131(13)00315-8

🔥 4. mTOR & AMPK Signaling

https://www.cell.com/fulltext/S0092-8674(11)00131-7

https://www.nature.com/articles/nrm3311

🧬 5. Epigenetics & Aging

https://www.nature.com/articles/nrg3604

https://genomebiology.biomedcentral.com/articles/10.1186/gb-2013-14-10-r115

🔋 6. Mitochondria & Oxidative Stress

https://www.cell.com/fulltext/S0092-8674(18)30386-9

https://www.ncbi.nlm.nih.gov/pmc/articles/PMC3156579/

🔬 7. Cellular Senescence

https://www.nature.com/articles/s41580-019-0124-5

https://www.annualreviews.org/doi/10.1146/annurev-pathol-020712-163927

🧪 8. Sex Hormones & Aging

https://www.nature.com/articles/nrendo.2015.6

https://www.nejm.org/doi/full/10.1056/NEJMoa1506119

🌙 9. Melatonin & Circadian Biology

https://www.sciencedirect.com/science/article/pii/S1568163716300785

https://www.nature.com/articles/nrn.2016.93

💻 10. Systems Biology & Databases

https://www.nature.com/articles/nrg.2017.62

https://genomics.senescence.info/genes/

https://www.nia.nih.gov/

Lifestyle, Diet, and Epigenetic Regulation of Aging: From Nutrients to Gene Expression

1. Introduction: Beyond "Good vs Bad Genes"

Aging is influenced not only by genetics but by how genes are regulated over time. Environmental exposures—including diet, toxins, and stress—modify gene expression through:

- DNA methylation
- Histone modification
- Non-coding RNAs

These epigenetic changes can:

- Suppress protective pathways
- Activate harmful signaling
- Accelerate biological aging

2. Processed Food, Sugar, and Fast Food

What happens biologically:

Highly processed diets rich in refined sugars, trans fats, and additives lead to:

- Chronic activation of mTOR signaling pathway
- Suppression of AMPK pathway
- Increased oxidative stress

Epigenetic effects:

- Increased DNA methylation of metabolic genes
- Activation of inflammatory gene networks

Key genes/pathways affected:

- INSR/IGF1 → insulin resistance
- SIRT1 → reduced longevity signaling
- **NF-κB → chronic inflammation (turned ON)**

3. Excess Fat, Oil, and Lipid Toxicity

Not all fats are equal. Excess saturated and trans fats:

- Promote mitochondrial dysfunction
- Increase lipid peroxidation

Gene-level effects:

- Upregulation of inflammatory genes (TNF-α, IL-6)
- Downregulation of mitochondrial genes (PGC-1α)

4. Carbohydrates and Glycation

High refined carbohydrate intake leads to:

- Formation of advanced glycation end products

Effects:

- DNA damage
- Protein crosslinking
- Epigenetic dysregulation

Genes impacted:

- RAGE receptor gene → inflammation
- FOXO genes → suppressed stress resistance

🧬 5. Protein Intake and Aging

- Moderate protein supports repair
- Excess protein → mTOR overactivation

Gene effects:

- Increased growth signaling
- Reduced autophagy genes (e.g., ATG family)

🧪 6. Microplastics and Environmental Toxins

Emerging evidence shows that microplastics and pollutants:

- Act as endocrine disruptors
- Generate oxidative stress

Epigenetic impact:

- Alter DNA methylation patterns
- Disrupt hormone-regulated gene expression

Affected pathways:

- Estrogen receptor signaling
- Stress-response genes

😰 7. Psychological Stress and Hormonal Aging

Chronic stress elevates cortisol hormone regulation, leading to:

- Telomere shortening
- Epigenetic drift

Genes impacted:

- TP53 (DNA repair)
- NR3C1 (glucocorticoid receptor)
- Inflammatory genes (IL-6, CRP)

🧬 8. Do These Factors Cause Mutations?

Important distinction:

✔️ YES:

- Oxidative stress → DNA damage
- Toxins → mutations (limited but real)

❌ BUT:

Most lifestyle effects act through:
👉 Epigenetic regulation, not permanent mutation

⚖️ 9. "Good" vs "Bad" Genes — Correct Scientific Framing

Instead of "good vs bad genes," use:

🟢 Protective Pathways (often suppressed with aging):

- Sirtuins (SIRT1) → longevity
- FOXO transcription factors → stress resistance
- Autophagy genes (ATG) → cellular cleanup

🟠 **Harmful Pathways (often activated):**

- NF-κB → inflammation
- mTOR → excessive growth signaling
- p16INK4a → cellular senescence

🔗 10. Link to Hallmarks of Aging

These lifestyle-driven changes connect directly to:

- Genomic instability
- Epigenetic alterations
- Loss of proteostasis
- Mitochondrial dysfunction
- Cellular senescence
- Chronic inflammation

👉 So yes, this chapter fits perfectly within the hallmark's framework

🌿 11. Positive Modifiers (Reversal Potential)

Lifestyle can also improve gene regulation:

- Caloric restriction → activates AMPK & SIRT1
- Exercise → improves mitochondrial genes
- Polyphenols (resveratrol) → epigenetic modulation
- Sleep → restores circadian gene expression

🧠 12. Conclusion

Aging is not dictated solely by genetic code but by how that code is read and regulated. Diet, environment, and lifestyle do not create "bad genes," but they can shift gene expression toward harmful or protective states through epigenetic mechanisms.

Understanding this dynamic regulation provides a powerful framework for interventions aimed at extending health span and delaying aging-related decline.

📊 **Table: Food → Epigenetic Effect → Genes/Pathways → Hallmarks of Aging**

Factor (Food/Lifestyle)	Epigenetic/Molecular Effect	Key Genes/Pathways Affected	Linked Hallmarks of Aging
Processed Food/Fast Food	**DNA methylation changes, ↑ inflammation**	**NF-κB ↑, SIRT1 ↓, AMPK ↓**	**Inflammation, Epigenetic alterations, Proteostasis loss**
Refined Sugar	**Glycation, oxidative stress**	**FOXO ↓, RAGE ↑, Insulin/IGF ↑**	**Genomic instability, Mitochondrial dysfunction**
Trans Fats/Excess Oils	**Lipid peroxidation, mitochondrial stress**	**PGC-1α ↓, TNF-α ↑**	**Mitochondrial dysfunction, Inflammation**

Factor (Food/Lifestyle)	Epigenetic/Molecular Effect	Key Genes/Pathways Affected	Linked Hallmarks of Aging
Excess Carbohydrates	↑ AGEs formation, insulin resistance	mTOR ↑, IGF-1 ↑	Deregulated nutrient sensing, Cellular senescence
Excess Protein (chronic high intake)	mTOR overactivation, ↓ autophagy	mTOR ↑, ATG genes ↓	Loss of proteostasis, Reduced autophagy
Ultra-processed foods (additives)	Epigenetic dysregulation	Histone modification changes	Epigenetic alterations
Microplastics/Toxins	DNA damage, endocrine disruption	Estrogen receptor disruption, oxidative genes ↑	Genomic instability, Hormonal dysregulation
Chronic Stress	Epigenetic drift, cortisol imbalance	NR3C1 ↓, TP53 ↓, IL-6 ↑	Telomere attrition, Inflammation
Sleep Deprivation	Circadian gene disruption	CLOCK genes ↓, SIRT1 ↓	Metabolic dysfunction, Epigenetic alterations
Sedentary Lifestyle	↓ mitochondrial biogenesis	AMPK ↓, PGC-1α ↓	Mitochondrial dysfunction, Stem cell exhaustion

🧠 **Interpretation**

👉 **Lifestyle does not create "bad genes," but shifts gene expression patterns**

👉 **Protective pathways ↓ and damage pathways ↑ → Aging accelerates**

🌿 📖 Storybook Version: Cell City – Junk Food vs Clean Food

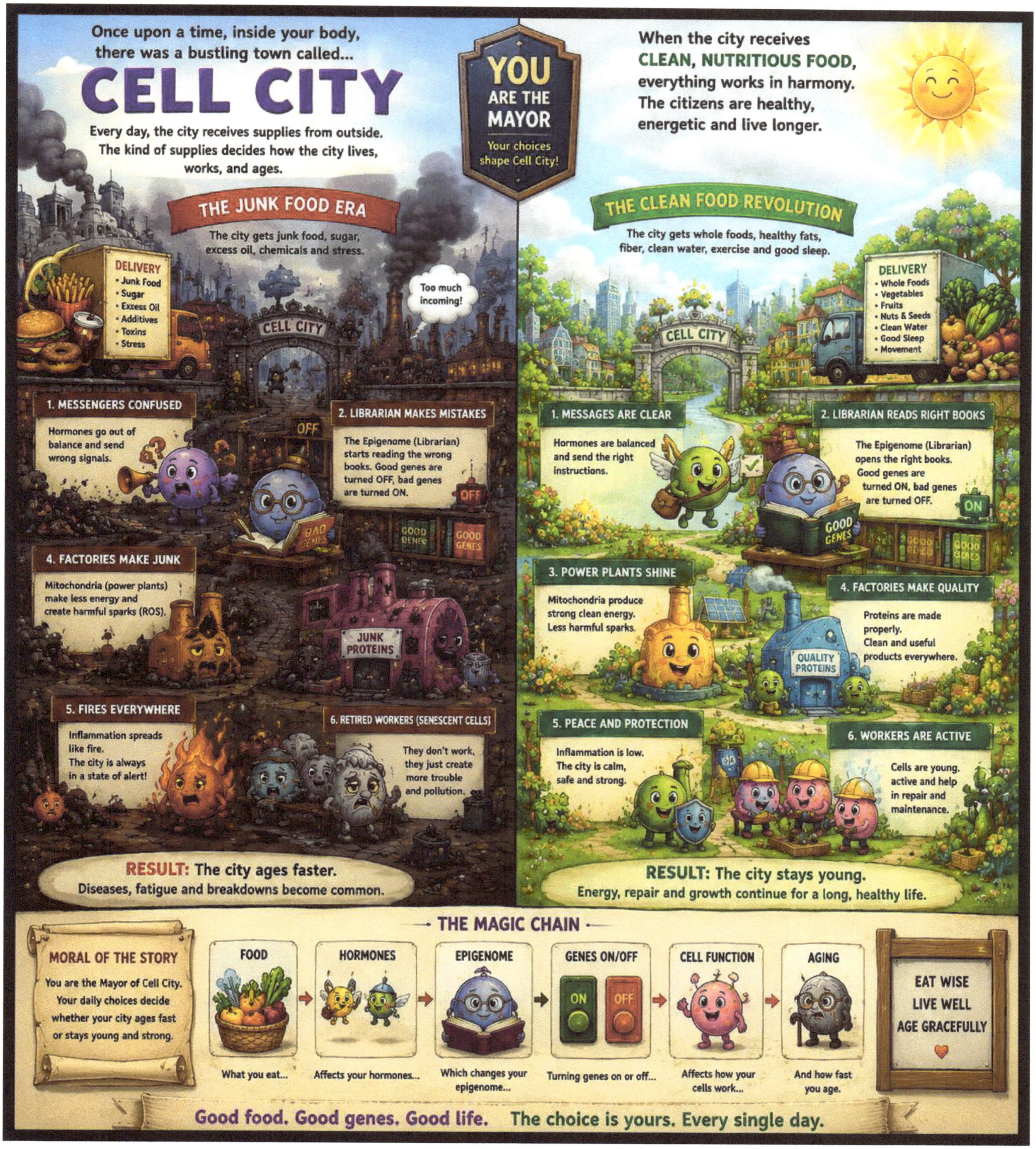

🌆 The Two Kinds of Fuel

In the great Cell City, everything depended on fuel.

The city had:

- 🏛️ A Library (DNA)
- 🧑‍🏫 A Librarian (Epigenome)

- 🏭 Factories (Proteins)
- ⚡ Power Plants (Mitochondria)
- 📡 Messengers (Hormones)

But there was one more thing…

👉 The Food Supply.

🍔 The Junk Food Era

One day, the city began receiving a new type of fuel:

- Fast food
- Sugary drinks
- Processed snacks

At first, nothing seemed wrong.

But slowly…

📡 **The Messengers Got Confused**

They started shouting:
👉 **"Grow! Grow! Grow!"**

Even when the city needed repair.

🏛️ **The Librarian Made Mistakes**

The epigenome began:

- Opening the wrong books
- Ignoring repair instructions

👉 **Important genes were turned OFF**
👉 **Harmful signals were turned ON**

⚡ **The Power Plants Started Failing**

Mitochondria began:

- Producing less energy
- Releasing harmful sparks (ROS)

The city lights dimmed.

🏭 **The Factories Produced Junk**

Proteins were:

- Misfolded
- Damaged

Trash piled up.

🔥 **Fires Broke Out Everywhere**

Inflammation spread like uncontrolled fire.

The city was always slightly burning.

🧓 **Workers Stopped Working**

Some workers became:
👉 **Senescent cells**

They didn't work…
They only complained.

🥗 The Clean Food Revolution

Then something changed.

The city started receiving better fuel:

- Fresh vegetables
- Balanced nutrients
- Clean water
- Proper rest

📡 Messages Became Clear Again

Hormones started saying:
👉 **"Repair. Restore. Clean."**

👩‍🏫 The Librarian Refocused

The epigenome:

- Opened the right books
- Activated repair genes

⚡ Power Plants Recovered

Mitochondria:

- Produced strong energy
- Reduced harmful sparks

🧹 The Cleaning Crew Returned

Autophagy restarted:

- Damaged parts removed
- New structures built

🌱 The Builders Came Back

Stem cells:

- Repaired tissues
- Restored the city

🌟 The Big Lesson

The city realized something powerful:

👉 It was not just the buildings (DNA)
👉 It was how the city was being run

And that depended on:

- Food
- Environment
- Stress
- Lifestyle

🧠 Summary

"Your genes are the blueprint—but your lifestyle decides how the blueprint is read."

🏙️ Cell City: How Food, Hormones, and the Epigenome Control Aging

🧭 1. The Big Idea: Aging is a Connected System

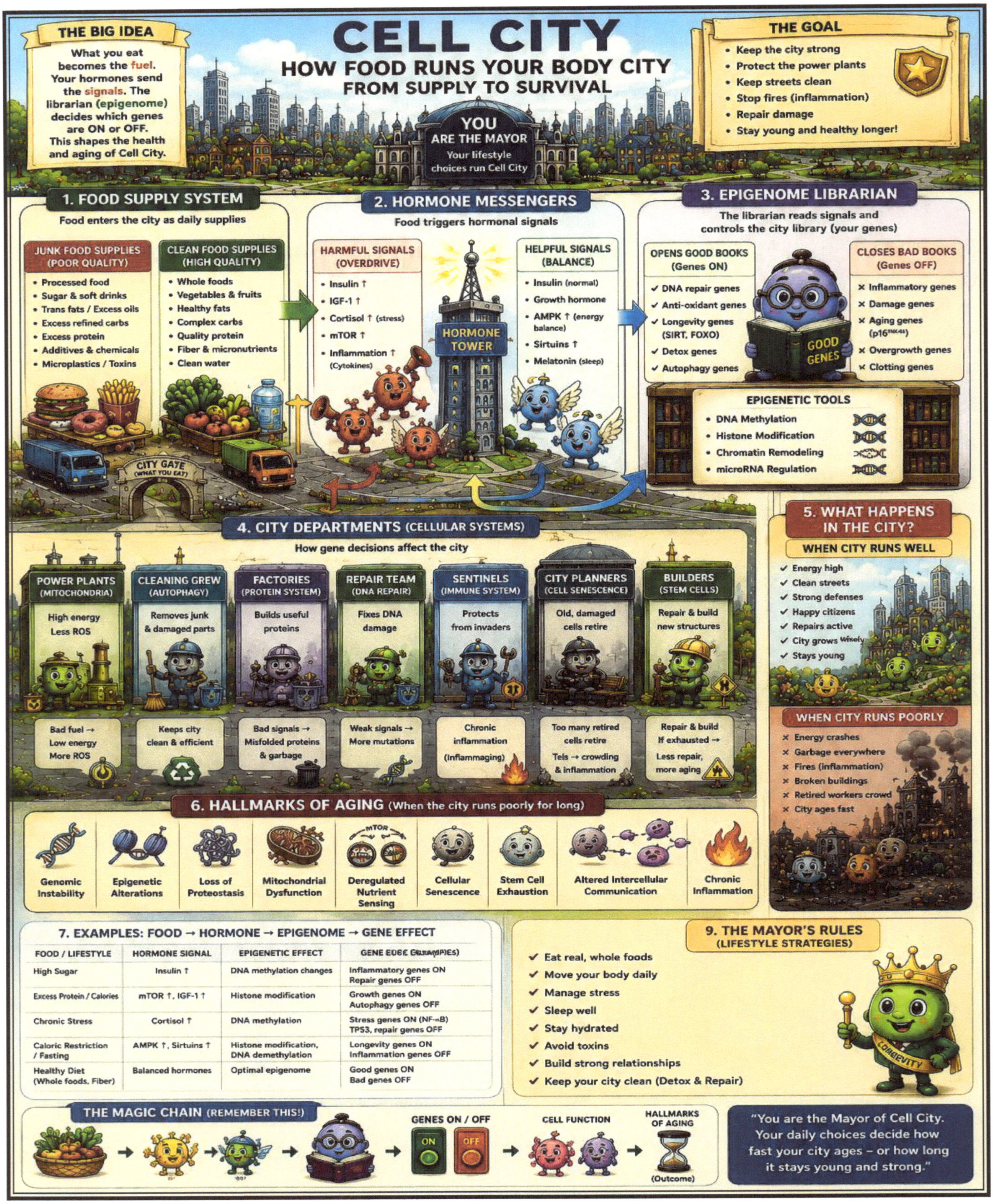

CELL CITY
HOW FOOD RUNS YOUR BODY CITY
FROM SUPPLY TO SURVIVAL
THE BIG IDEA
What you eat becomes the fuel. Your hormones send the signals. The librarian (epigenome) decides which genes are ON or OFF. This shapes the health and aging of Cell City.
YOU ARE THE MAYOR
Your lifestyle choices run Cell City
THE GOAL
• Keep the city strong
• Protect the power plants
• Keep streets clean
• Stop fires (inflammation)
• Repair damage
• Stay young and healthy longer!
1. FOOD SUPPLY SYSTEM
Food enters the city as daily supplies
JUNK FOOD SUPPLIES (POOR QUALITY)
• Processed food
• Sugar & soft drinks
• Trans fats / Excess oils
• Excess refined carbs
• Excess protein
• Additives & chemicals
• Microplastics / Toxins
CLEAN FOOD SUPPLIES (HIGH QUALITY)
• Whole foods
• Vegetables & fruits
• Healthy fats
• Complex carbs
• Quality protein
• Fiber & micronutrients
• Clean water
CITY GATE (WHAT YOU EAT)
2. HORMONE MESSENGERS
Food triggers hormonal signals
HARMFUL SIGNALS (OVERDRIVE)
• Insulin ↑
• IGF-1 ↑
• Cortisol ↑ (stress)
• mTOR ↑
• Inflammation ↑ (Cytokines)
HORMONE TOWER
HELPFUL SIGNALS (BALANCE)
• Insulin (normal)
• Growth hormone
• AMPK ↑ (energy balance)
• Sirtuins ↑
• Melatonin (sleep)
3. EPIGENOME LIBRARIAN
The librarian reads signals and controls the city library (your genes)
OPENS GOOD BOOKS (Genes ON)
✓ DNA repair genes
✓ Anti-oxidant genes
✓ Longevity genes (SIRT, FOXO)
✓ Detox genes
✓ Autophagy genes
GOOD GENES
CLOSES BAD BOOKS (Genes OFF)
× Inflammatory genes
× Damage genes
× Aging genes (p16INK4a)
× Overgrowth genes
× Clotting genes
EPIGENETIC TOOLS
• DNA Methylation
• Histone Modification
• Chromatin Remodeling
• microRNA Regulation
4. CITY DEPARTMENTS (CELLULAR SYSTEMS)
How gene decisions affect the city
POWER PLANTS (MITOCHONDRIA)
High energy Less ROS
Bad fuel → Low energy More ROS
CLEANING CREW (AUTOPHAGY)
Removes junk & damaged parts
Keeps city clean & efficient
FACTORIES (PROTEIN SYSTEM)
Builds useful proteins
Bad signals → Misfolded proteins & garbage
REPAIR TEAM (DNA REPAIR)
Fixes DNA damage
Weak signals → More mutations
SENTINELS (IMMUNE SYSTEM)
Protects from invaders
Chronic inflammation (Inflammaging)
CITY PLANNERS (CELL SENESCENCE)
Old, damaged cells retire
Too many retired cells retire
Tels → crowding & inflammation
BUILDERS (STEM CELLS)
Repair & build new structures
Repair & build If exhausted → Less repair, more aging
5. WHAT HAPPENS IN THE CITY?
WHEN CITY RUNS WELL
✓ Energy high
✓ Clean streets
✓ Strong defenses
✓ Happy citizens
✓ Repairs active
✓ City grows wisely
✓ Stays young
WHEN CITY RUNS POORLY
× Energy crashes
× Garbage everywhere
× Fires (inflammation)
× Broken buildings
× Retired workers crowd
× City ages fast
6. HALLMARKS OF AGING (When the city runs poorly for long)
Genomic Instability
Epigenetic Alterations
Loss of Proteostasis
Mitochondrial Dysfunction
Deregulated Nutrient Sensing
Cellular Senescence
Stem Cell Exhaustion
Altered Intercellular Communication
Chronic Inflammation
7. EXAMPLES: FOOD → HORMONE → EPIGENOME → GENE EFFECT
FOOD / LIFESTYLE | HORMONE SIGNAL | EPIGENETIC EFFECT | GENE EFFECT (EXAMPLES)
High Sugar | Insulin ↑ | DNA methylation changes | Inflammatory genes ON Repair genes OFF
Excess Protein / Calories | mTOR ↑, IGF-1 ↑ | Histone modification | Growth genes ON Autophagy genes OFF
Chronic Stress | Cortisol ↑ | DNA methylation | Stress genes ON (NF-κB) TP53, repair genes OFF
Caloric Restriction / Fasting | AMPK ↑, Sirtuins ↑ | Histone modification, DNA demethylation | Longevity genes ON Inflammation genes OFF
Healthy Diet (Whole foods, Fiber) | Balanced hormones | Optimal epigenome | Good genes ON Bad genes OFF
9. THE MAYOR'S RULES (LIFESTYLE STRATEGIES)
✓ Eat real, whole foods
✓ Move your body daily
✓ Manage stress
✓ Sleep well
✓ Stay hydrated
✓ Avoid toxins
✓ Build strong relationships
✓ Keep your city clean (Detox & Repair)
LONGEVITY
THE MAGIC CHAIN (REMEMBER THIS!)
GENES ON / OFF
ON
OFF
CELL FUNCTION
HALLMARKS OF AGING
(Outcome)
"You are the Mayor of Cell City. Your daily choices decide how fast your city ages – or how long it stays young and strong."

Diagram beautifully captures a key concept:

👉 Aging is not caused by one factor

👉 It is a network process driven by:

Food → Hormones → Epigenome → Cellular Function → Hallmarks of Aging

Think of it as a control chain inside your body, where each level influences the next.

2. The Supply System: Food Enters the City

In *Cell City*, food is the supply system.

Two types of supply:

Clean Fuel (Healthy Inputs)

- Whole foods, fiber, omega-3 fats
- Vitamins, antioxidants
- Balanced proteins and carbs

Effects:

- **Stable metabolism**
- **Low inflammation**
- **Efficient repair systems**

Toxic Supply (Unhealthy Inputs)

- Processed food, sugar, trans fats
- Microplastics, toxins, alcohol excess

Effects:

- Oxidative stress
- Inflammation
- Metabolic overload

3. Hormones: The Messengers of the City

After food enters, the hormonal system acts like communication signals.

Key Hormones in Your Diagram:

- Insulin/IGF-1 → nutrient sensing
- Cortisol → stress signal
- Growth hormone → repair & regeneration
- Estrogen/Testosterone → tissue maintenance
- Melatonin → circadian rhythm

These hormones tell the city:

- "Grow" (mTOR activation)
- "Repair" (AMPK activation)
- "Store energy"
- "Fight stress"

! What Happens with Bad Inputs?

Unhealthy food + stress leads to:

- Chronic high insulin
- Elevated cortisol
- Reduced repair signals

Result: Hormonal imbalance

🛂 4. The Epigenome: The Librarian of the City

This is the core control system.

- DNA = Library (instructions)
- Epigenome = Librarian (decision maker)

👉 **Hormones directly influence the epigenome:**

- DNA methylation
- Histone modification
- Chromatin remodelling

🧠 **Key Concept:**

The epigenome decides:

- Which genes turn ON
- Which genes turn OFF
- When and how strongly

⚠️ **Under Stress & Poor Diet:**

The librarian becomes confused:

- Good genes → turned OFF
- Harmful pathways → turned ON

👉 **This is epigenetic dysregulation**

🔬 5. From Epigenome to Hallmarks of Aging

Once gene control is disturbed, it affects all hallmarks of aging:

🧬 **Genomic Instability**

- ROS damages DNA
- Poor repair due to faulty signaling

🧵 **Telomere Attrition**

- Chronic stress hormones shorten telomeres

🧪 **Epigenetic Alterations**

- Direct result of environmental + hormonal signals

🧹 **Loss of Proteostasis**

- Misfolded proteins accumulate
- Poor cleanup systems

🔋 **Mitochondrial Dysfunction**

- Energy drops
- ROS increases → vicious cycle

🍽️ **Deregulated Nutrient Sensing**

- mTOR overactive (growth mode always ON)
- AMPK suppressed (repair mode OFF)

👴 **Cellular Senescence**

- Cells stop dividing
- Release inflammatory signals (SASP)

Stem Cell Exhaustion

- Reduced regeneration capacity

🔥 **Chronic Inflammation (Inflammaging)**

- Persistent low-grade inflammation

🧠 **Altered Communication**

- Cells stop "talking" properly

🔄 6. The Vicious Cycle

Diagram also shows an important loop:

👉 **Bad food → Hormonal imbalance**
→ Epigenetic errors
→ Cellular damage
→ More inflammation
→ Further hormonal disruption

This creates a self-amplifying aging cycle

🌿 7. The Positive Loop (Reversal Possibility)

The same pathway can work in reverse:

Healthy lifestyle:

- Balanced diet
- Fasting/caloric restriction
- Exercise
- Good sleep

👉 **Leads to:**

- Better hormone signaling
- Stable epigenome
- Activation of repair genes

Result:

- Improved mitochondrial function
- Reduced inflammation
- Slower aging

🧠 8. The Core Message of the Diagram

👉 You are not just "aging" passively
👉 You are constantly programming your biology

One-Line Summary:

"Food shapes hormones, hormones guide the epigenome, and the epigenome controls how fast or slow your body ages."

9. Story Version (For Memory)

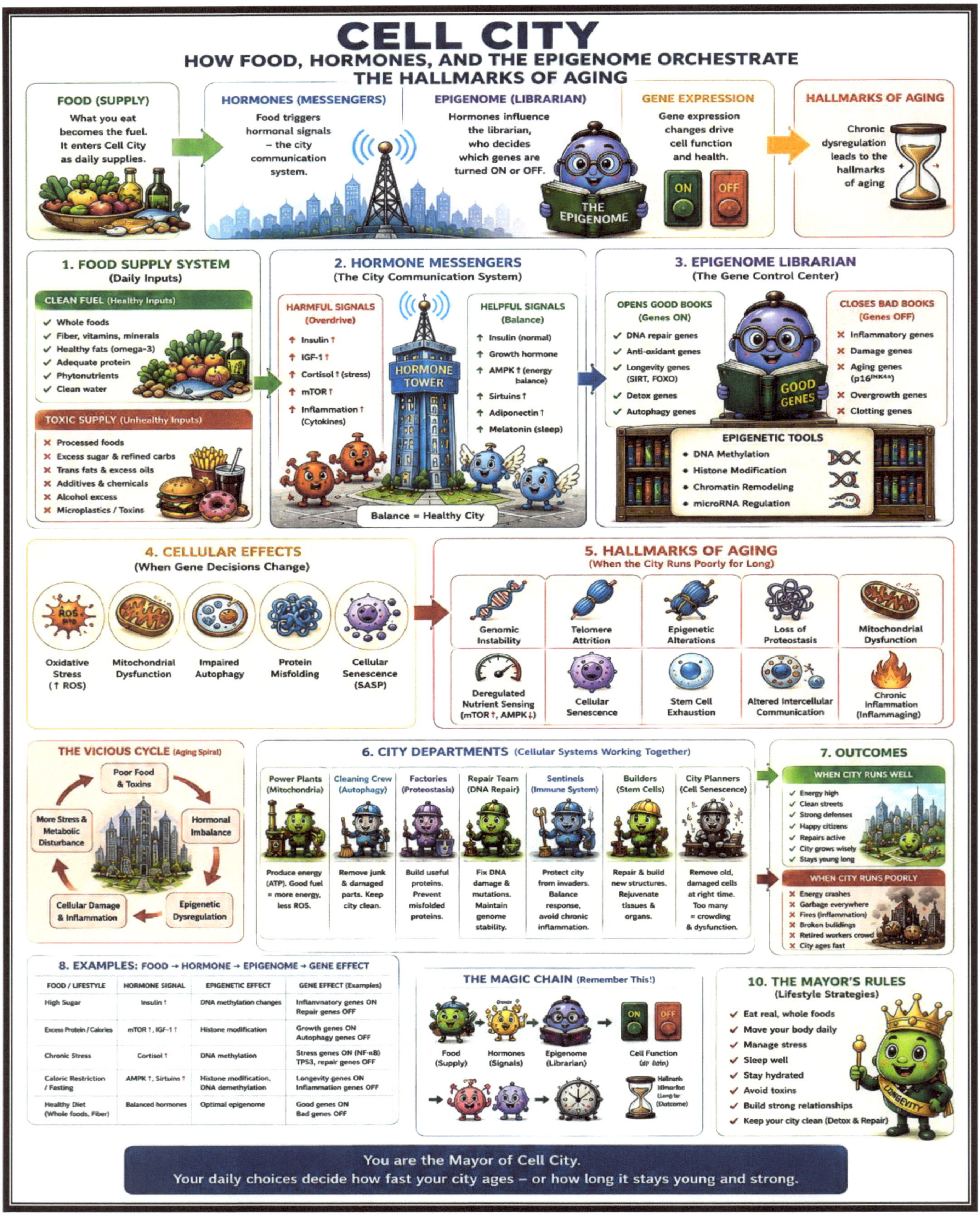
CELL CITY
HOW FOOD, HORMONES, AND THE EPIGENOME ORCHESTRATE THE HALLMARKS OF AGING
FOOD (SUPPLY)
What you eat becomes the fuel. It enters Cell City as daily supplies.
HORMONES (MESSENGERS)
Food triggers hormonal signals – the city communication system.
EPIGENOME (LIBRARIAN)
Hormones influence the librarian, who decides which genes are turned ON or OFF.
THE EPIGENOME
GENE EXPRESSION
Gene expression changes drive cell function and health.
ON
OFF
HALLMARKS OF AGING
Chronic dysregulation leads to the hallmarks of aging
1. FOOD SUPPLY SYSTEM
(Daily Inputs)
CLEAN FUEL (Healthy Inputs)
✓ Whole foods
✓ Fiber, vitamins, minerals
✓ Healthy fats (omega-3)
✓ Adequate protein
✓ Phytonutrients
✓ Clean water
TOXIC SUPPLY (Unhealthy Inputs)
✗ Processed foods
✗ Excess sugar & refined carbs
✗ Trans fats & excess oils
✗ Additives & chemicals
✗ Alcohol excess
✗ Microplastics / Toxins
2. HORMONE MESSENGERS
(The City Communication System)
HARMFUL SIGNALS (Overdrive)
↑ Insulin ↑
↑ IGF-1 ↑
↑ Cortisol ↑ (stress)
↑ mTOR ↑
↑ Inflammation ↑ (Cytokines)
HORMONE TOWER
HELPFUL SIGNALS (Balance)
↑ Insulin (normal)
↑ Growth hormone
↑ AMPK ↑ (energy balance)
↑ Sirtuins ↑
↑ Adiponectin ↑
↑ Melatonin (sleep)
Balance = Healthy City
3. EPIGENOME LIBRARIAN
(The Gene Control Center)
OPENS GOOD BOOKS (Genes ON)
✓ DNA repair genes
✓ Anti-oxidant genes
✓ Longevity genes (SIRT, FOXO)
✓ Detox genes
✓ Autophagy genes
GOOD GENES
CLOSES BAD BOOKS (Genes OFF)
✗ Inflammatory genes
✗ Damage genes
✗ Aging genes (p16INK4a)
✗ Overgrowth genes
✗ Clotting genes
EPIGENETIC TOOLS
• DNA Methylation
• Histone Modification
• Chromatin Remodeling
• microRNA Regulation
4. CELLULAR EFFECTS
(When Gene Decisions Change)
ROS
Oxidative Stress (↑ ROS)
Mitochondrial Dysfunction
Impaired Autophagy
Protein Misfolding
Cellular Senescence (SASP)
5. HALLMARKS OF AGING
(When the City Runs Poorly for Long)
Genomic Instability
Telomere Attrition
Epigenetic Alterations
Loss of Proteostasis
Mitochondrial Dysfunction
Deregulated Nutrient Sensing (mTOR ↑, AMPK ↓)
Cellular Senescence
Stem Cell Exhaustion
Altered Intercellular Communication
Chronic Inflammation (Inflammaging)
THE VICIOUS CYCLE (Aging Spiral)
Poor Food & Toxins
Hormonal Imbalance
Epigenetic Dysregulation
Cellular Damage & Inflammation
More Stress & Metabolic Disturbance
6. CITY DEPARTMENTS (Cellular Systems Working Together)
Power Plants (Mitochondria)
Produce energy (ATP). Good fuel = more energy, less ROS.
Cleaning Crew (Autophagy)
Remove junk & damaged parts. Keep city clean.
Factories (Proteostasis)
Build useful proteins. Prevent misfolded proteins.
Repair Team (DNA Repair)
Fix DNA damage & mutations. Maintain genome stability.
Sentinels (Immune System)
Protect city from invaders. Balance response, avoid chronic inflammation.
Builders (Stem Cells)
Repair & build new structures. Rejuvenate tissues & organs.
City Planners (Cell Senescence)
Remove old, damaged cells at right time. Too many = crowding & dysfunction.
7. OUTCOMES
WHEN CITY RUNS WELL
✓ Energy high
✓ Clean streets
✓ Strong defenses
✓ Happy citizens
✓ Repairs active
✓ City grows wisely
✓ Stays young long
WHEN CITY RUNS POORLY
✗ Energy crashes
✗ Garbage everywhere
✗ Fires (inflammation)
✗ Broken buildings
✗ Retired workers crowd
✗ City ages fast
8. EXAMPLES: FOOD → HORMONE → EPIGENOME → GENE EFFECT
FOOD / LIFESTYLE | HORMONE SIGNAL | EPIGENETIC EFFECT | GENE EFFECT (Examples)
High Sugar | Insulin ↑ | DNA methylation changes | Inflammatory genes ON, Repair genes OFF
Excess Protein / Calories | mTOR ↑, IGF-1 ↑ | Histone modification | Growth genes ON, Autophagy genes OFF
Chronic Stress | Cortisol ↑ | DNA methylation | Stress genes ON (NF-κB), TP53, repair genes OFF
Caloric Restriction / Fasting | AMPK ↑, Sirtuins ↑ | Histone modification, DNA demethylation | Longevity genes ON, Inflammation genes OFF
Healthy Diet (Whole foods, Fiber) | Balanced hormones | Optimal epigenome | Good genes ON, Bad genes OFF
THE MAGIC CHAIN (Remember This!)
Food (Supply)
Hormones (Signals)
Epigenome (Librarian)
ON
OFF
Cell Function
10. THE MAYOR'S RULES
(Lifestyle Strategies)
✓ Eat real, whole foods
✓ Move your body daily
✓ Manage stress
✓ Sleep well
✓ Stay hydrated
✓ Avoid toxins
✓ Build strong relationships
✓ Keep your city clean (Detox & Repair)
LONGEVITY
You are the Mayor of Cell City.
Your daily choices decide how fast your city ages – or how long it stays young and strong.

Inside your body is a city.

- Food = supplies entering the city
- Hormones = messengers delivering instructions
- Epigenome = librarian controlling decisions
- Cells = workers executing tasks

When:

- Supplies are poor
- Messages are confusing
- The librarian makes mistakes

👉 **The city slowly falls into disorder (aging)**

But when:

- Supplies are clean
- Signals are balanced
- The librarian is precise

👉 **The city thrives and stays young longer**

📚 **Scientific References**

🧬 **Epigenetics, Food, Lifestyle & Aging**

1. **Epigenetics and Aging (PMC)**
   https://pmc.ncbi.nlm.nih.gov/articles/PMC4966880/
2. **Epigenetic Regulation of Ageing – Nature Reviews**
   https://www.nature.com/articles/nrm4048
3. **The Ageing Epigenome and its Rejuvenation**
   https://www.nature.com/articles/s41580-019-0204-5
4. **Epigenetics Linking Nutrition to Aging**
   https://pmc.ncbi.nlm.nih.gov/articles/PMC5503416/
5. **Dietary Lifestyle, Inflammaging & Epigenetics**
   https://link.springer.com/article/10.1186/s13148-015-0068-2
6. **DNA Methylation & Human Disease**
   https://www.nature.com/articles/s12276-020-00497-4
7. **Hallmarks of Aging (Original Framework)**
   https://www.cell.com/fulltext/S0092-8674(13)00645-4
8. **Hallmarks of Aging: Expanding Universe**
   https://www.cell.com/cell/fulltext/S0092-8674(22)01570-7
9. **Gene Expression Hallmarks of Cellular Ageing**
   https://link.springer.com/article/10.1007/s10522-018-9750-z
10. **Epigenetic Timeline & Environmental Factors**
    https://clinicalepigeneticsjournal.biomedcentral.com/articles/10.1186/s13148-020-00893-7
11. **Epigenetic Aging & Dietary Regulation**
    https://www.sciencedirect.com/science/article/pii/S0955286325003183
12. **Age-Associated Epigenetic Alterations**
    https://www.mdpi.com/2073-4409/11/3/468

Further Reading and Scientific References

- Nature Reviews Molecular Cell Biology – Epigenetic Regulation of Aging
- Cell – Hallmarks of Aging (2013, 2023)
- Clinical Epigenetics – Environmental Factors and Epigenetic Aging
- PMC – Epigenetics and Aging
- Springer – Dietary Lifestyle, Inflammaging & Epigenetics
- Nature Reviews – The Ageing Epigenome and Rejuvenation

Assessing the Hallmarks of Aging: Role of Genetic and Biochemical Testing

Introduction: Measuring Aging Beyond Chronological Time

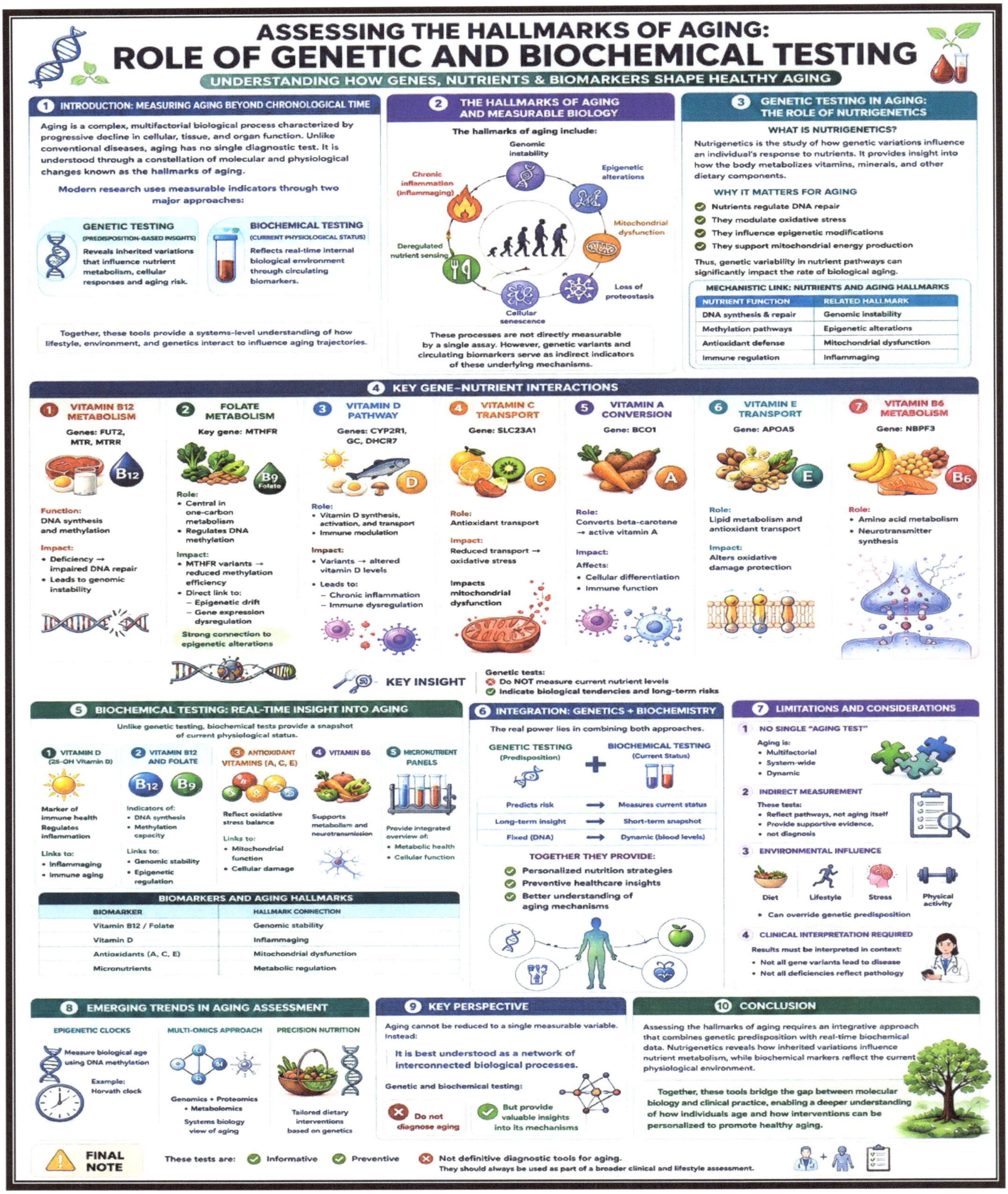

Aging is a complex, multifactorial biological process characterized by progressive decline in cellular, tissue, and organ function. Unlike conventional diseases such as diabetes or hypertension, aging does not have a single diagnostic biomarker or clinical test. Instead, it is understood through a constellation of molecular and physiological changes collectively described as the **hallmarks of aging**.

Modern biomedical research increasingly focuses on identifying measurable indicators that reflect these hallmarks. Two major approaches have emerged:

Genetic testing (predisposition-based insights)

Biochemical testing (current physiological status)

Together, these tools provide a systems-level understanding of how individuals age and how lifestyle, environment, and genetics interact to influence aging trajectories.

🧬 The Hallmarks of Aging and Measurable Biology

The hallmarks of aging include:

Genomic instability

Epigenetic alterations

Mitochondrial dysfunction

Loss of proteostasis

Cellular senescence

Deregulated nutrient sensing

Chronic inflammation (inflammaging)

These processes are not directly measurable through a single assay. However, **genetic variants and circulating biomarkers serve as indirect indicators** of these underlying mechanisms.

🧬 Genetic Testing in Aging: The Role of Nutrigenetics

🧠 What is Nutrigenetics?

Nutrigenetics is the study of how genetic variations influence an individual's response to nutrients. It provides insight into how the body metabolizes vitamins, minerals, and other dietary components.

This is highly relevant to aging because:

Nutrients regulate **DNA repair**

They modulate **oxidative stress**

They influence **epigenetic modifications**

They support **mitochondrial energy production**

Thus, genetic variability in nutrient pathways can significantly impact the rate of biological aging.

🔬 Mechanistic Link: Nutrients and Aging Hallmarks

Nutrient Function	Related Hallmark
DNA synthesis & repair	Genomic instability
Methylation pathways	Epigenetic alterations
Antioxidant defence	Mitochondrial dysfunction
Immune regulation	Inflammaging

🧪 Key Gene–Nutrient Interactions

1. Vitamin B12 Pathway

🧬 **Genes involved:**

FUT2

MTR

MTRR

👉 These genes control how your body absorbs, activates, and uses Vitamin B12.

🔄 **Step-by-Step: What These Genes Actually Do**

🚪 **FUT2 – Entry Gate (Gut level)**

👉 Controls how well Vitamin B12 is absorbed from food

Food → B12 enters intestine

FUT2 helps absorption into bloodstream

⚠️ If gene is less active:

Poor B12 absorption

Even with good diet → levels may be low

⚙️ **MTR – DNA Builder**

👉 Uses Vitamin B12 to make DNA

B12 → used in DNA synthesis

Helps build new cells

⚠️ If MTR is inefficient:

DNA production slows

Cells cannot repair properly

🔧 **MTRR – Repair Technician**

👉 Keeps MTR working properly

Recycles MTR enzyme

Maintains continuous DNA synthesis

⚠️ If MTRR is weak:

MTR stops working efficiently

DNA repair becomes poor

🎯 **So What's the "Benefit" of These Genes?**

👉 These genes determine how well your body **uses Vitamin B12 for DNA repair**

Gene	Role	Effect if not optimal
FUT2	Absorption	Low B12 levels
MTR	DNA synthesis	Poor DNA formation
MTRR	Maintenance	Weak repair system

🧠 **Why This Matters for Aging**

👉 Vitamin B12 is critical for:

DNA repair

Cell division

Nervous system function

🔗 **Final Connection**

Gene variation

↓

Vitamin B12 deficiency/inefficiency

↓

Poor DNA repair

↓

Mutation accumulation

↓

Faster aging (Genomic Instability)

💡 **Easy Analogy**

FUT2 → gate allowing raw material in 🚪

MTR → worker building DNA 🧱

MTRR → mechanic fixing the worker 🔧

👉 If any fails → DNA construction collapses

2. Folate Pathway

Gene involved:

MTHFR

👉 Controls how your body **activates folate and regulates genes**

🔄 **Step-by-Step**

⚙️ **MTHFR – Activation & Control Center**

👉 Converts folate into active form used for methylation

Folate → active folate

Used for gene regulation (methylation)

⚠️ If MTHFR is less active:

Folate not activated properly

Methylation becomes inefficient

🧠 **Why This Matters for Aging**

Methylation controls:

Gene ON/OFF

Cell identity

Protein production

🔗 **Final Connection**

Gene variation
↓
Poor methylation
↓
Genes misregulated
↓
Abnormal cell Behavior
↓
Faster aging (Epigenetic alterations)

💡 **Easy Analogy**

MTHFR = volume control knob 🎚️ for genes

👉 If broken → genes too loud/too silent

3. ☀️ Vitamin D Pathway

🧬 **Genes involved:**

CYP2R1

GC

DHCR7

These genes don't "give a benefit" directly — instead, they **control how your body makes, activates, and uses Vitamin D**.

🔄 **Step-by-Step: What These Genes Actually Do**

🧪 **DHCR7 – Starting Point (Skin level)**

👉 Controls how much Vitamin D your body can produce from sunlight

Sunlight hits skin → Vitamin D precursor is made

DHCR7 regulates this process

⚠️ If gene is less active:

Less Vitamin D is produced

Even with sunlight, levels may stay low

⚙️ **CYP2R1 – Activation in Liver**

👉 Converts Vitamin D into its usable form

Raw Vitamin D → converted to **25-OH Vitamin D** (blood test form)

⚠️ If CYP2R1 is inefficient:

Vitamin D stays inactive

Blood levels appear low

🚚 **GC Gene – Transport System**

👉 Carries Vitamin D in the blood

Acts like a **delivery protein (Vitamin D Binding Protein)**

Moves Vitamin D to tissues (bones, immune cells)

⚠️ If GC is altered:

Vitamin D may not reach cells properly

Functional deficiency occurs

🎯 **So What's the "Benefit" of These Genes?**

👉 These genes **determine how well your body handles Vitamin D**

Gene	Role	Effect if not optimal
DHCR7	Production	Low Vitamin D synthesis
CYP2R1	Activation	Poor conversion
GC	Transport	Poor delivery to cells

🧠 **Why This Matters for Aging**

Vitamin D is NOT just for bones — it affects aging pathways:

🛡️ **Immune Regulation**

Helps control inflammation
👉 Prevents **chronic inflammation (inflammaging)**

🔥 **Inflammation Control**

Low Vitamin D → higher inflammatory cytokines

👉 Leads to:

Tissue damage

Faster aging

🧬 **Cellular Protection**

Supports:

DNA repair

Cellular signaling

🔗 **Final Connection (Very Important)**

👉 These genes → control Vitamin D → affects aging pathways

Flow:

Gene variation
↓
Vitamin D imbalance
↓
Immune dysfunction + inflammation
↓
Faster aging (inflammaging)

💡 **Easy Analogy**

Think of Vitamin D like a **delivery package**:

DHCR7 → factory producing the package 📦

CYP2R1 → packaging & activation center ⚙️

GC → delivery truck 🚚

👉 If any step fails → package never reaches destination

⚠️ **Key Insight**

These genes do NOT directly cause disease

They influence **risk and efficiency**

👉 That's why:

Some people have low Vitamin D despite sunlight

Some need higher supplementation

🧠 **Final Takeaway**

👉 The "benefit" is not the gene itself
👉 The benefit is **efficient Vitamin D metabolism**

And that directly supports:

Immune health

Inflammation control

Healthy aging

4. Vitamin C Pathway

🧬 Gene involved:

SLC23A1

👉 Controls how Vitamin C enters cells

🔄 **Step-by-Step**

🚪 SLC23A1 – Transport Gate

👉 Moves Vitamin C from blood → inside cells

⚠️ If gene is less active:

Less Vitamin C enters cells

Antioxidant defence drops

🎯 **Benefit**

👉 Determines how well your body uses antioxidants

🧠 **Why This Matters for Aging**

Vitamin C protects against:

Free radicals

Oxidative damage

🔗 **Final Connection**

Gene variation
↓
Low Vitamin C inside cells
↓
Oxidative stress increases
↓
Mitochondria damaged
↓
Faster aging (Mitochondrial dysfunction)

💡 **Analogy**

SLC23A1 = security gate letting antioxidants in 🚪

👉 If closed → cells unprotected

5. Vitamin A Pathway

🧬 Gene involved:

BCO1

🔄 **Step-by-Step**

🔄 **BCO1 – Converter Machine**

👉 Converts plant carotene → active Vitamin A

⚠️ If inefficient:

Cannot convert beta-carotene

Functional Vitamin A deficiency

🎯 **Benefit**

👉 Determines how well your body **produces active Vitamin A**

🧠 **Why It Matters**

Vitamin A controls:

Cell growth

Tissue repair

Immune system

🔗 **Final Connection**

Gene variation

↓

Low active Vitamin A

↓

Poor cell differentiation

↓

Weak tissue repair

↓

Faster aging

💡 **Analogy**

BCO1 = **machine converting raw food → usable nutrient** 🔄

6. Vitamin E Pathway

🧬 Gene involved:

APOA5

🔄 **Step-by-Step**

🚚 APOA5 – Fat Transport System

👉 Moves Vitamin E through blood with lipids

⚠️ **If altered:**

Vitamin E not delivered properly

Cells lose protection

🎯 **Benefit**

👉 Determines how well your body protects cells from damage

🧠 **Why It Matters**

Vitamin E:

Protects cell membranes

Prevents oxidative damage

🔗 **Final Connection**

Gene variation
↓
Low Vitamin E delivery
↓
Cell membrane damage
↓
Oxidative stress
↓
Faster aging

💡 **Analogy**

APOA5 = **delivery truck for fat-based antioxidants** 🚚

7. Vitamin B6 Pathway

🧬 Gene involved:

NBPF3

🔄 **Step-by-Step**

⚙️ NBPF3 – Metabolic Coordinator

👉 Supports metabolism and neurotransmitter production

⚠️ **If inefficient:**

Poor amino acid metabolism

Neurotransmitter imbalance

🎯 **Benefit**

👉 Determines how well your body maintains metabolism & brain function

🧠 **Why It Matters**

Vitamin B6 is needed for:

Brain health

Energy metabolism

🔗 **Final Connection**

Gene variation
↓
Metabolic imbalance
↓
Cell stress
↓
Functional decline
↓
Faster aging

💡 **Analogy**

NBPF3 = control system managing metabolism 🧠⚙️

🧠 **FINAL MASTER SUMMARY (Same as Vitamin D logic)**

👉 All genes follow ONE pattern:

Gene efficiency
↓
Nutrient handling
↓
Cellular function
↓
Aging pathway affected

🎯 **MOST IMPORTANT TAKEAWAY**

👉 **Genes do NOT directly give benefits**
👉 **They control how efficiently your body uses nutrients**

🎯 **Key Insight**

Genetic tests:

❌ Do NOT measure current nutrient levels

✅ Indicate **biological tendencies and long-term risks**

🩸 **Biochemical Testing: Real-Time Insight into Aging**

Unlike genetic testing, biochemical tests provide a **snapshot of current physiological status**.

🧪 **Key Biomarkers**

1. Vitamin D (25-OH Vitamin D)

Marker of immune health

Regulates inflammation

👉 Links to:

Inflammaging

Immune aging

2. Vitamin B12 and Folate

Indicators of:

DNA synthesis

Methylation capacity

👉 Links to:

Genomic stability

Epigenetic regulation

3. Antioxidant Vitamins (A, C, E)

Reflect oxidative stress balance

👉 Links to:

Mitochondrial function

Cellular damage

4. Vitamin B6

Supports metabolism and neurotransmission

5. Micronutrient Panels

Provide integrated overview of:

Metabolic health

Cellular function

🔬 Biomarkers and Aging Hallmarks

Biomarker	Hallmark Connection
Vitamin B12/Folate	Genomic stability
Vitamin D	Inflammaging
Antioxidants	Mitochondrial dysfunction
Micronutrients	Metabolic regulation

🔗 Integration: Genetics + Biochemistry

The real power lies in combining both approaches:

Genetic Testing	Biochemical Testing
Predicts risk	Measures current status
Long-term insight	Short-term snapshot
Fixed (DNA)	Dynamic (blood levels)

👉 Together they provide:

Personalized nutrition strategies

Preventive healthcare insights

Better understanding of aging mechanisms

⚠️ Limitations and Considerations

1. No Single "Aging Test"

Aging is:

Multifactorial

System-wide

Dynamic

2. Indirect Measurement

These tests:

Reflect **pathways**, not aging itself

Provide **supportive evidence**, not diagnosis

3. Environmental Influence

Diet

Lifestyle

Stress

Physical activity

👉 Can override genetic predisposition

4. Clinical Interpretation Required

Results must be interpreted in context:

Not all gene variants lead to disease

Not all deficiencies reflect pathology

🧠 **Emerging Trends in Aging Assessment**

🔬 **Epigenetic Clocks**

Measure biological age using DNA methylation

Example: Horvath clock

🧬 **Multi-omics Approach**

Genomics + proteomics + metabolomics

Systems biology view of aging

🧪 **Precision Nutrition**

Tailored dietary interventions based on genetics

🎯 **Key Perspective**

Aging cannot be reduced to a single measurable variable. Instead:

👉 It is best understood as a **network of interconnected biological processes**

Genetic and biochemical testing:

Do not diagnose aging

But provide **valuable insights into its mechanisms**

📌 **Conclusion**

Assessing the hallmarks of aging requires an integrative approach that combines genetic predisposition with real-time biochemical data. Nutrigenetics reveals how inherited variations influence nutrient metabolism, while biochemical markers reflect the current physiological environment.

Together, these tools bridge the gap between molecular biology and clinical practice, enabling a deeper understanding of how individuals age and how interventions can be personalized to promote healthy aging.

⚠️ **Final Note**

These tests are:

✔️ Informative

✔️ Preventive

❌ Not definitive diagnostic tools for aging

They should always be used as part of a **broader clinical and lifestyle assessment**.

📚 **Scientific References**

López-Otín C, Blasco MA, Partridge L, Serrano M, Kroemer G. The Hallmarks of Aging. *Cell*. 2013.

Aunan JR, Watson MM, Hagland HR, Søreide K. Molecular and biological hallmarks of ageing. *Br J Surg*. 2016.

Horvath S, Raj K. DNA methylation-based biomarkers and the epigenetic clock theory of ageing. *Nat Rev Genet*. 2018.

Frenk S, Houseley J. Gene expression hallmarks of cellular ageing. *Biogerontology*. 2018.

Li Y, Tian X, Luo J, et al. Molecular mechanisms of aging and anti-aging strategies. *Cell Commun Signal*. 2024.

Frontiers in Nutrition. Nutrigenetics and personalized nutrition. 2020.

WHO, NIH, and related biomarker studies on aging and molecular assessment.

These references collectively support the scientific basis for nutrigenetics, biochemical testing, epigenetic aging, and the molecular hallmarks of aging.

Epigenetic Reprogramming and OSK — Resetting the Biology of Aging

From Damage to Information Loss: A Paradigm Shift

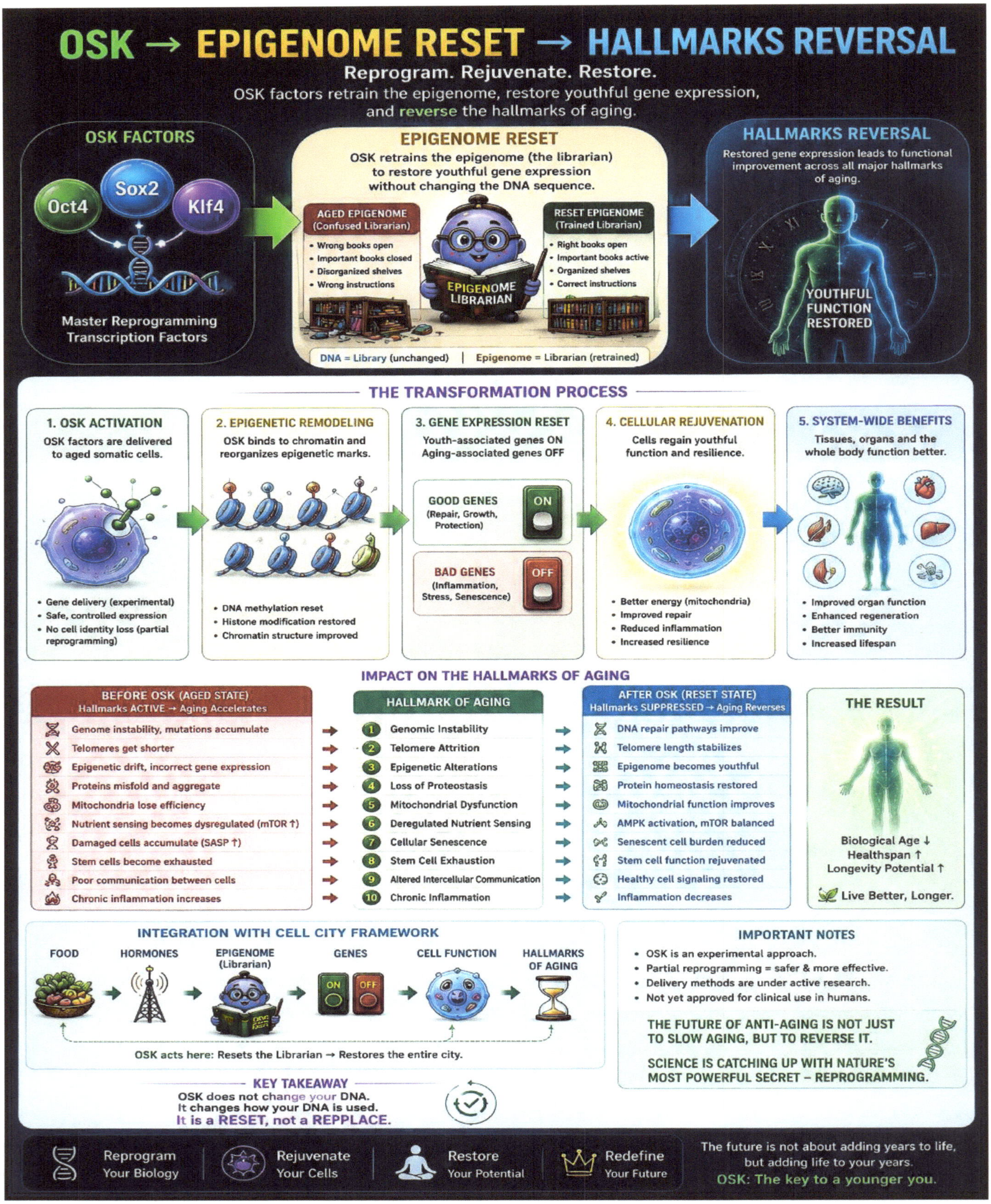

For decades, aging was viewed primarily as the accumulation of molecular damage—DNA mutations, oxidative stress, and cellular wear. However, emerging evidence suggests a deeper layer:

👉 Aging may be driven not only by damage, but by loss of epigenetic information.

This concept reframes aging as a reversible biological state, opening the door to interventions that restore youthful function rather than merely slowing decline.

At the centre of this revolution lies a powerful biological tool:

The OSK Reprogramming Factors

The term **"OSK genes"** refers to a specific set of three transcription factors:

🧬 **OSK = Oct4 + Sox2 + Klf4**

These are part of the famous **Yamanaka factors**, discovered by **Shinya Yamanaka**, which can reprogram adult cells back into a youthful, stem-cell-like state.

📏 **What Are OSK Factors?**

OSK refers to three transcription factors:

- **Oct4 (POU5F1)**
- **Sox2**
- **Klf4**

These proteins regulate gene expression and cellular identity. They were originally identified as part of the **Yamanaka factors**, discovered by Shinya Yamanaka, which can convert adult somatic cells into **induced pluripotent stem cells (iPSCs)**.

🔬 **Why only OSK (and not OSKM)?**

The original set included:

- **c-Myc** (oncogenic risk)

Modern aging research focuses on **OSK alone** to enable **safer partial reprogramming**, avoiding tumor formation.

🔬 **What each gene does**

1. Oct4 (POU5F1)

- Maintains pluripotency (ability of a cell to become any cell type)
- Keeps cells in an undifferentiated, "youthful" state

2. Sox2

- Works with Oct4 to regulate gene expression for stemness
- Important for self-renewal and neural development

3. Klf4

- Controls cell proliferation and differentiation
- Has roles in DNA repair, stress response, and survival

📏 **Why OSK is important in aging research**

Originally, the full set of Yamanaka factors (OSKM = Oct4, Sox2, Klf4, c-Myc) could completely reprogram cells into induced pluripotent stem cells (iPSCs).

👉 **But there was a problem:**

- **c-Myc increases cancer risk**

So, researchers now focus on OSK (without c-Myc) for safer partial reprogramming.

🔁 OSK and Aging

OSK is now being studied for:

🔹 **1. Epigenetic Resetting**

- Restores youthful gene expression patterns
- Reverses epigenetic drift (your "librarian confusion" concept)

🔹 **2. Cellular Rejuvenation**

- **Improves:**
  - DNA repair
  - Mitochondrial function
  - Cellular resilience

🔹 **3. Reversal of Aging Markers**

In animal studies:

- Vision restoration (optic nerve damage reversed)
- Tissue repair improved
- Biological age markers reduced

🧠 Simple "Cell City" Analogy

- **OSK = Master Reset Button** 🧠
- **It tells the librarian (epigenome):**
  👉 **"Go back to original settings and read the correct books again"**

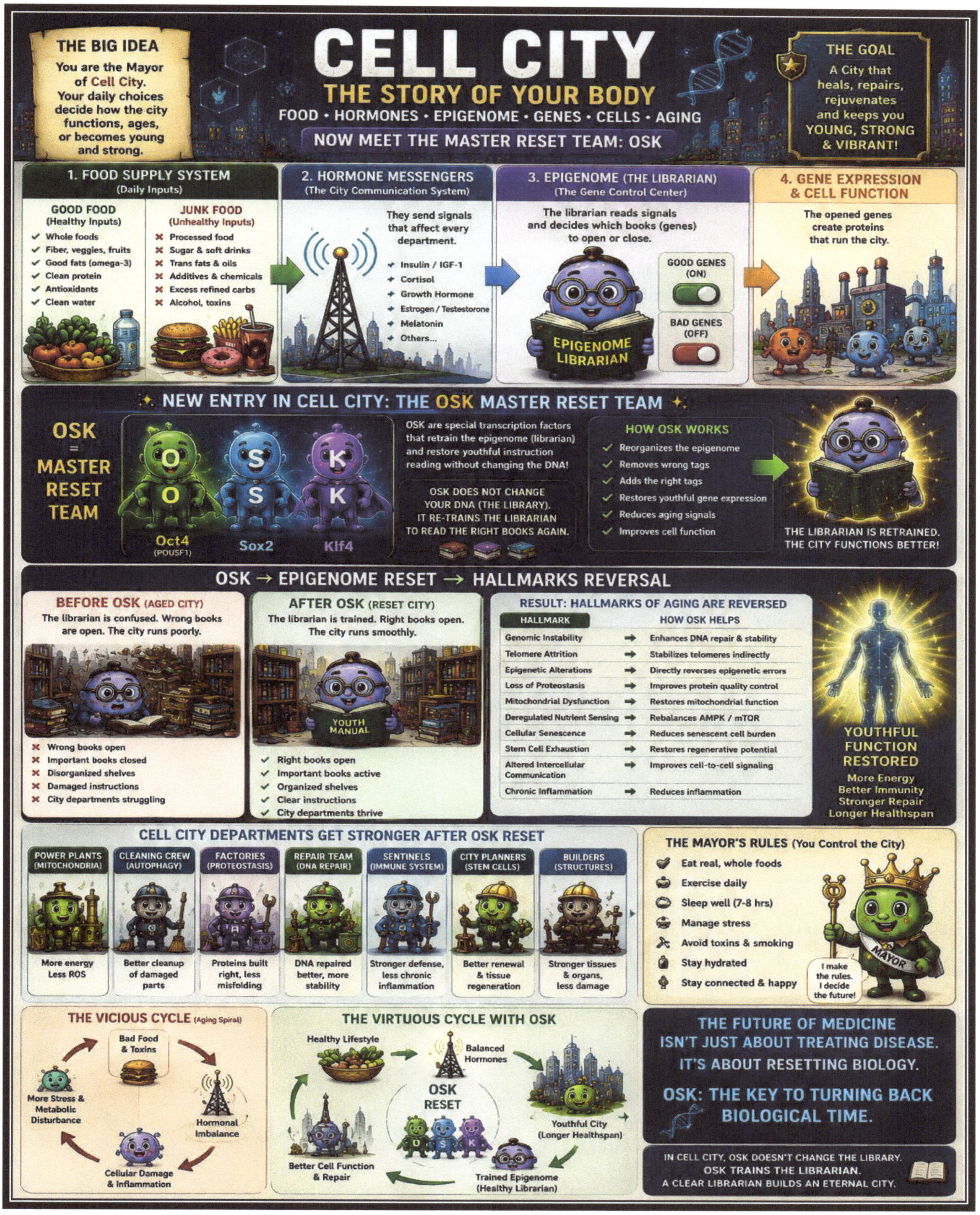
THE BIG IDEA
You are the Mayor of Cell City. Your daily choices decide how the city functions, ages, or becomes young and strong.
CELL CITY
THE STORY OF YOUR BODY
FOOD • HORMONES • EPIGENOME • GENES • CELLS • AGING
NOW MEET THE MASTER RESET TEAM: OSK
THE GOAL
A City that heals, repairs, rejuvenates and keeps you YOUNG, STRONG & VIBRANT!
1. FOOD SUPPLY SYSTEM
(Daily Inputs)
GOOD FOOD
(Healthy Inputs)
Whole foods
Fiber, veggies, fruits
Good fats (omega-3)
Clean protein
Antioxidants
Clean water
JUNK FOOD
(Unhealthy Inputs)
Processed food
Sugar & soft drinks
Trans fats & oils
Additives & chemicals
Excess refined carbs
Alcohol, toxins
2. HORMONE MESSENGERS
(The City Communication System)
They send signals that affect every department.
Insulin / IGF-1
Cortisol
Growth Hormone
Estrogen / Testestorone
Melatonin
Others...
3. EPIGENOME (THE LIBRARIAN)
(The Gene Control Center)
The librarian reads signals and decides which books (genes) to open or close.
GOOD GENES (ON)
BAD GENES (OFF)
EPIGENOME LIBRARIAN
4. GENE EXPRESSION & CELL FUNCTION
The opened genes create proteins that run the city.
NEW ENTRY IN CELL CITY: THE OSK MASTER RESET TEAM
OSK = MASTER RESET TEAM
Oct4 (POU5F1)
Sox2
Klf4
OSK are special transcription factors that retrain the epigenome (librarian) and restore youthful instruction reading without changing the DNA!
OSK DOES NOT CHANGE YOUR DNA (THE LIBRARY). IT RE-TRAINS THE LIBRARIAN TO READ THE RIGHT BOOKS AGAIN.
HOW OSK WORKS
Reorganizes the epigenome
Removes wrong tags
Adds the right tags
Restores youthful gene expression
Reduces aging signals
Improves cell function
THE LIBRARIAN IS RETRAINED. THE CITY FUNCTIONS BETTER!
OSK → EPIGENOME RESET → HALLMARKS REVERSAL
BEFORE OSK (AGED CITY)
The librarian is confused. Wrong books are open. The city runs poorly.
Wrong books open
Important books closed
Disorganized shelves
Damaged instructions
City departments struggling
AFTER OSK (RESET CITY)
The librarian is trained. Right books open. The city runs smoothly.
YOUTH MANUAL
Right books open
Important books active
Organized shelves
Clear instructions
City departments thrive
RESULT: HALLMARKS OF AGING ARE REVERSED
HALLMARK | HOW OSK HELPS
Genomic Instability → Enhances DNA repair & stability
Telomere Attrition → Stabilizes telomeres indirectly
Epigenetic Alterations → Directly reverses epigenetic errors
Loss of Proteostasis → Improves protein quality control
Mitochondrial Dysfunction → Restores mitochondrial function
Deregulated Nutrient Sensing → Rebalances AMPK / mTOR
Cellular Senescence → Reduces senescent cell burden
Stem Cell Exhaustion → Restores regenerative potential
Altered Intercellular Communication → Improves cell-to-cell signaling
Chronic Inflammation → Reduces inflammation
YOUTHFUL FUNCTION RESTORED
More Energy
Better Immunity
Stronger Repair
Longer Healthspan
CELL CITY DEPARTMENTS GET STRONGER AFTER OSK RESET
POWER PLANTS (MITOCHONDRIA) — More energy Less ROS
CLEANING CREW (AUTOPHAGY) — Better cleanup of damaged parts
FACTORIES (PROTEOSTASIS) — Proteins built right, less misfolding
REPAIR TEAM (DNA REPAIR) — DNA repaired better, more stability
SENTINELS (IMMUNE SYSTEM) — Stronger defense, less chronic inflammation
CITY PLANNERS (STEM CELLS) — Better renewal & tissue regeneration
BUILDERS (STRUCTURES) — Stronger tissues & organs, less damage
THE MAYOR'S RULES (You Control the City)
Eat real, whole foods
Exercise daily
Sleep well (7-8 hrs)
Manage stress
Avoid toxins & smoking
Stay hydrated
Stay connected & happy
I make the rules. I decide the future!
MAYOR
THE VICIOUS CYCLE (Aging Spiral)
Bad Food & Toxins
Hormonal Imbalance
Cellular Damage & Inflammation
More Stress & Metabolic Disturbance
THE VIRTUOUS CYCLE WITH OSK
Healthy Lifestyle
Balanced Hormones
Youthful City (Longer Healthspan)
Trained Epigenome (Healthy Librarian)
Better Cell Function & Repair
OSK RESET
THE FUTURE OF MEDICINE ISN'T JUST ABOUT TREATING DISEASE. IT'S ABOUT RESETTING BIOLOGY.
OSK: THE KEY TO TURNING BACK BIOLOGICAL TIME.
IN CELL CITY, OSK DOESN'T CHANGE THE LIBRARY. OSK TRAINS THE LIBRARIAN. A CLEAR LIBRARIAN BUILDS AN ETERNAL CITY.

So instead of:
❌ **Wrong genes ON → aging**
You get:
✅ **Correct genes ON → rejuvenation**

🔁 Mechanism: How OSK Reprograms Cellular Age

Epigenetic Resetting

OSK does not primarily "repair" DNA—it reorganizes how DNA is read.

- Restores youthful DNA methylation patterns
- Reverses histone modifications associated with aging
- Improves chromatin structure and accessibility

👉 **framework:**

- DNA = Library (unchanged)
- Epigenome = Librarian (confused with age)
- OSK = Retraining the librarian

Restoration of Gene Expression Programs

Aging alters transcriptional networks. OSK helps:

- Reactivate youth-associated genes
- Suppress pro-inflammatory and stress genes
- Restore cellular identity

Functional Rejuvenation

Downstream effects include:

- Improved mitochondrial efficiency
- Enhanced DNA repair capacity
- Reduced oxidative stress
- Increased cellular resilience

Restoration of Gene Expression Programs

Aging alters transcriptional networks. OSK helps:

- Reactivate youth-associated genes
- Suppress pro-inflammatory and stress genes
- Restore cellular identity

Functional Rejuvenation

Downstream effects include:

- Improved mitochondrial efficiency
- Enhanced DNA repair capacity
- Reduced oxidative stress
- Increased cellular resilience

🔗 OSK and the Hallmarks of Aging

OSK acts upstream, influencing multiple hallmarks simultaneously:

Hallmark	OSK Effect
Genomic instability	Improves DNA repair pathways
Epigenetic alterations	Directly reversed
Telomere attrition	Indirect stabilization
Loss of proteostasis	Improved protein regulation
Mitochondrial dysfunction	Enhanced energy metabolism
Deregulated nutrient sensing	Rebalanced signaling
Cellular senescence	Reduced senescent burden
Stem cell exhaustion	Restores regenerative capacity
Altered communication	Reduces inflammation

👉 **Key Insight:**
OSK is not targeting one hallmark—it acts at the control layer above all hallmarks.

🧪 Partial vs Full Reprogramming

❌ Full Reprogramming

- Cells revert to embryonic state (iPSCs)
- Loss of identity
- High tumor risk

✅ Partial Reprogramming (OSK Approach)

- Cells remain differentiated
- Epigenetic age is reduced
- Function improves without losing identity

👉 **This is the most promising strategy for anti-aging interventions.**

🧠 Experimental Evidence

🔬 Animal Studies

- Restoration of vision in aged mice
- Improved tissue repair
- Reversal of epigenetic aging markers

🧬 Cellular Studies

- Reset of DNA methylation clocks
- Improved cellular function and longevity markers

🏙 6. Cell City Analogy: "Resetting the Librarian"

In *Cell City*:

- 📚 DNA = The Library (intact)
- 👩‍🏫 Epigenome = The Librarian (confused with age)
- 🧬 OSK = The Master Reset Training Program

What OSK does:

- Retrains the librarian
- Reorganizes the shelves
- Reopens the correct instruction manuals

👉 **Result:**

- Good genes ON
- Harmful genes OFF
- City functions restored

⚙️ Integration with Systems Biology

OSK interacts with multiple biological layers:

🔹 **Hormonal Systems**

- Improves sensitivity to insulin, growth factors
- May indirectly influence longevity pathways (AMPK, mTOR)

🔹 **Metabolism**

- Restores energy balance
- Reduces ROS production

🔹 **Immune System**

- Reduces chronic inflammation
- Improves immune surveillance

🔹 **Microbiome (emerging area)**

- Potential indirect effects via systemic signaling

⚠️ Limitations and Risks

Despite its promise:

- Not yet widely tested in humans
- Long-term safety unknown
- Risk of uncontrolled cell growth if misregulated
- Delivery systems (viral vectors, gene therapy) still evolving

👉 **OSK remains experimental, not clinical standard.**

🔮 Future Directions

- Precision epigenetic reprogramming therapies
- Non-genetic approaches to mimic OSK effects
- **Combination strategies:**
    - Lifestyle + epigenetic modulation
    - Bioinformatics-guided interventions
- **Integration into personalized longevity medicine**

🧾 Key Takeaways

- Aging may be driven by epigenetic information loss
- OSK provides a method to reset biological age
- Acts at a master regulatory level, influencing all hallmarks

- **Represents a shift from:**
  - ❌ **Slowing aging**
  - ✅ **Potentially reversing aging processes**

🧠 **One-Line Summary**

👉 *"OSK does not rebuild the cell—it reminds the cell how to be young again."*

🔑 **Concept Integration**

Food → Hormones → Epigenome → Hallmarks → Aging
⬇️
OSK acts here → Epigenome Reset → System-wide Rejuvenation

📚 **Scientific References**

🧬 **OSK/Yamanaka Factors**

https://lifespan.io/topic/yamanaka-factors/

🧠 **Epigenetic Rejuvenation**

https://epigeneticsandchromatin.biomedcentral.com/articles/10.1186/s13072-018-0244-7

🔬 **Cellular Reprogramming (Nature Review)**

https://www.nature.com/articles/nrg3473

🧪 **Aging Reversal Study (PubMed)**

https://pubmed.ncbi.nlm.nih.gov/37437248/

🧬 **Epigenetics & Aging (Nature)**

https://www.nature.com/articles/s41392-022-01211-8

🧫 **Stem Cell Epigenome & Aging**

https://academic.oup.com/hmg/article/29/R2/R236/5879701

🧬 **Chromatin Remodelling (PMC)**

https://www.ncbi.nlm.nih.gov/pmc/articles/PMC7857421/

ORAC, Free Radicals, Antioxidants, and Aging

Understanding the Science, Claims, Limitations, and Clinical Reality

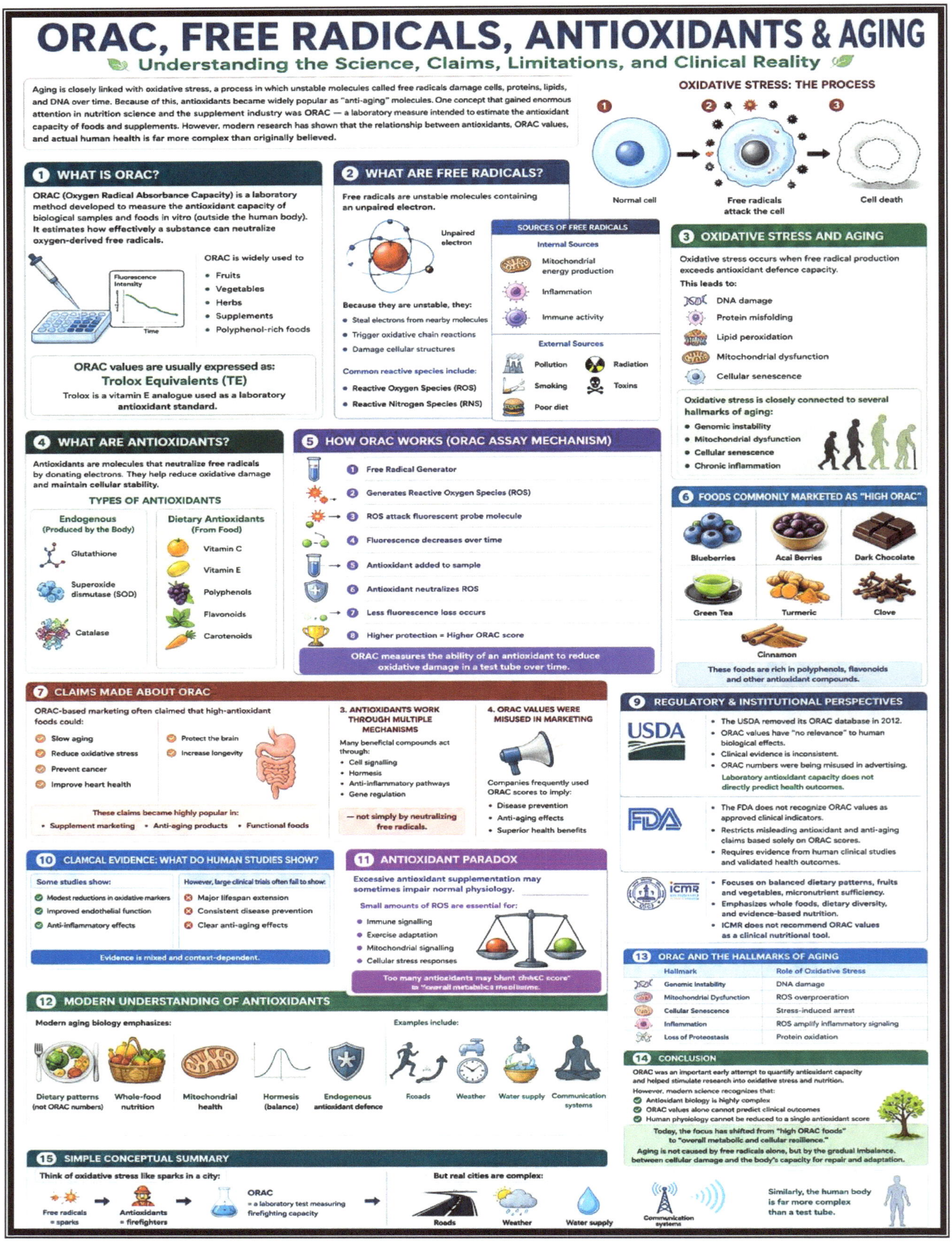

Introduction

Aging is closely linked with oxidative stress, a process in which unstable molecules called free radicals damage cells, proteins, lipids, and DNA over time. Because of this, antioxidants became widely popular as "anti-aging" molecules.

One concept that gained enormous attention in nutrition science and the supplement industry was ORAC — a laboratory measure intended to estimate the antioxidant capacity of foods and supplements.

However, modern research has shown that the relationship between antioxidants, ORAC values, and actual human health is far more complex than originally believed.

What is ORAC?

ORAC Definition

ORAC (Oxygen Radical Absorbance Capacity) is a laboratory method developed to measure the antioxidant capacity of biological samples and foods *in vitro* (outside the human body).

It estimates how effectively a substance can neutralize oxygen-derived free radicals.

The ORAC assay was developed in the 1990s and became widely used to compare:

- Fruits
- Vegetables
- Herbs
- Supplements
- Polyphenol-rich foods

ORAC values are usually expressed as:

Trolox Equivalents (TE)

Trolox is a vitamin E analogue used as a laboratory antioxidant standard.

What Are Free Radicals?

Free radicals are unstable molecules containing an unpaired electron.

Because they are unstable, they:

- Steal electrons from nearby molecules
- Trigger oxidative chain reactions
- Damage cellular structures

Common reactive species include:

- Reactive Oxygen Species (ROS)
- Reactive Nitrogen Species (RNS)

Sources of Free Radicals

Internal Sources

- Mitochondrial energy production
- Inflammation
- Immune activity

External Sources

- Pollution
- Radiation
- Smoking
- Toxins
- Poor diet

🧬 Oxidative Stress and Aging

Oxidative stress occurs when free radical production exceeds antioxidant defence capacity.

This contributes to:

- DNA damage
- Protein misfolding
- Lipid peroxidation
- Mitochondrial dysfunction
- Cellular senescence

Oxidative stress is closely connected to several hallmarks of aging:

- Genomic instability
- Mitochondrial dysfunction
- Cellular senescence
- Chronic inflammation

🛡️ What Are Antioxidants?

Antioxidants are molecules that neutralize free radicals by donating electrons.

They help reduce oxidative damage and maintain cellular stability.

⚙️ Types of Antioxidants

Endogenous (Produced by the Body)

- Glutathione
- Superoxide dismutase (SOD)
- Catalase

Dietary Antioxidants

- Vitamin C
- Vitamin E
- Polyphenols
- Flavonoids
- Carotenoids

🔄 How ORAC Works (Flow Diagram)

🧪 ORAC Assay Mechanism

Free Radical Generator
↓
Generates Reactive Oxygen Species (ROS)
↓
ROS attack fluorescent probe molecule
↓
Fluorescence decreases over time
↓
Antioxidant added to sample
↓
Antioxidant neutralizes ROS
↓
Less fluorescence loss occurs
↓
Higher protection = Higher ORAC score

🍓 Foods Commonly Marketed as "High ORAC"

Foods often promoted for high ORAC values include:

- Blueberries
- Acai berries
- Dark chocolate
- Green tea
- Turmeric
- Clove
- Cinnamon

📈 Claims Made About ORAC

ORAC-based marketing often claimed that high-antioxidant foods could:

- Slow aging
- Reduce oxidative stress
- Prevent cancer
- Improve heart health
- Protect the brain
- Increase longevity

These claims became highly popular in:

- Supplement marketing
- Anti-aging products
- Functional foods

⚠️ Scientific Limitations of ORAC

Over time, major scientific concerns emerged.

❌ 1. ORAC is an *In Vitro* Test

ORAC measures antioxidant activity in a test tube — not inside the human body.

Human physiology is far more complex:

- Digestion
- Absorption
- Metabolism
- Bioavailability
- Tissue distribution

…all influence antioxidant Behavior.

👉 **A food with high ORAC in the lab may have little biological effect in humans.**

❌ 2. Bioavailability Problem

Many polyphenols:

- Are poorly absorbed
- Rapidly metabolized
- Quickly eliminated

Therefore:

👉 **High ORAC ≠ high biological activity**

❌ 3. Antioxidants Work Through Multiple Mechanisms

Many beneficial compounds act through:

- Cell signaling
- Hormesis

- Anti-inflammatory pathways
- Gene regulation

—not simply by neutralizing free radicals.

❌ 4. ORAC Values Were Misused in Marketing

Food and supplement companies frequently used ORAC scores to imply:

- Disease prevention
- Anti-aging effects
- Superior health benefits

without strong clinical evidence.

🏛 USDA Position on ORAC

The United States Department of Agriculture removed its ORAC database in 2012.

The USDA stated that:

- ORAC values had "no relevance" to human biological effects
- Clinical evidence was inconsistent
- ORAC numbers were being misused in advertising

The USDA emphasized that:
👉 laboratory antioxidant capacity does not directly predict health outcomes.

🏛 FDA Perspective

The U.S. Food and Drug Administration does not recognize ORAC values as approved clinical indicators of antioxidant benefit.

The FDA generally restricts:

- misleading antioxidant claims
- unsupported anti-aging claims
- disease-prevention claims based solely on ORAC scores

The FDA requires:

- evidence from human clinical studies
- validated health outcomes

before health claims can be made.

🇮🇳 ICMR Perspective

The Indian Council of Medical Research focuses on:

- balanced dietary patterns
- fruits and vegetables
- micronutrient sufficiency

rather than ORAC scoring systems.

Current nutritional guidance from ICMR emphasizes:

- whole foods
- dietary diversity
- evidence-based nutrition

ICMR does not officially recommend ORAC values as a clinical nutritional tool.

🧪 Clinical Evidence: What Do Human Studies Show?

Clinical studies on antioxidant supplementation have produced mixed results.

Some studies show:

- modest reductions in oxidative markers
- improved endothelial function
- anti-inflammatory effects

However, large clinical trials often fail to show:

- major lifespan extension
- consistent disease prevention
- clear anti-aging effects

⚠️ Antioxidant Paradox

Interestingly:
👉 excessive antioxidant supplementation may sometimes impair normal physiology.

Reactive oxygen species are not always harmful.

Small amounts of ROS are essential for:

- immune signaling
- exercise adaptation
- mitochondrial signaling
- cellular stress responses

Excessive antioxidant intake may blunt these adaptive mechanisms.

🌱 Modern Understanding of Antioxidants

Modern aging biology now emphasizes:

- dietary patterns rather than ORAC numbers
- whole-food nutrition
- mitochondrial health
- hormesis
- endogenous antioxidant defence systems

Examples include:

- Exercise
- Caloric moderation
- Plant-rich diets
- Sleep
- Stress regulation

🧬 ORAC and the Hallmarks of Aging

Oxidative stress intersects with multiple hallmarks of aging:

Hallmark	Role of Oxidative Stress
Genomic Instability	**DNA damage**
Mitochondrial Dysfunction	**ROS overproduction**
Cellular Senescence	**Stress-induced arrest**
Inflammation	**ROS amplify inflammatory signaling**
Loss of Proteostasis	**Protein oxidation**

🧾 Conclusion

ORAC was an important early attempt to quantify antioxidant capacity and helped stimulate research into oxidative stress and nutrition.

However, modern science recognizes that:

- antioxidant biology is highly complex
- ORAC values alone cannot predict clinical outcomes
- human physiology cannot be reduced to a single antioxidant score

Today, the focus has shifted from:
👉 "high ORAC foods"

to:
👉 "overall metabolic and cellular resilience."

Aging is not caused by free radicals alone, but by the gradual imbalance between cellular damage and the body's capacity for repair and adaptation.

🌟 Simple Conceptual Summary

Think of oxidative stress like sparks in a city:

- **Free radicals = sparks**
- **Antioxidants = firefighters**
- **ORAC = a laboratory test measuring firefighting capacity**

But real cities are complex:

- Roads
- Weather
- Water supply
- Communication systems

Similarly, the human body is far more complex than a test tube.

📚 Scientific References

- **Harman D. *Journal of Gerontology.* 1956.**
- **Finkel T, Holbrook NJ. *Nature.* 2000.**
- **Jomova K et al. *Archives of Toxicology.* 2023.**
- **USDA ORAC database withdrawal statements.**
- **MDPI review on antioxidant assays.**

1. Free Radical Theory of Aging

Denham Harman proposed the original free radical theory of aging, suggesting that reactive oxygen species (ROS) contribute to cellular damage and aging.

Harman D. Aging: A theory based on free radical and radiation chemistry. *Journal of Gerontology.* 1956;11(3):298–300.

2. Oxidative Stress and Aging Biology

Toren Finkel and Nikki J. Holbrook reviewed how oxidative stress influences aging and lifespan regulation.

Finkel T, Holbrook NJ. Oxidants, oxidative stress and the biology of ageing. *Nature.* 2000;408(6809):239–247.
DOI: 10.1038/35041687

3. Reactive Oxygen Species and Chronic Disease

This review explains the role of ROS, oxidative stress, antioxidants, and their relationship with chronic diseases and aging.

Jomova K, Raptova R, Alomar SY, et al. Reactive oxygen species, toxicity, oxidative stress, and antioxidants: chronic diseases and aging. *Archives of Toxicology.* 2023;97:2499–2574.
DOI: 10.1007/s00204-023-03562-9

4. Mitochondrial Oxidative Stress in Aging

This paper discusses mitochondrial ROS production and mitochondrial dysfunction in aging and health span.

Dai DF, Chiao YA, Marcinek DJ, et al. Mitochondrial oxidative stress in aging and health span. *Longevity & Health span.* 2014;3(1):6.
DOI: 10.1186/2046-2395-3-6

5. Oxidative Stress and Antioxidant Supplementation

A comprehensive overview of oxidative stress, antioxidants, and aging-related diseases.

Martemucci G, Portincasa P, Di Ciaula A, et al. Oxidative stress, aging, antioxidant supplementation and their impact on human health: An overview. *Mechanisms of Ageing and Development.* 2022;206:111707.
DOI: 10.1016/j.mad.2022.111707

6. Antioxidants and Cellular Senescence

This review explains how oxidative stress contributes to cellular senescence and age-related pathology.

Varesi A, Chirumbolo S, Campagnoli LIM, et al. The Role of Antioxidants in the Interplay between Oxidative Stress and Senescence. *Antioxidants.* 2022;11(7):1224.
DOI: 10.3390/antiox11071224

7. Antioxidants and Age-Related Diseases

Review article discussing oxidative stress, inflammaging, and antioxidant mechanisms.

Tan BL, Norhaizan ME, Liew WPP, Rahman HS. Antioxidant and Oxidative Stress: A Mutual Interplay in Age-Related Diseases. *Frontiers in Pharmacology.* 2018;9:1162.
DOI: 10.3389/fphar.2018.01162

8. Polyphenols, Oxidative Stress, and Anti-Aging

Explains the antioxidant role of dietary polyphenols in aging biology.

Rolt A, Cox LS. Structural basis of the anti-ageing effects of polyphenolics: mitigation of oxidative stress. *BMC Chemistry.* 2020;14:50.
DOI: 10.1186/s13065-020-00696-0

9. Free Radical Theory and Antioxidant Supplements

A systematic review discussing the evidence and limitations of antioxidant supplementation.

Buehler BA. The Free Radical Theory of Aging and Antioxidant Supplements: A Systematic Review. *Journal of Alternative and Complementary Medicine.* 2012;18(4):313–321.
DOI: 10.1177/2156587212441939

🌿 Biochemical Decline in Aging: From Mitochondrial Dysfunction to Targeted Nutritional Support

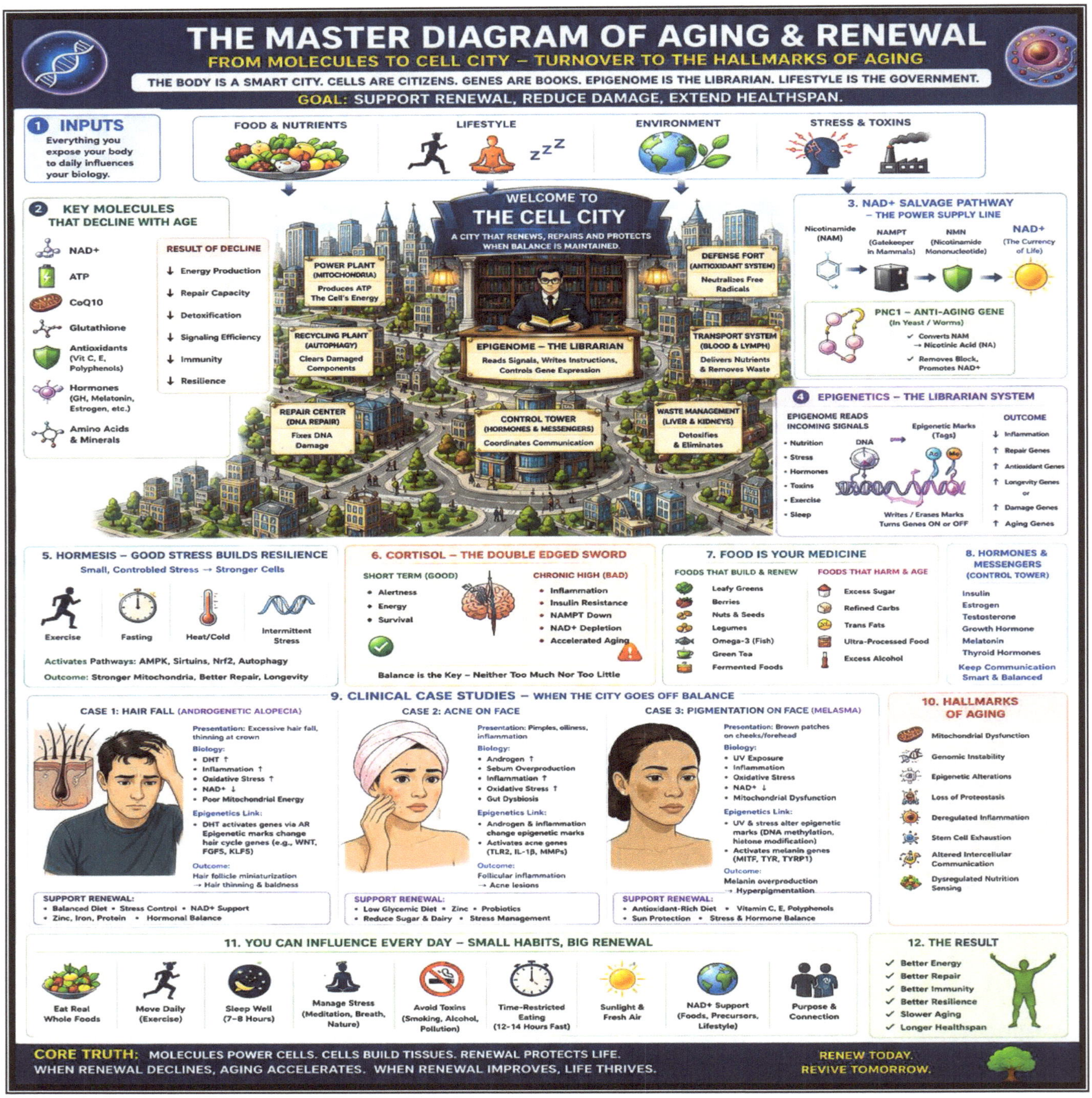

🧬 Foundation: What Changes with Aging

Explain decline in:

- NAD+
- Glutathione
- Mitochondrial efficiency
- Hormonal signaling
- Cellular repair mechanisms

👉 **Connect to:**

- Oxidative stress
- Inflammation
- Poor energy metabolism

Introduction

Aging is a multifactorial biological process characterized not only by the passage of time but by progressive decline in cellular and biochemical function. While chronological aging is inevitable, biological aging is influenced by molecular, metabolic, and environmental factors.

Recent advances in biomedical research highlight that many age-related disorders originate from **early biochemical dysfunction**, often preceding clinical disease by years or decades. Among these, mitochondrial impairment, oxidative stress, and disruption of cellular repair systems play a central role.

This chapter integrates concepts from mitochondrial biology, biochemistry, and nutritional science to present a structured understanding of how aging-related biochemical decline may be supported through targeted, evidence-based interventions—without overstating therapeutic claims.

⚙ **Mechanism: Why Diseases Start**

simple chain:

Aging → Cellular decline → Biochemical imbalance → Organ dysfunction → Clinical symptoms

Example:

- **Mitochondrial dysfunction → ↓ ATP → ↑ ROS → inflammation → tissue damage**

⚙ **Biochemical Hallmarks of Aging**

Aging is associated with measurable declines in key biochemical systems:

Mitochondrial Dysfunction

Mitochondria are central to energy production (ATP synthesis). With age:

- ATP production decreases
- Reactive oxygen species (ROS) increase
- Mitochondrial DNA damage accumulates

This leads to impaired cellular energy metabolism and increased oxidative stress.

⚙ **Oxidative Stress and Redox Imbalance**

An imbalance between ROS and antioxidant defences results in:

- Lipid peroxidation
- Protein damage
- DNA mutations

Key antioxidant systems such as glutathione decline with age.

⚙ **Decline in Cellular Repair Mechanisms**

- Reduced DNA repair capacity
- Impaired autophagy
- Altered protein folding and degradation

⚙ **Epigenetic Alterations**

Changes in DNA methylation, histone modification, and gene expression influence:

- Inflammation
- Metabolism
- Longevity pathways

⚙️Metabolic Dysregulation

- Insulin resistance
- Altered lipid metabolism
- Chronic low-grade inflammation (inflammaging)

🔬 From Biochemical Dysfunction to Disease

The progression from aging to disease follows a logical cascade:

Aging → Cellular Dysfunction → Biochemical Imbalance → Tissue Damage → Clinical Disease

Example:

- Mitochondrial dysfunction → ↓ ATP + ↑ ROS
- Leads to oxidative stress → inflammation
- Results in cellular damage → organ dysfunction

This framework emphasizes that disease often begins at the biochemical level, long before symptoms appear.

📉 Role of Nutrients in Human Biochemistry

Nutrients are fundamental to biochemical processes and function as:

- **Cofactors** (e.g., vitamins and minerals in enzymatic reactions)
- **Substrates** (e.g., amino acids, fatty acids)
- **Signaling molecules** (e.g., influencing gene expression and metabolism)

It is important to emphasize:

Nutrients and bioactive compounds support physiological pathways but do not function as standalone cures for disease.

Their role is to **optimize biochemical function**, particularly in the presence of deficiencies or increased physiological demand.

👉Age-Related Decline in Key Molecules

Several critical molecules decline with age:

- NAD^+ (cellular energy and repair)
- Glutathione (antioxidant defence)
- Coenzyme Q10 (mitochondrial function)
- Melatonin (circadian and antioxidant role)

This decline contributes to reduced cellular resilience and increased susceptibility to disease.

👉Clinical Approach: When and How to Intervene

A scientific and responsible approach to nutritional intervention requires:

Stepwise Framework

1. **Identify Symptoms**
   (e.g., fatigue, hair loss, metabolic issues)
2. **Conduct Laboratory Evaluation**
   Examples:
   - Vitamin levels (B12, D)
   - Iron studies (ferritin)
   - Metabolic markers (glucose, insulin)
3. **Identify Deficiency or Dysfunction**
   - Nutrient deficiency
   - Mitochondrial impairment
   - Hormonal imbalance

4. **Targeted Intervention**

- Dietary modification
- Lifestyle changes
- Supplementation (if required)

📘 Conceptual Framework: Integrated View

A simplified model:

Aging → Biochemical Decline → Pathway Dysfunction → Early Symptoms → Clinical Detection → Targeted Support → Functional Improvement

This framework highlights that interventions aim to **restore function**, not to claim disease reversal.

Scientific Considerations and Limitations

- Nutritional interventions should be **evidence-based and individualized**
- Supplementation without assessment may be ineffective or harmful
- Clinical conditions require **medical diagnosis and treatment**

🎯 Conclusion

Aging is fundamentally a biochemical process influenced by mitochondrial function, oxidative stress, and metabolic regulation. Understanding these pathways provides an opportunity for early intervention through targeted nutritional and lifestyle strategies.

However, the role of such interventions must be framed appropriately:

The goal is not to cure disease, but to support biological systems, correct deficiencies, and enhance physiological resilience.

This integrative approach bridges fundamental biochemistry with practical health strategies, offering a scientifically grounded perspective on healthy aging.

⚠️ Important Scientific Disclaimer

- Supplements support biology
- They do **NOT** cure diseases
- Medical supervision is required

📊 MASTER FLOWCHART

Aging
↓
Biochemical Decline
(NAD+, Glutathione, Mitochondria)
↓
Pathway Dysfunction
↓
Early Symptoms
↓
Lab Testing
↓
Targeted Intervention
(Diet + Nutrients)
↓
Improved Function (not cure)

Key Takeaways 👉

- Aging involves measurable biochemical decline
- Mitochondrial dysfunction is central to many age-related changes
- Nutrients support, but do not replace, medical treatment
- Laboratory-guided interventions are essential
- Early biochemical correction may improve long-term health outcomes

Energy Metabolism in Humans: Fuel Selection, Tissue Specificity, and Homeostatic Regulation

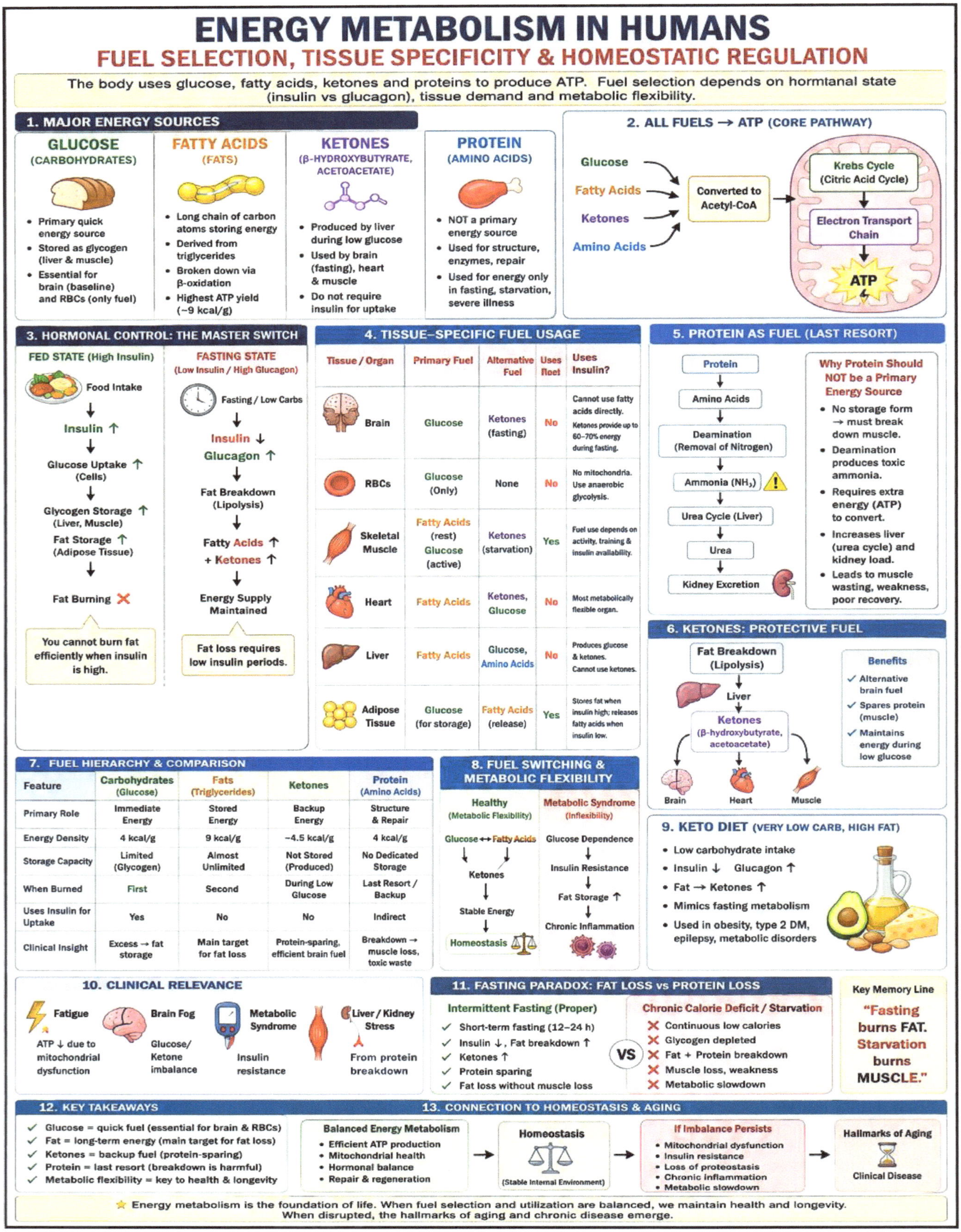

1. Introduction

The human body maintains energy balance through a highly regulated system that utilizes **glucose, fatty acids, ketones, and proteins** to generate ATP. This process is tightly controlled by hormonal signals—primarily **insulin (fed state)** and **low insulin/glucagon (fasting state)**.

Energy metabolism is not uniform; different tissues have **specific fuel preferences**, and this flexibility is essential for maintaining **homeostasis** and adapting to physiological stress.

2. What is ATP and Why It Matters

ATP (Adenosine Triphosphate) is the universal energy currency of the cell.

All fuels—carbohydrates, fats, proteins, and ketones—are ultimately converted into ATP via:

- Glycolysis
- Citric Acid (Krebs) Cycle
- Electron Transport Chain

3. Major Energy Sources

3.1 Glucose (Carbohydrates)

- Primary **quick energy source**
- Stored as **glycogen** (liver & muscle)
- Essential for:
    - Brain (baseline)
    - RBCs (only fuel)

3.2 Fatty Acids (Fats)

What is a Fatty Acid?

A **fatty acid** is a long chain of carbon atoms that stores energy in chemical bonds.

- Derived from **triglycerides**
- Broken down via **β-oxidation**
- Produces **highest ATP per gram (~9 kcal/g)**

3.3 Proteins (Amino Acids)

Proteins are **not primary energy sources**.

- Used mainly for:
    - Structure
    - Enzymes
    - Repair

Used for energy only when:

- Fasting
- Starvation
- Severe illness

3.4 Ketones

- Produced by liver during **low glucose**
- Used by:
    - Brain (fasting)
    - Heart
    - Muscle

🧠 4. Tissue-Specific Fuel Usage

🧠 Brain

- Primary: Glucose
- Fasting: Ketones (up to 60–70%)

👉 Cannot use fatty acids directly

🩸 Red Blood Cells (RBCs)

- Only fuel: **Glucose**

👉 Reason:

- No mitochondria
- Use **anaerobic glycolysis**

💪 Skeletal Muscle

- Rest: Fatty acids
- Exercise: Glucose
- Starvation: Ketones

🧡 Heart

- Primary: Fatty acids
- Also uses: Ketones, glucose

👉 Most metabolically flexible organ

🏭 Liver

- Uses: Fatty acids
- Produces: Glucose & ketones

👉 Cannot use ketones

🧈 Adipose Tissue

- Stores fat (insulin-driven)
- Releases fatty acids (fasting)

📊 5. Summary Table

Tissue	Primary Fuel	Alternative	Special Note
Brain	Glucose	Ketones	No fatty acids
RBCs	Glucose	None	No mitochondria
Muscle	Fat/Glucose	Ketones	Activity-dependent
Heart	Fatty acids	Ketones/Glucose	Highly flexible
Liver	Fatty acids	Glucose/Amino acids	Produces ketones

🔁 6. Flowchart: Energy Production

🔬 All Fuels → ATP

Glucose/Fat/Protein/Ketones
↓
Converted to Acetyl-CoA
↓
Krebs Cycle (Mitochondria)
↓
Electron Transport Chain
↓
ATP ⚡

⚖️ 7. Role of Insulin (Fed vs Fasting State)

🍽️ Fed State (High Insulin)

Food Intake
↓
Insulin ↑
↓
Glucose Uptake ↑
↓
Glycogen Storage + Fat Storage
↓
Reduced Fat Burning

🔥 Fasting State (Low Insulin)

Fasting/Low Carbs
↓
Insulin ↓ | Glucagon ↑
↓
Fat Breakdown (Lipolysis)
↓
Fatty Acids + Ketones
↓
Energy Supply Maintained

Understanding Insulin: The Master Switch

🍽️ When Insulin is HIGH (Fed State)

- Glucose enters cells
- Liver stores glycogen
- Excess glucose → fat (lipogenesis)
- Fat burning is **blocked**

👉 Key Point:

You cannot burn fat efficiently when insulin is high.

🔥 When Insulin is LOW (Fasting State)

- Fat breakdown (lipolysis) starts
- Fatty acids released

- Liver produces ketones
- Body shifts to **fat-burning mode**

👉 **Key Point:**

Fat loss requires **low insulin periods**

🧬 8. Is Protein Used for Energy?

✅ **YES — But Not Preferred**

🔁 **Flowchart: Protein as Fuel**

Protein
↓
Amino Acids
↓
Liver (Gluconeogenesis)
↓
Glucose
↓
ATP

⚠️ **Key Points**

- Used only in **energy deficit**
- Leads to **muscle breakdown**
- Produces **nitrogen waste (urea)**

🔥 9. Fuel Switching: The Key to Fat Loss

🧠 **Healthy Body = Metabolic Flexibility**

Ability to switch between:

- Glucose (fed)
- Fat (fasting)

❌ **Metabolic Syndrome = Inflexibility**

- Always dependent on glucose
- Cannot access fat stores
- Frequent hunger + fatigue

🧬 10. Role of Each Fuel in Weight Loss

🍞 **Glucose**

- Needed for:
  - Brain
  - RBCs

👉 Excess → stored as fat

🧈 **Fat (Stored Energy)**

- Primary fuel during fasting
- Largest energy reserve

👉 **Target for fat loss**

🔥 Add-On: Ketones & Keto Diet

Component	Definition	Role	When Activated	Clinical Meaning
🔥 Ketones	Molecules (β-hydroxybutyrate, acetoacetate) made in liver	Alternative fuel	Low glucose/ fasting	Brain energy backup
🥑 Keto Diet	Very low-carb, high-fat diet	Promotes ketone production	Low insulin state	Mimics fasting metabolism

🔥 Ketones

- Produced when fat is used
- Efficient brain fuel

👉 Sign of **fat metabolism activation**

🧬 Protein

🧠 Core Principle

The human body is not designed to use protein as a primary fuel because protein has essential structural and functional roles, and its breakdown for energy creates metabolic stress and clinical consequences.

⚛️ Biochemical Limitation: No Storage Form

Unlike glucose and fat:

- **Carbohydrates → stored as glycogen**
- **Fat → stored as triglycerides**
- **Protein →** ❌ ***no dedicated storage form***
- Preserves muscle
- Used only when:
  - Severe deficit
  - Poor nutrition

👉 Excess breakdown = **muscle loss**

👉 Therefore:

Using protein for energy = breaking down **functional tissue (muscle, enzymes, organs)**

Energy Production from Protein is Metabolically Costly

🔁 Pathway

Protein
↓
Amino Acids
↓
Deamination (removal of nitrogen)
↓
Carbon skeleton → Glucose or Krebs cycle
↓
ATP

⚠️ Clinical Issue

Deamination Produces Toxic Ammonia (NH_3)

- Ammonia is neurotoxic
- Must be converted to urea in liver

🔁 Urea Cycle Burden

Ammonia (toxic)
↓
Liver (Urea Cycle)
↓
Urea
↓
Kidney Excretion

🩺 **Clinical Relevance:**

- Increased liver workload
- Increased kidney load
- Risk in:
  - CKD patients
  - Liver disease

👉 **Key Concept:**

Protein requires **extra energy (ATP cost)** to convert into usable fuel → **metabolic inefficiency**

🎯 Key Takeaways

- Glucose = quick fuel
- Fat = long-term energy
- Ketones = backup fuel
- Protein = last resort

👉 **Homeostasis depends on fuel flexibility**

Final Integration Diagram

Fuel Intake (Glucose, Fat, Protein)
↓
Hormonal Control (Insulin/Glucagon)
↓
Energy Pathways (ATP Production)
↓
Mitochondrial Function ⚡
↓

IF BALANCED → Homeostasis ⚖️

↓
Healthy Aging

IF IMBALANCED → Dysfunction ❌

↓
Hallmarks of Aging
↓
Clinical Disease

Summary

The type, availability, and utilization of metabolic fuels determine mitochondrial efficiency and cellular balance. When this system is disrupted, it initiates and accelerates the hallmarks of aging, ultimately manifesting as clinical disease.

📊 Master Integrated Table: Energy Sources, Tissue Usage & Metabolic Hierarchy

Tissue/Feature	Primary Fuel	Alternative Fuel	Uses Insulin?	Role in Body	Energy Density	Storage	When Used	Clinical Insight
🧠 Brain	Glucose	Ketones (fasting)	No	High-energy organ	4 kcal/g (glucose)	Limited	First	Cannot use fat directly → needs glucose or ketones
🩸 RBCs	Glucose ONLY	None	No	Oxygen transport	4 kcal/g	None	Always	No mitochondria → cannot use fat/ketones
💪 Muscle	Fat (rest), Glucose (active)	Ketones	Yes	Movement & metabolism	Mixed	Moderate	Flexible	Key site of insulin resistance
❤️ Heart	Fatty acids	Ketones, Glucose	No	Continuous work	9 kcal/g (fat)	High	Continuous	Most energy-efficient organ
🏭 Liver	Fatty acids	Glucose, Amino acids	No	Metabolic control	Mixed	Moderate	Always active	Produces ketones, cannot use them
🧈 Adipose	Fat storage	Glucose (for storage)	Yes	Energy reservoir	9 kcal/g	Very High	Storage state	Central in obesity
🍞 Carbohydrates	Glucose	—	Yes	Immediate energy	4 kcal/g	Limited (glycogen)	First	Prevents protein breakdown
🧈 Fats	Fatty acids	Ketones (via liver)	No	Long-term energy	9 kcal/g	Almost unlimited	Second	Main fat-loss target
🧬 Protein	Amino acids	Glucose (via liver)	Indirect	Structure & repair	4 kcal/g	❌ None	Last resort	

Fasting burns fat, starvation burns muscle - Fuel Switching in Fasting vs Starvation

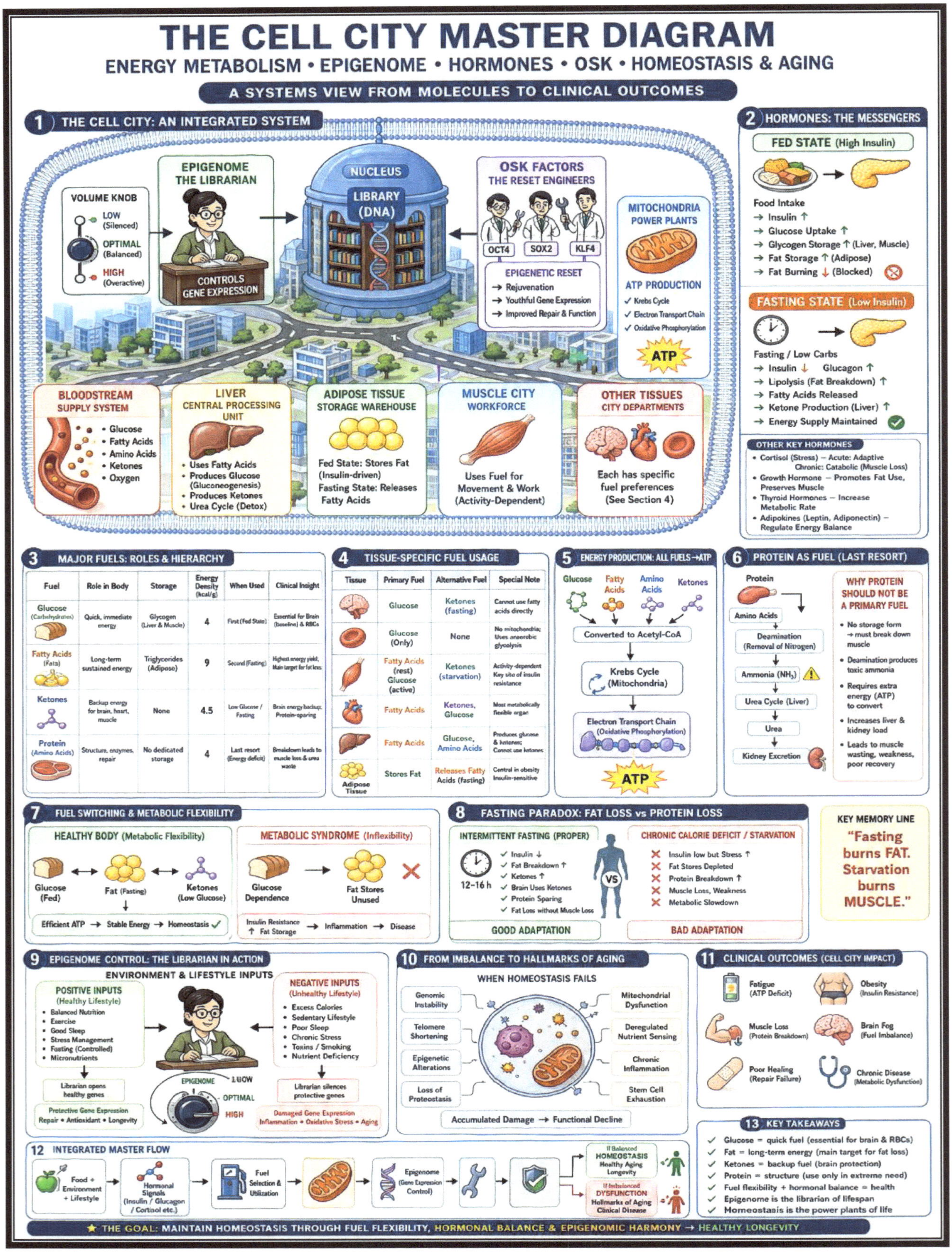

🧠 1. The Root of the Confusion

Situation	What Happens
❌ Chronic calorie deficit	Protein breakdown (bad)
✅ Intermittent fasting (proper)	Fat burning + protein sparing (good)

🔥 2. The Key Difference = ADAPTATION + DURATION

❌ A. Chronic Calorie Deficit (Danger Zone)

Low Calories (continuous)
↓
Glycogen Depleted
↓
Fat + Protein Breakdown
↓
Muscle Loss ⚠️

👉 Happens in:

- Crash dieting
- Undereating daily
- Poor nutrition

✅ B. Intermittent Fasting (Controlled Physiology)

Short Fasting (12–16 hrs)
↓
Insulin ↓
↓
Fat Breakdown ↑
↓
Ketones ↑
↓
Protein Sparing ✅

👉 Key Point:

Intermittent fasting works because the body **switches to fat and ketones BEFORE breaking protein.**

🧬 3. The Role of Ketones

🔁 Without Ketones

Low Glucose
↓
Body Needs Energy
↓
Protein Breakdown ⚠️

🔁 With Ketones (Fasting Adaptation)

Low Glucose
↓
Fat Breakdown
↓
Ketones Produced
↓
Brain Uses Ketones
↓
Protein Breakdown ↓ ✅

👉 Ketones act as a **protein-sparing mechanism**

⚖️ 4. Time Matters (Very Important)

⏱️ Short-Term Fasting (Safe)

- Uses glycogen → fat → ketones
- Minimal protein loss

⏱️ Prolonged Starvation (Danger)

- Fat stores ↓
- Body forced to use protein

👉 So:

Duration	Effect
12–24 hrs	Fat burning
24–72 hrs	Ketones ↑
Prolonged	Protein breakdown ↑

🧠 5. Why Intermittent Fasting is NOT Muscle Wasting

Because:

- Growth hormone ↑
- Insulin ↓ (fat burning)
- Ketones ↑ (brain fuel)

👉 Net effect:

Body protects muscle and uses **fat instead**

⚠️ 6. When Intermittent Fasting CAN Cause Protein Loss

❌ Wrong Way

- Very low calories overall
- No protein intake
- Excess stress
- Over-exercise

🔁 **Result**

Fasting + Undernutrition
↓
No energy reserve
↓
Protein breakdown ⚠️

🧠 **7. Clinical Interpretation**

🩺 **Scenario 1: Healthy IF**

- Adequate nutrition
- Controlled fasting

👉 Result:

- Fat loss
- Protein preserved

🩺 **Scenario 2: Crash Diet**

- Continuous deficit
- Poor nutrition

👉 Result:

- Muscle loss
- Metabolic slowdown

🔗 **8. CONNECTION TO HALLMARKS OF AGING**

Protein used as fuel
↓
Proteostasis disruption
↓
Misfolded proteins ↑
↓
Cellular stress ↑
↓
Hallmarks of Aging:
• Loss of proteostasis
• Mitochondrial dysfunction
• Inflammation
↓
Clinical disease

🔗 **Link to Hallmarks of Aging**

✅ **Proper Fasting**

- Improves:
  - Autophagy
  - Mitochondrial function
  - Insulin sensitivity

❌ Chronic Undereating

- Causes:
  - Loss of proteostasis
  - Muscle loss
  - Frailty

🎯 9. Final Simple Explanation

Intermittent fasting and protein breakdown are not contradictory concepts. Short-term fasting promotes a metabolic switch from glucose to fat and ketone utilization, which protects muscle protein. In contrast, chronic calorie deficiency without adequate nutrition forces the body into a catabolic state where protein is used as a backup fuel. Thus, the difference lies not in fasting itself, but in duration, nutritional adequacy, and metabolic adaptation.

⚖️ The Core Principle (Very Important)

👉 Protein as a nutrient (good, essential) vs Protein used as fuel (stress response, not ideal)

Once we separate these, the paradox disappears.

👉 Eating protein ≠ body using protein for energy

- When the body **uses protein for energy** → it means:
  - Energy shortage (calorie deficit, illness, starvation)
  - Muscle breakdown (catabolism)
  - Metabolic stress
- When you **eat protein properly** → it is used for:
  - Muscle maintenance
  - Enzymes & hormones
  - Hair, skin, nails (keratin, collagen)
  - Immune function

Proteins are not just structural—they are **direct precursors of many hormones**. But here's the key clarification:

👉 Some hormones ARE proteins
👉 Some hormones are MADE FROM amino acids (derived from proteins)

Protein-Based Hormones (Peptide/Protein Hormones)

These hormones are literally made of proteins (chains of amino acids).

🩺 Major Protein Hormones

- Insulin → regulates blood glucose
- Glucagon → raises blood glucose
- Growth Hormone (GH) → growth, metabolism
- Prolactin → milk production
- ADH (Vasopressin) → water balance (kidney)
- Oxytocin → uterine contraction, bonding

👉 Clinical point:
If protein intake is very low → synthesis of these hormones can be affected.

Amino Acid–Derived Hormones

These are not full proteins, but are made from single amino acids (from dietary protein).

A. From Tyrosine

- Thyroid hormones (T3, T4)
- Dopamine
- Norepinephrine
- Epinephrine (Adrenaline)

👉 Roles:

- Metabolism
- Stress response
- Brain function

B. From Tryptophan

- Serotonin → mood, sleep
- Melatonin → circadian rhythm

👉 **Clinical link:**

- Low protein → mood issues, sleep disturbance

Hormones NOT Made from Protein (Important Contrast)

Not all hormones come from protein.

Type	Made From	Examples
🧬 **Protein hormones**	**Amino acids**	**Insulin, GH**
⚡ **Amino acid-derived**	**Single amino acid**	**Thyroid, adrenaline**
🧈 **Steroid hormones**	**Cholesterol (fat)**	**Cortisol, estrogen, testosterone**

👉 **This is why:**

- Low fat → hormone issues (steroids)
- Low protein → peptide + neurotransmitter issues

📚 **Scientific References**

🔬 **Energy Metabolism & ATP**

1. http://www.ncbi.nlm.nih.gov/books/NBK22436/
2. http://www.ncbi.nlm.nih.gov/books/NBK26882/

🍞 **Glucose Metabolism**

3. http://www.ncbi.nlm.nih.gov/books/NBK22436/
4. http://pubmed.ncbi.nlm.nih.gov/21372343/

🧈 **Fatty Acid Metabolism**

5. http://www.ncbi.nlm.nih.gov/books/NBK556002/
6. http://pubmed.ncbi.nlm.nih.gov/24789821/

🔥 **Ketone Bodies**

7. http://www.ncbi.nlm.nih.gov/books/NBK22414/
8. http://pubmed.ncbi.nlm.nih.gov/19641727/

🧬 **Protein & Amino Acid Metabolism**

9. http://www.ncbi.nlm.nih.gov/books/NBK22436/
10. http://pubmed.ncbi.nlm.nih.gov/20307394/

🧠 **Tissue-Specific Metabolism**

11. http://pubmed.ncbi.nlm.nih.gov/17683933/
12. http://pubmed.ncbi.nlm.nih.gov/24655533/

⚖️ **Hormonal Regulation (Insulin & Glucagon)**

13. http://www.ncbi.nlm.nih.gov/books/NBK279012/
14. http://pubmed.ncbi.nlm.nih.gov/25471307/

🔁 **Fasting & Metabolic Switching**

15. http://pubmed.ncbi.nlm.nih.gov/28446414/
16. http://pubmed.ncbi.nlm.nih.gov/29951594/

💪 **Protein Catabolism**

17. http://pubmed.ncbi.nlm.nih.gov/22570379/
18. http://pubmed.ncbi.nlm.nih.gov/11348563/

🧬 **Aging & Metabolism**

19. http://pubmed.ncbi.nlm.nih.gov/23746838/
20. http://pubmed.ncbi.nlm.nih.gov/19187778/

🧬 **Peptide/Protein Hormones**

21. http://www.ncbi.nlm.nih.gov/books/NBK279054/
22. http://www.ncbi.nlm.nih.gov/books/NBK278938/
23. http://www.ncbi.nlm.nih.gov/books/NBK538259/

🧪 **Amino Acid–Derived Hormones**

🧠 **Tyrosine-Derived**

24. http://www.ncbi.nlm.nih.gov/books/NBK279031/
25. http://www.ncbi.nlm.nih.gov/books/NBK285556/

IGF1 - The Paradox of Growth vs Longevity

Why the same signals that build the body may also accelerate its aging?

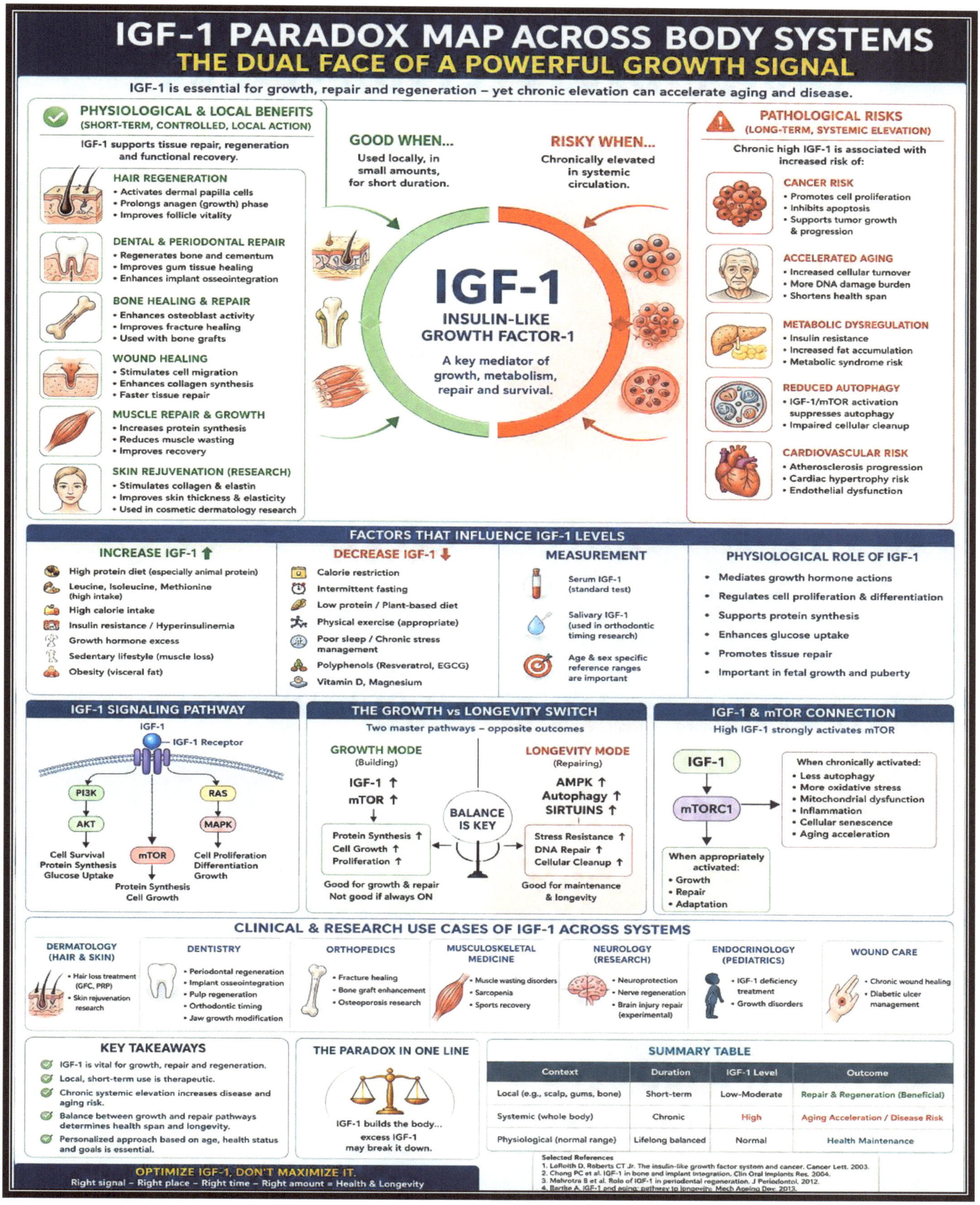

IGF-1 (Insulin-like Growth Factor 1) is a peptide hormone that plays a key role in:

- cell growth and proliferation
- tissue repair and regeneration
- protein synthesis
- overall body development

👉 It is called "insulin-like" because its structure is similar to insulin, but its function is mainly related to growth and development.

💡 Simple definition

"IGF-1 is a growth-promoting hormone that mediates the effects of growth hormone and regulates cell growth, repair, and metabolism in the human body."

🏭 Which Organ Produces IGF-1?

🟢 Primary Organ: Liver

👉 The **liver** is the main organ that produces IGF-1.

- Growth Hormone (GH) from the pituitary gland stimulates the liver
- The liver then releases IGF-1 into the bloodstream

💡 Flow:
Pituitary (GH) → Liver → IGF-1 → Body tissues

🟡 Secondary (Local) Production

IGF-1 is also produced in small amounts by other tissues for **local action**:

- muscles 💪
- bones 🦴
- skin 🧴
- brain 🧠
- kidneys

👉 This is called:
"Paracrine/Autocrine IGF-1" (local effect)

🧠 Simple Analogy

- Pituitary gland = "Commander"
- Liver = "Factory"
- IGF-1 = "Growth messenger"

🎯 One-Line Summary

"IGF-1 is a growth-regulating hormone primarily produced by the liver under the stimulation of growth hormone, with additional local production in various tissues for repair and regeneration."

Growth is often associated with health, stronger muscles, thicker hair, faster recovery, and youthful skin—all are signs of a body that is actively building, repairing, and regenerating itself. At the center of this biological activity lies a powerful network of growth signals, among which **Insulin-like Growth Factor 1 (IGF-1)** plays a central role.

Yet, a deeper examination reveals a striking paradox:

The very pathways that promote growth and vitality in the short term may, when persistently activated, accelerate aging and increase disease risk.

Understanding IGF-1: The Growth Signal

IGF-1 is a hormone primarily produced in response to growth hormone. It acts as a key regulator of:

- cellular growth and proliferation
- protein synthesis
- tissue repair and regeneration

In physiological terms, IGF-1 is essential for:

- childhood growth
- muscle maintenance
- wound healing

In simple language:

IGF-1 tells the body to grow, build, and multiply.

The Dual Nature of Growth Signals

The biological effects of IGF-1 are not inherently harmful. In fact, they are necessary for survival. However, problems arise when these signals are **chronically elevated**.

Short-Term/Controlled Activation

- tissue repair
- muscle growth
- improved recovery
- follicle stimulation (e.g., hair growth)

Long-Term/Chronic Elevation

- increased cellular proliferation
- reduced apoptosis (cell death)
- higher probability of abnormal cell survival

This creates an environment where:

Damaged or mutated cells are more likely to survive and multiply.

IGF-1 and Cancer Risk

Multiple studies have linked elevated systemic IGF-1 levels with an increased risk of certain cancers. The mechanism is not that IGF-1 "causes" cancer directly, but rather that it:

- promotes rapid cell division
- inhibits natural cellular cleanup
- supports survival of abnormal cells

In this sense:

IGF-1 acts as a "fertile ground" rather than a direct trigger.

The Longevity Trade-Off

From an evolutionary perspective, the body balances two competing priorities:

Growth Mode

- driven by IGF-1 and mTOR pathways
- focused on building and reproduction

Repair Mode

- driven by AMPK and autophagy
- focused on maintenance and longevity

These two modes cannot be maximally active at the same time.

When growth pathways are high, repair pathways are suppressed.
When repair pathways are active, growth slows down.

This trade-off forms the foundation of the growth–longevity paradox.

🥩 Diet, Protein, and IGF-1

Dietary patterns significantly influence IGF-1 levels.

High intake of:

- animal protein
- branched-chain amino acids (leucine, isoleucine)
- methionine

can stimulate:

- IGF-1 production
- mTOR activation

However, it is important to distinguish between:

- **Physiological elevation** (within normal range)
- **Pathological elevation** (disease-level excess)

Not all increases in IGF-1 are harmful—context and magnitude matter.

💉 Clinical Paradox: Growth Factors in Hair Therapy

An interesting contradiction emerges in modern clinical practice.

Treatments such as:

- Growth Factor Concentrate (GFC)
- platelet-rich plasma (PRP)

are widely used in hair restoration.

These therapies involve:

- localized delivery of growth signals
- activation of follicular stem cells
- improved blood flow and regeneration

At first glance, this appears contradictory:

If growth factors can increase cancer risk, why are they used therapeutically?

🧠 Resolving the Paradox

The answer lies in **context, scale, and duration.**

🔹 Systemic IGF-1

- circulates throughout the body
- long-term exposure
- affects multiple organs

🔹 Local Growth Factor Therapy

- applied to a specific area (e.g., scalp)
- short-lived effect
- tightly localized action

Localized, temporary stimulation supports regeneration,
while chronic systemic elevation may promote disease.

🦷 **Dental Uses**

🧹 **Gum Disease Repair**

- In severe gum disease → bone and tissue get damaged
- IGF-1 helps:
  - regrow bone
  - repair supporting tissue

🦴 **Dental Implants**

- When bone is weak → implant may fail
- IGF-1 is used with bone graft

👉 helps implant "stick" strongly to bone

🧬 **Tooth Repair (Pulp Therapy)**

- When tooth is damaged
- IGF-1 activates stem cells

👉 helps form new dentin

🧠 **Summary**

"IGF-1 is like a growth signal that tells teeth, bone, and gums when to repair and grow."

🏥 **MORE Medical Use Cases of IGF-1**

Now expanding beyond hair + dental 👇

💪 **1. Muscle Wasting Disorders**

Used in:

- cachexia
- muscle loss diseases

👉 helps:

- muscle growth
- recovery

🦴 **2. Bone Healing & Fractures**

- used with bone grafts
- improves healing

👉 especially in:

- fractures
- osteoporosis research

🧠 **3. Brain & Nerve Repair (Emerging)**

- studied in:
  - neurodegeneration
  - brain injury

👉 helps:

- neuron survival
- repair pathways

👶 4. Growth Disorders in Children

Approved use in:

- IGF-1 deficiency

👉 helps:

- height growth
- development

❤️ 5. Wound Healing

- used in chronic wounds

👉 helps:

- tissue repair
- faster healing

🧴 6. Skin & Anti-Aging Research

- improves collagen
- enhances skin repair

👉 used in:

- cosmetic dermatology (research level)

💇 7. Hair (Your Original Context)

- follicle activation
- growth phase stimulation

🟠 SAME MOLECULE — TWO OUTCOMES

🟢 When IGF-1 is USED LOCALLY

- hair growth
- bone repair
- gum healing
- wound recovery

👉 **beneficial**

🟠 When IGF-1 is CHRONICALLY HIGH SYSTEMICALLY

- cancer risk
- faster aging
- reduced autophagy

👉 **harmful**

🧠 Summary

"IGF-1 is not good or bad by itself—its impact depends on where, how long, and how much it acts in the body."

Context	Effect
Local + short-term	Healing & regeneration
Systemic + long-term	Aging & disease risk

📚 Scientific References

1. Pollak M. Insulin-like growth factor physiology and cancer risk. *Eur J Cancer*. 2000;36(10):1224–1228.
2. Renehan AG, Zwahlen M, Minder C, O'Dwyer ST, Shalet SM, Egger M. Insulin-like growth factor (IGF)-I, IGF binding protein-3, and cancer risk: systematic review and meta-regression analysis. *Lancet*. 2004;363(9418):1346–1353.
3. Laplante M, Sabatini DM. mTOR signaling in growth control and disease. *Cell*. 2012;149(2):274–293.
4. Kenyon CJ. The genetics of ageing. *Nature*. 2010;464(7288):504–512.

🥩 Diet, Protein & IGF-1

5. Levine ME, Suarez JA, Brandhorst S, et al. Low protein intake is associated with a major reduction in IGF-1, cancer, and overall mortality in the 65 and younger but not older population. *Cell Metab*. 2014;19(3):407–417.
6. Fontana L, Partridge L, Longo VD. Extending healthy life span—from yeast to humans. *Science*. 2010;328(5976):321–326.

💇 Hair & Growth Factor Research

7. Gentile P, Garcovich S. Advances in regenerative medicine for hair loss: growth factors and platelet-rich plasma. *Dermatol Surg*. 2019;45(4):503–515.

🦷 Dental & Bone Regeneration

8. Lynch SE, de Castilla GR, Williams RC, et al. The effects of short-term application of a combination of platelet-derived and insulin-like growth factors on periodontal wound healing. *J Periodontol*. 1991;62(7):458–467.
9. Giannobile WV. Periodontal tissue engineering by growth factors. *Bone*. 1996;19(1 Suppl):23S–37S.

💪🧠 Muscle, Brain & Repair

10. Florini JR, Ewton DZ, Coolican SA. Growth hormone and the insulin-like growth factor system in myogenesis. *Endocr Rev*. 1996;17(5):481–517.
11. Dyer AH, Vahdatpour C, Sanfeliu A, Tropea D. The role of insulin-like growth factor 1 (IGF-1) in brain development, maturation and neuroplasticity. *Neuroscience*. 2016;325:89–99.

🧡 Metabolic Effects

12. Clemmons DR. Role of IGF-1 in controlling glucose homeostasis. *Horm Res*. 2004;62(Suppl 1):77–82.

🌿 Integration of Hallmarks of Aging in Cancer Biology: Pathways, Mechanisms, and Clinical Relevance

Aging is characterized by a gradual decline in cellular and physiological function, leading to increased susceptibility to chronic diseases, including cancer. The concept of the *hallmarks of aging* has provided a structured framework to explain the molecular basis of aging. Interestingly, many of these hallmarks overlap with mechanisms that drive cancer development.

Cancer can be viewed as a pathological state in which normal cellular processes—such as growth, repair, and survival—are dysregulated. Integrating aging biology with cancer research enables a systems-level understanding of disease progression and therapeutic targeting.

Hallmark of Aging	Pathway/Target	Therapeutic Strategy	Major Cancer Types	Key Concept (Exam Point)
Genomic Instability	DNA repair (PARP)	DNA repair targeting	Breast (BRCA), Ovarian	Targets defective DNA repair
	DNA replication	Cytotoxic therapy	Many solid tumors	Induces lethal DNA damage
Epigenetic Alterations	DNA methylation	Epigenetic modulation	AML, MDS	Reverses abnormal gene silencing
	Histone modification	Chromatin regulation	T-cell lymphoma	Restores gene expression
Deregulated Nutrient Sensing	mTOR pathway	Growth pathway inhibition	Renal, Breast	↓ Growth, ↑ Autophagy
	PI3K/AKT	Survival pathway inhibition	Leukemia, Lymphoma	Blocks survival signaling
Uncontrolled Proliferation	Cell cycle (CDK4/6)	Cell cycle inhibition	Breast cancer	Stops cell cycle progression
Apoptosis Resistance	BCL-2 pathway	Apoptosis induction	CLL, AML	Promotes cancer cell death
Loss of Proteostasis	Autophagy/lysosome	Autophagy modulation	Experimental (many cancers)	Affects protein clearance
	Proteasome	Protein degradation targeting	Multiple Myeloma	Blocks protein degradation
Mitochondrial Dysfunction	Metabolism	Metabolic modulation	Multiple (research)	Alters tumor energy supply
Cellular Senescence	Senescent cell survival	Senescence targeting	Experimental	Removes dysfunctional cells
Inflammaging	Cytokines (IL-6, TNF)	Anti-inflammatory strategy	Colon, liver cancers	Reduces chronic inflammation
Altered Intercellular Communication	Immune checkpoints	Immune modulation	Melanoma, Lung	Reactivates immune response
	Angiogenesis	Vascular targeting	Colon, renal	Reduces tumor blood supply
Stem Cell Exhaustion/ Renewal	Stemness pathways	Differentiation therapy	Acute Promyelocytic Leukemia	Promotes cellular maturation

Cancer Biology Through Hallmarks of Aging

🧬 Genomic Instability

🧠 Core Principle

Cancer begins when DNA damage accumulates beyond repair capacity.

🔬 Mechanism

DNA damage
↓
Defective repair
↓
Mutations accumulate
↓
Oncogene activation/Tumor suppressor loss

🎯 Key Points

- DNA = Instruction manual 📖
- Damage = Wrong instructions ❌
- Repair failure = Permanent errors

👉 Result: **Cancer initiation**

🎚️ Epigenetic Alterations

🧠 Core Principle

Gene expression becomes dysregulated without changing DNA sequence.

⚛️ Concept

- DNA = Digital code 💿
- Epigenome = Volume control 🎚️ (analog)

🔬 Mechanism

Epigenetic drift
↓
Wrong gene expression levels
↓
Oncogenes ↑/Tumor suppressors ↓

🎯 Key Points

- Not ON/OFF ❌
- It's a spectrum 🔈🔉🔊
- Cell forgets its identity

👉 Result: **Cell behaves abnormally**

⚙️ Deregulated Nutrient Sensing

🧠 Core Principle

Growth pathways remain constantly activated.

🔬 Pathway

Insulin/IGF-1
↓
PI3K–AKT
↓
mTOR activation

🎯 **Key Points**

- Growth switch stuck ON ⚙️
- Autophagy OFF 🧹❌
- Cells grow even when not needed

👉 Result: **Uncontrolled growth**

🔁 **Uncontrolled Proliferation**

🧠 **Core Principle**

Cell cycle checkpoints fail.

🔬 **Mechanism**

Checkpoint failure
↓
Continuous division
↓
Tumor expansion

🎯 **Key Points**

- Normal = controlled division
- Cancer = endless division 🔁

👉 Result: **Tumor mass formation**

🛑 **Apoptosis Resistance**

🧠 **Core Principle**

Damaged cells refuse to die.

🔬 **Mechanism**

Apoptosis signals blocked
↓
Survival of abnormal cells

🎯 **Key Points**

- Normal = delete damaged cells 🗑️
- Cancer = survival of damaged cells ❌

👉 Result: **Accumulation of abnormal cells**

🧹 **Loss of Proteostasis**

🧠 **Core Principle**

Protein quality control system fails.

🔬 **Mechanism**

Misfolded proteins
↓
Poor clearance
↓
Accumulation

🎯 **Key Points**

- Cell = factory 🏭
- Defective products accumulate ❌
- Cleaning system weak 🧹

👉 Result: **Cell dysfunction**

🪫 **Mitochondrial Dysfunction**

🧠 **Core Principle**

Energy system becomes abnormal.

🔬 **Mechanism**

Mitochondrial damage
↓
↓ ATP + ↑ ROS
↓
Metabolic shift

🎯 **Key Points**

- Battery weak 🪫❌
- Energy inefficient
- Cancer uses alternative fuel

👉 Result: **Metabolic reprogramming**

🧟 **Cellular Senescence**

🧠 **Core Principle**

Cells stop dividing but remain metabolically active.

🔬 **Mechanism**

Damage
↓
Cell cycle arrest
↓
SASP release

🎯 **Key Points**

- Zombie cells 🧟
- Not dividing but harmful
- Release inflammatory signals

👉 Result: **Tumor-promoting environment**

🔥 **Inflammaging**

🧠 **Core Principle**

Chronic inflammation drives cancer progression.

🔬 **Mechanism**

Cytokines (IL-6, TNF)
↓
DNA damage + signaling
↓
Tumor promotion

🎯 **Key Points**

- Slow fire 🔥
- Continuous damage
- Supports tumor growth

👉 Result: **Cancer progression**

📡 **Altered Intercellular Communication**

🧠 **Core Principle**

Cells stop communicating properly.

🔬 **Mechanism**

Signal disruption
↓
Immune evasion
↓
Tumor survival

🎯 **Key Points**

- Messages distorted 📩❌
- Immune system confused
- Tumor hides

👉 Result: **Immune escape**

👷 **Stem Cell Dysfunction**

🧠 **Core Principle**

Repair system becomes defective.

🔬 **Mechanism**

Stem cell exhaustion
↓
Abnormal self-renewal
↓
Cancer stem cells

🎯 **Key Points**

- Repair engineers 👷 decrease
- Some become rogue
- Drive recurrence

👉 Result: **Tumor initiation + relapse**

🎯 **FINAL INTEGRATION**

👉 Cancer = ⚙️ Growth ON + 🧹 Cleaning OFF + 🧟 No death (cells that should die but do NOT die) + 🔥 Inflammation + 📡 Signal failure

📚 **Scientific References**

López-Otín C, Blasco MA, Partridge L, Serrano M, Kroemer G. The hallmarks of aging. *Cell*. 2013;153(6):1194–1217.

Hanahan D, Weinberg RA. Hallmarks of cancer: the next generation. *Cell*. 2011;144(5):646–674.

Saxton RA, Sabatini DM. mTOR signaling in growth, metabolism, and disease. *Cell*. 2017;168(6):960–976.

Baylin SB, Jones PA. Epigenetic determinants of cancer. *Cold Spring Harb Perspect Biol*. 2016;8(1):a019505.

Campisi J. Aging, cellular senescence, and cancer. *Annu Rev Physiol*. 2013;75:685–705.

Franceschi C, Campisi J. Chronic inflammation (inflammaging) and its potential contribution to age-associated diseases. *J Gerontol A Biol Sci Med Sci*. 2014;69(Suppl 1):S4–S9.

Vander Heiden MG, Cantley LC, Thompson CB. Understanding the Warburg effect: the metabolic requirements of cell proliferation. *Science*. 2009;324(5930):1029–1033.

Loss of Cellular Identity

Every cell in the body contains the same DNA, yet each cell uses only the instructions relevant to its specific role. A skin cell follows “skin” instructions, a brain cell follows “thinking” instructions, and a kidney cell follows “filtration” instructions.

This can be understood by imagining the body as a highly organized system:

- **DNA = the complete instruction manual**
- **Cells = specialized workers**
    - A **skin cell** uses skin instructions
    - A **brain cell** uses thinking instructions
    - A **kidney cell** uses filtration instructions
- **The Job Role:** Each cell reads only the chapter required for its specific function
- **Regulatory proteins = bookmarks** that tell each cell which part of the manual to read

In a healthy state, these “bookmarks” ensure that each cell reads the correct instructions and performs its function precisely.

However, with aging—and especially under conditions of chronic stress, overeating, and continuous high activity—this system begins to lose precision. Scientist describes this state as **“burning the candle at both ends,”** where the body is constantly pushed toward output and growth without adequate time for repair.

Under these conditions, DNA undergoes repeated minor damage. During repair, the regulatory proteins (the “bookmarks”) temporarily leave their positions to fix the damage. The critical problem arises when these proteins do not return exactly to their original locations.

As a result, the cell loses clarity about which instructions to follow.

- A skin cell may begin using instructions not meant for skin
- A brain cell may lose precision in its specialized function

Importantly, cells do not transform into other cell types—but they begin to function incorrectly and lose their specialization.

This process is known as **ex-differentiation**, meaning a gradual loss of cellular identity and functional precision.

At the same time, chronic overextension suppresses key longevity pathways such as **sirtuins**, which are essential for DNA repair and maintaining the organization of the epigenome—the system that controls which genes are turned on or off.

Over time, this leads to **epigenetic disorganization (epigenetic noise)**, where the cellular instruction system becomes increasingly imprecise.

The result is a progressive decline in the accuracy of gene expression, causing cells to lose their identity, efficiency, and specialized function.

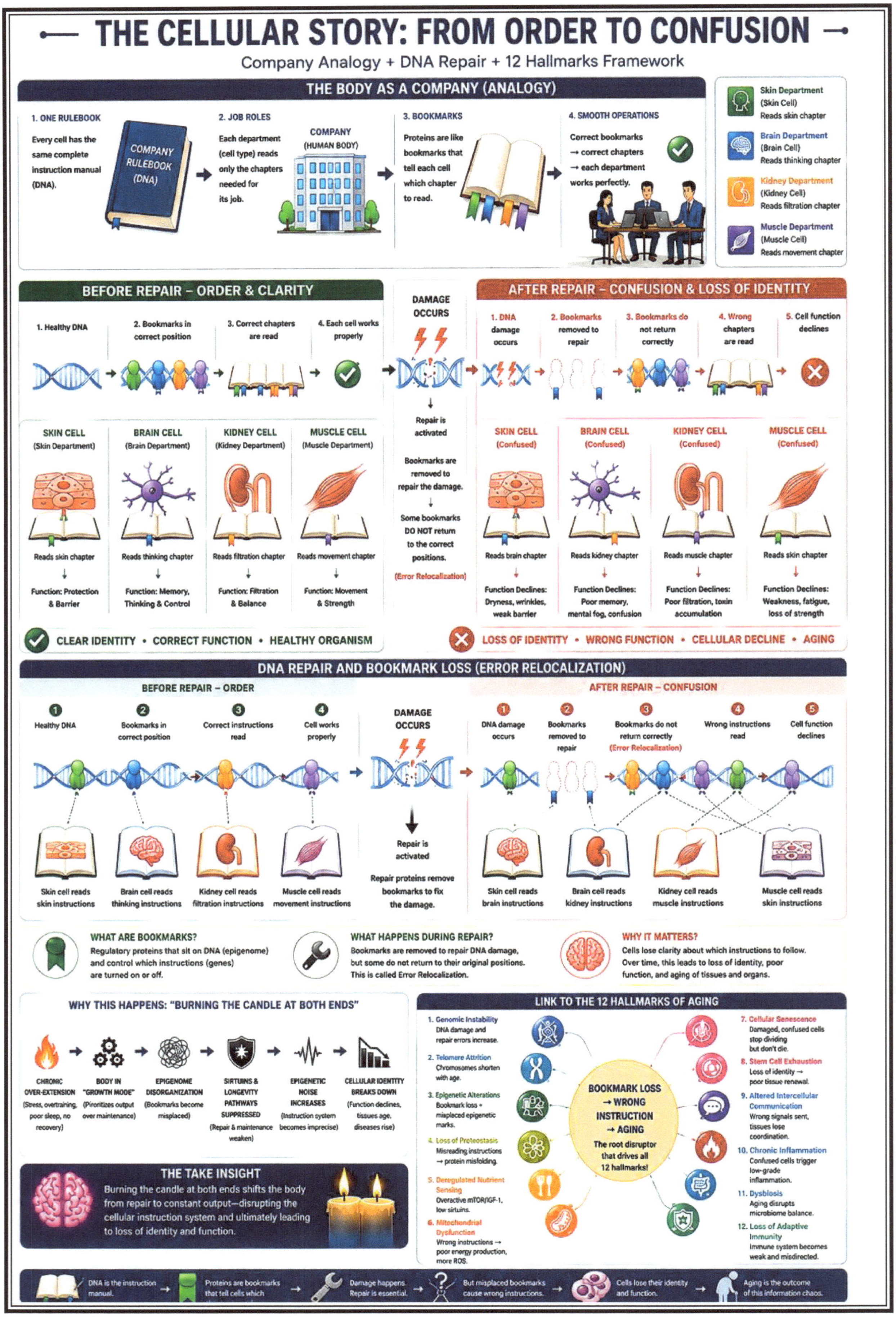
THE CELLULAR STORY: FROM ORDER TO CONFUSION
Company Analogy + DNA Repair + 12 Hallmarks Framework
THE BODY AS A COMPANY (ANALOGY)
1. ONE RULEBOOK
Every cell has the same complete instruction manual (DNA).
COMPANY RULEBOOK (DNA)
2. JOB ROLES
Each department (cell type) reads only the chapters needed for its job.
COMPANY (HUMAN BODY)
3. BOOKMARKS
Proteins are like bookmarks that tell each cell which chapter to read.
4. SMOOTH OPERATIONS
Correct bookmarks → correct chapters → each department works perfectly.
Skin Department (Skin Cell) Reads skin chapter
Brain Department (Brain Cell) Reads thinking chapter
Kidney Department (Kidney Cell) Reads filtration chapter
Muscle Department (Muscle Cell) Reads movement chapter
BEFORE REPAIR – ORDER & CLARITY
1. Healthy DNA
2. Bookmarks in correct position
3. Correct chapters are read
4. Each cell works properly
DAMAGE OCCURS
Repair is activated
Bookmarks are removed to repair the damage.
Some bookmarks DO NOT return to the correct positions.
(Error Relocalization)
AFTER REPAIR – CONFUSION & LOSS OF IDENTITY
1. DNA damage occurs
2. Bookmarks removed to repair
3. Bookmarks do not return correctly
4. Wrong chapters are read
5. Cell function declines
SKIN CELL (Skin Department)
Reads skin chapter
Function: Protection & Barrier
BRAIN CELL (Brain Department)
Reads thinking chapter
Function: Memory, Thinking & Control
KIDNEY CELL (Kidney Department)
Reads filtration chapter
Function: Filtration & Balance
MUSCLE CELL (Muscle Department)
Reads movement chapter
Function: Movement & Strength
SKIN CELL (Confused)
Reads brain chapter
Function Declines: Dryness, wrinkles, weak barrier
BRAIN CELL (Confused)
Reads kidney chapter
Function Declines: Poor memory, mental fog, confusion
KIDNEY CELL (Confused)
Reads muscle chapter
Function Declines: Poor filtration, toxin accumulation
MUSCLE CELL (Confused)
Reads skin chapter
Function Declines: Weakness, fatigue, loss of strength
CLEAR IDENTITY • CORRECT FUNCTION • HEALTHY ORGANISM
LOSS OF IDENTITY • WRONG FUNCTION • CELLULAR DECLINE • AGING
DNA REPAIR AND BOOKMARK LOSS (ERROR RELOCALIZATION)
BEFORE REPAIR – ORDER
1 Healthy DNA
2 Bookmarks in correct position
3 Correct instructions read
4 Cell works properly
DAMAGE OCCURS
Repair is activated
Repair proteins remove bookmarks to fix the damage.
AFTER REPAIR – CONFUSION
1 DNA damage occurs
2 Bookmarks removed to repair
3 Bookmarks do not return correctly (Error Relocalization)
4 Wrong instructions read
5 Cell function declines
Skin cell reads skin instructions
Brain cell reads thinking instructions
Kidney cell reads filtration instructions
Muscle cell reads movement instructions
Skin cell reads brain instructions
Brain cell reads kidney instructions
Kidney cell reads muscle instructions
Muscle cell reads skin instructions
WHAT ARE BOOKMARKS?
Regulatory proteins that sit on DNA (epigenome) and control which instructions (genes) are turned on or off.
WHAT HAPPENS DURING REPAIR?
Bookmarks are removed to repair DNA damage, but some do not return to their original positions. This is called Error Relocalization.
WHY IT MATTERS?
Cells lose clarity about which instructions to follow. Over time, this leads to loss of identity, poor function, and aging of tissues and organs.
WHY THIS HAPPENS: "BURNING THE CANDLE AT BOTH ENDS"
CHRONIC OVER-EXTENSION (Stress, overtraining, poor sleep, no recovery)
BODY IN "GROWTH MODE" (Prioritizes output over maintenance)
EPIGENOME DISORGANIZATION (Bookmarks become misplaced)
SIRTUINS & LONGEVITY PATHWAYS SUPPRESSED (Repair & maintenance weaken)
EPIGENETIC NOISE INCREASES (Instruction system becomes imprecise)
CELLULAR IDENTITY BREAKS DOWN (Function declines, tissues age, diseases rise)
THE TAKE INSIGHT
Burning the candle at both ends shifts the body from repair to constant output—disrupting the cellular instruction system and ultimately leading to loss of identity and function.
LINK TO THE 12 HALLMARKS OF AGING
1. Genomic Instability DNA damage and repair errors increase.
2. Telomere Attrition Chromosomes shorten with age.
3. Epigenetic Alterations Bookmark loss + misplaced epigenetic marks.
4. Loss of Proteostasis Misreading instructions → protein misfolding.
5. Deregulated Nutrient Sensing Overactive mTOR/IGF-1, low sirtuins.
6. Mitochondrial Dysfunction Wrong instructions → poor energy production, more ROS.
BOOKMARK LOSS → WRONG INSTRUCTION → AGING
The root disruptor that drives all 12 hallmarks!
7. Cellular Senescence Damaged, confused cells stop dividing but don't die.
8. Stem Cell Exhaustion Loss of identity → poor tissue renewal.
9. Altered Intercellular Communication Wrong signals sent, tissues lose coordination.
10. Chronic Inflammation Confused cells trigger low-grade inflammation.
11. Dysbiosis Aging disrupts microbiome balance.
12. Loss of Adaptive Immunity Immune system becomes weak and misdirected.
DNA is the instruction manual.
Proteins are bookmarks that tell cells which
Damage happens. Repair is essential.
But misplaced bookmarks cause wrong instructions.
Cells lose their identity and function.
Aging is the outcome of this information chaos.

Homeostasis - The Biology of Balance

Homeostasis = the body's ability to maintain internal balance despite stress

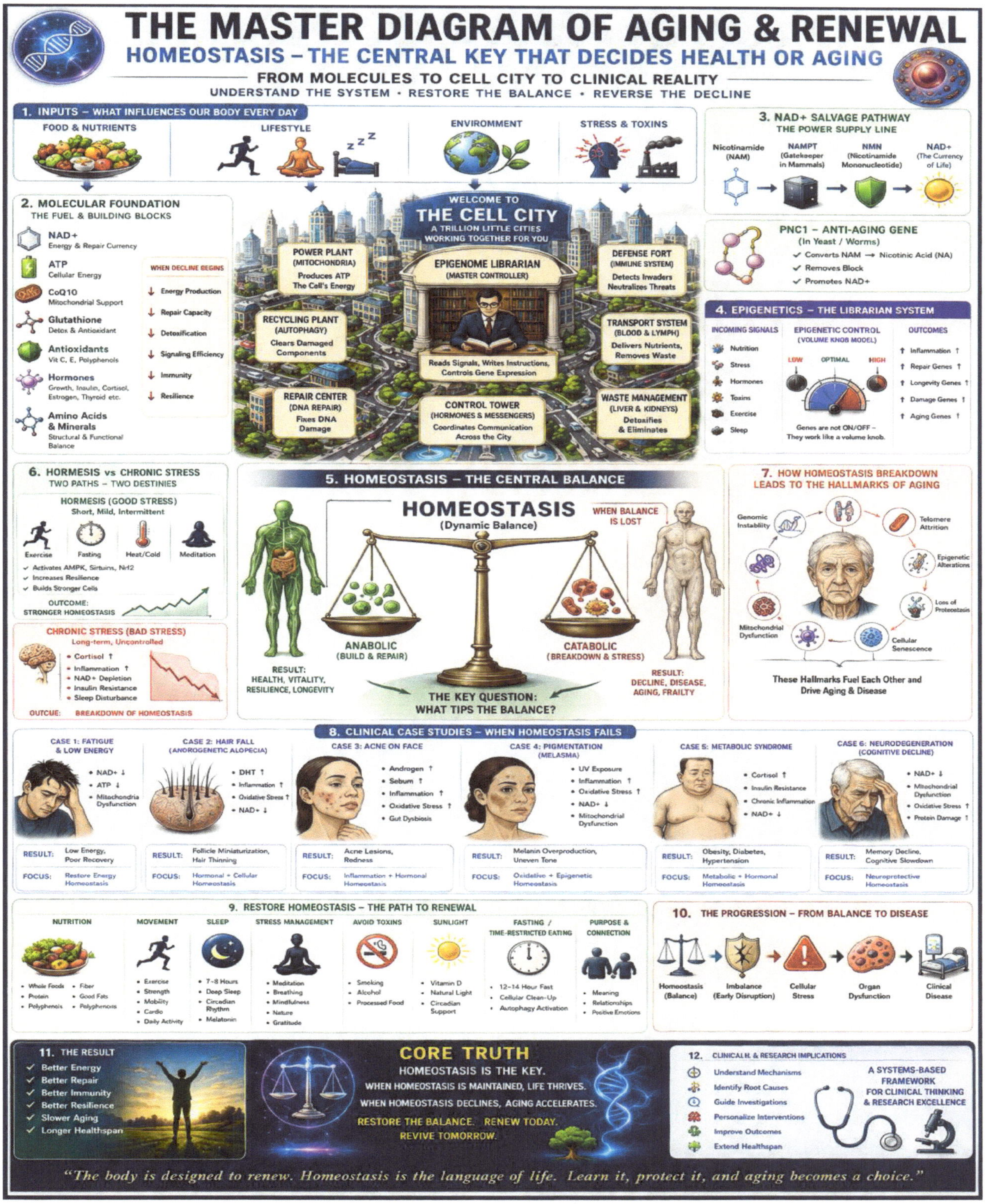

1. Introduction

Biological systems are inherently designed to maintain internal stability despite continuous external and internal challenges. This dynamic equilibrium, known as homeostasis, is essential for survival, optimal cellular function, and long-term health.

Aging can be conceptualized not merely as the passage of time, but as a progressive decline in the body's ability to maintain homeostasis. This decline manifests at multiple biological levels—from molecular imbalance to cellular dysfunction and ultimately to clinical disease.

This chapter presents a systems-level integrative model, connecting molecular biology, epigenetics, metabolism, and clinical observations under the central concept of homeostasis.

2. Definition of Homeostasis

Homeostasis refers to:

The ability of a biological system to maintain a stable internal environment through coordinated physiological, cellular, and molecular processes.

This regulation involves:

- Energy balance
- Redox equilibrium
- Hormonal signaling
- Gene expression control
- Cellular repair and regeneration

3. Multi-Level Organization of Homeostasis

Homeostasis operates across interconnected biological layers:

3.1 Molecular Level

Key molecules essential for homeostasis include:

- NAD^+ (cellular repair and signaling)
- ATP (energy currency)
- Antioxidants (redox balance)
- Hormones (systemic regulation)

Age-Related Changes:

- Decline in NAD^+ and ATP
- Increased oxidative stress
- Hormonal imbalance

3.2 Cellular Level

Cells maintain function through:

- Mitochondrial activity
- DNA repair mechanisms
- Proteostasis
- Autophagy

Age-Related Changes:

- Mitochondrial dysfunction
- Accumulation of DNA damage
- Impaired protein quality control

3.3 Epigenetic Regulation (The "Librarian" Example)

Gene expression is regulated by the epigenome, which functions as a dynamic control system.

Genes are not simply "on" or "off," but are expressed along a continuum depending on cellular needs.

Influencing Factors:

- Nutrition
- Stress
- Sleep
- Environmental exposure

Age-Related Changes:

- Epigenetic drift
- Dysregulated gene expression
- Reduced adaptive capacity

3.4 Hormonal and Signaling Networks

Hormones and signaling molecules coordinate communication between systems.

Balanced State:

- Efficient signaling
- Coordinated physiological response

Imbalance:

- Chronic cortisol elevation
- Insulin resistance
- Impaired metabolic signaling

3.5 Cell Turnover and Regeneration

Homeostasis depends on continuous renewal:

- Stem cell function
- Tissue regeneration
- Removal of damaged cells

Age-Related Changes:

- Slower cell turnover
- Stem cell exhaustion
- Accumulation of senescent cells

4. Integrated Flow of Homeostasis

A simplified systems model can be represented as:

Inputs (Nutrition, Lifestyle, Environment, Stress)

↓

Molecular Balance (NAD^+, ATP, Hormones)

↓

Cellular Function (Mitochondria, DNA Repair, Proteostasis)

↓

Gene Regulation (Epigenetic Control)

↓

Tissue Function (Cell Turnover and Regeneration)

↓

HOMEOSTASIS (Dynamic Balance)
↓
Loss of Balance →
Hallmarks of Aging →
Clinical Disease

⚖️ 5. Hormesis and Stress: Dual Role in Homeostasis

Stress plays a critical role in modulating homeostasis.

✅ 5.1 Hormesis (Adaptive Stress)

- Mild, intermittent stress
- Activates repair pathways (AMPK, sirtuins, Nrf2)
- Enhances resilience

Outcome:

Improved homeostasis and increased biological robustness

❌ 5.2 Chronic Stress (Cortisol Dysregulation)

- Persistent stress exposure
- Sustained cortisol elevation
- Impaired recovery

Outcome:

- Metabolic imbalance
- Inflammation
- Accelerated aging

🧬 6. Loss of Homeostasis and the Hallmarks of Aging

The hallmarks of aging can be understood as manifestations of disrupted homeostasis:

- Genomic instability
- Telomere attrition
- Epigenetic alterations
- Loss of proteostasis
- Mitochondrial dysfunction
- Cellular senescence
- Stem cell exhaustion
- Altered intercellular communication

These processes are interconnected and self-reinforcing, leading to progressive physiological decline.

🩺 7. Clinical Correlates of Homeostatic Failure

The loss of homeostasis manifests clinically across multiple systems:

🧠 7.1 Fatigue and Reduced Energy

- NAD^+ decline
- Mitochondrial dysfunction

🧴 7.2 Skin Aging and Impaired Repair

- Reduced cellular turnover
- Increased oxidative stress

7.3 Neurodegeneration

- Impaired neuronal repair
- Energy deficiency

7.4 Metabolic Disorders

- Hormonal dysregulation
- Insulin resistance
- Chronic inflammation

7.5 Longevity Mechanisms (Experimental Models)

In lower organisms:

- Activation of stress-response genes (e.g., PNC1)
- Increased NAD^+ availability
- Enhanced survival pathways

These findings highlight the evolutionary conservation of homeostatic regulation in aging.

8. A Systems-Level Clinical Framework

Understanding aging through homeostasis allows a structured interpretation:

- Symptoms → reflect disrupted balance
- Molecular changes → underlying drivers
- Cellular dysfunction → mechanistic link

This approach supports:

- Integrated biological understanding
- Mechanism-based clinical reasoning
- Hypothesis generation in research

9. Scientific Considerations

- Homeostasis is dynamic, not static
- Biological systems are complex and nonlinear
- Individual variability influences outcomes
- Not all changes are reversible

Interpretations should remain grounded in evidence-based scientific principles.

10. Conclusion

Aging can be understood as a progressive loss of biological homeostasis, where disturbances at the molecular level propagate through cellular systems, leading to functional decline and disease.

This integrative model provides a unifying framework that connects:

- Molecular biology
- Epigenetic regulation
- Cellular function
- Clinical manifestations

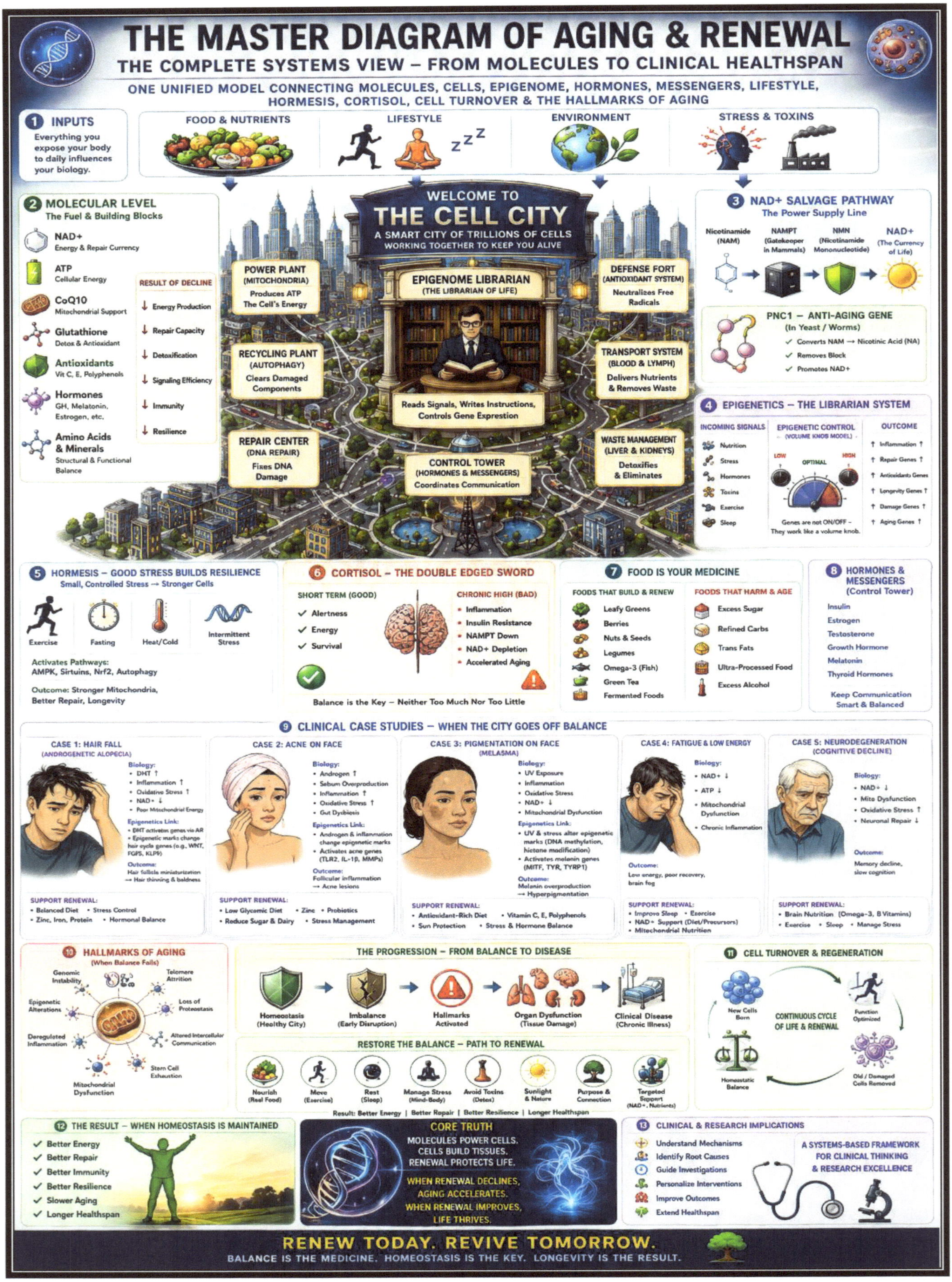
THE MASTER DIAGRAM OF AGING & RENEWAL
THE COMPLETE SYSTEMS VIEW – FROM MOLECULES TO CLINICAL HEALTHSPAN
ONE UNIFIED MODEL CONNECTING MOLECULES, CELLS, EPIGENOME, HORMONES, MESSENGERS, LIFESTYLE, HORMESIS, CORTISOL, CELL TURNOVER & THE HALLMARKS OF AGING
1 INPUTS
Everything you expose your body to daily influences your biology.
FOOD & NUTRIENTS
LIFESTYLE
ENVIRONMENT
STRESS & TOXINS
2 MOLECULAR LEVEL
The Fuel & Building Blocks
NAD+
Energy & Repair Currency
ATP
Cellular Energy
CoQ10
Mitochondrial Support
Glutathione
Detox & Antioxidant
Antioxidants
Vit C, E, Polyphenols
Hormones
GH, Melatonin, Estrogen, etc.
Amino Acids & Minerals
Structural & Functional Balance
RESULT OF DECLINE
↓ Energy Production
↓ Repair Capacity
↓ Detoxification
↓ Signaling Efficiency
↓ Immunity
↓ Resilience
WELCOME TO
THE CELL CITY
A SMART CITY OF TRILLIONS OF CELLS WORKING TOGETHER TO KEEP YOU ALIVE
POWER PLANT (MITOCHONDRIA)
Produces ATP
The Cell's Energy
EPIGENOME LIBRARIAN (THE LIBRARIAN OF LIFE)
DEFENSE FORT (ANTIOXIDANT SYSTEM)
Neutralizes Free Radicals
RECYCLING PLANT (AUTOPHAGY)
Clears Damaged Components
TRANSPORT SYSTEM (BLOOD & LYMPH)
Delivers Nutrients & Removes Waste
Reads Signals, Writes Instructions, Controls Gene Expression
REPAIR CENTER (DNA REPAIR)
Fixes DNA Damage
CONTROL TOWER (HORMONES & MESSENGERS)
Coordinates Communication
WASTE MANAGEMENT (LIVER & KIDNEYS)
Detoxifies & Eliminates
3 NAD+ SALVAGE PATHWAY
The Power Supply Line
Nicotinamide (NAM)
NAMPT (Gatekeeper in Mammals)
NMN (Nicotinamide Mononucleotide)
NAD+ (The Currency of Life)
PNC1 – ANTI-AGING GENE
(In Yeast / Worms)
✓ Converts NAM → Nicotinic Acid (NA)
✓ Removes Block
✓ Promotes NAD+
4 EPIGENETICS – THE LIBRARIAN SYSTEM
INCOMING SIGNALS
Nutrition
Stress
Hormones
Toxins
Exercise
Sleep
EPIGENETIC CONTROL (VOLUME KNOB MODEL)
LOW
OPTIMAL
HIGH
Genes are not ON/OFF – They work like a volume knob.
OUTCOME
↑ Inflammation ↑
↑ Repair Genes ↑
↑ Antioxidants Genes
↑ Longevity Genes ↑
↑ Damage Genes ↑
↑ Aging Genes ↑
5 HORMESIS – GOOD STRESS BUILDS RESILIENCE
Small, Controlled Stress → Stronger Cells
Exercise
Fasting
Heat/Cold
Intermittent Stress
Activates Pathways: AMPK, Sirtuins, Nrf2, Autophagy
Outcome: Stronger Mitochondria, Better Repair, Longevity
6 CORTISOL – THE DOUBLE EDGED SWORD
SHORT TERM (GOOD)
✓ Alertness
✓ Energy
✓ Survival
CHRONIC HIGH (BAD)
• Inflammation
• Insulin Resistance
• NAMPT Down
• NAD+ Depletion
• Accelerated Aging
Balance is the Key – Neither Too Much Nor Too Little
7 FOOD IS YOUR MEDICINE
FOODS THAT BUILD & RENEW
Leafy Greens
Berries
Nuts & Seeds
Legumes
Omega-3 (Fish)
Green Tea
Fermented Foods
FOODS THAT HARM & AGE
Excess Sugar
Refined Carbs
Trans Fats
Ultra-Processed Food
Excess Alcohol
8 HORMONES & MESSENGERS (Control Tower)
Insulin
Estrogen
Testosterone
Growth Hormone
Melatonin
Thyroid Hormones
Keep Communication Smart & Balanced
9 CLINICAL CASE STUDIES – WHEN THE CITY GOES OFF BALANCE
CASE 1: HAIR FALL (ANDROGENETIC ALOPECIA)
Biology:
• DHT ↑
• Inflammation ↑
• Oxidative Stress ↑
• NAD+ ↓
• Poor Mitochondrial Energy
Epigenetics Link:
• DHT activates genes via AR
• Epigenetic marks change hair cycle genes (e.g., WNT, FGF5, KLF9)
Outcome:
Hair follicle miniaturization → Hair thinning & baldness
SUPPORT RENEWAL:
• Balanced Diet • Stress Control
• Zinc, Iron, Protein • Hormonal Balance
CASE 2: ACNE ON FACE
Biology:
• Androgen ↑
• Sebum Overproduction
• Inflammation ↑
• Oxidative Stress ↑
• Gut Dysbiosis
Epigenetics Link:
• Androgen & inflammation change epigenetic marks
• Activates acne genes (TLR2, IL-1β, MMPs)
Outcome:
Follicular inflammation → Acne lesions
SUPPORT RENEWAL:
• Low Glycemic Diet • Zinc • Probiotics
• Reduce Sugar & Dairy • Stress Management
CASE 3: PIGMENTATION ON FACE (MELASMA)
Biology:
• UV Exposure
• Inflammation
• Oxidative Stress
• NAD+ ↓
• Mitochondrial Dysfunction
Epigenetics Link:
• UV & stress alter epigenetic marks (DNA methylation, histone modification)
• Activates melanin genes (MITF, TYR, TYRP1)
Outcome:
Melanin overproduction → Hyperpigmentation
SUPPORT RENEWAL:
• Antioxidant-Rich Diet • Vitamin C, E, Polyphenols
• Sun Protection • Stress & Hormone Balance
CASE 4: FATIGUE & LOW ENERGY
Biology:
• NAD+ ↓
• ATP ↓
• Mitochondrial Dysfunction
• Chronic Inflammation
Outcome:
Low energy, poor recovery, brain fog
SUPPORT RENEWAL:
• Improve Sleep • Exercise
• NAD+ Support (Diet/Precursors)
• Mitochondrial Nutrition
CASE 5: NEURODEGENERATION (COGNITIVE DECLINE)
Biology:
• NAD+ ↓
• Mito Dysfunction
• Oxidative Stress ↑
• Neuronal Repair ↓
Outcome:
Memory decline, slow cognition
SUPPORT RENEWAL:
• Brain Nutrition (Omega-3, B Vitamins)
• Exercise • Sleep • Manage Stress
10 HALLMARKS OF AGING
(When Balance Fails)
Genomic Instability
Telomere Attrition
Epigenetic Alterations
Loss of Proteostasis
Deregulated Inflammation
Altered Intercellular Communication
Mitochondrial Dysfunction
Stem Cell Exhaustion
THE PROGRESSION – FROM BALANCE TO DISEASE
Homeostasis (Healthy City)
Imbalance (Early Disruption)
Hallmarks Activated
Organ Dysfunction (Tissue Damage)
Clinical Disease (Chronic Illness)
RESTORE THE BALANCE – PATH TO RENEWAL
Nourish (Real Food)
Move (Exercise)
Rest (Sleep)
Manage Stress (Mind-Body)
Avoid Toxins (Detox)
Sunlight & Nature
Purpose & Connection
Targeted Support (NAD+, Nutrients)
Result: Better Energy | Better Repair | Better Resilience | Longer Healthspan
11 CELL TURNOVER & REGENERATION
New Cells Born
Function Optimized
CONTINUOUS CYCLE OF LIFE & RENEWAL
Homeostatic Balance
Old / Damaged Cells Removed
12 THE RESULT – WHEN HOMEOSTASIS IS MAINTAINED
✓ Better Energy
✓ Better Repair
✓ Better Immunity
✓ Better Resilience
✓ Slower Aging
✓ Longer Healthspan
CORE TRUTH
MOLECULES POWER CELLS.
CELLS BUILD TISSUES.
RENEWAL PROTECTS LIFE.
WHEN RENEWAL DECLINES, AGING ACCELERATES.
WHEN RENEWAL IMPROVES, LIFE THRIVES.
13 CLINICAL & RESEARCH IMPLICATIONS
Understand Mechanisms
Identify Root Causes
Guide Investigations
Personalize Interventions
Improve Outcomes
Extend Healthspan
A SYSTEMS-BASED FRAMEWORK FOR CLINICAL THINKING & RESEARCH EXCELLENCE
RENEW TODAY. REVIVE TOMORROW.
BALANCE IS THE MEDICINE. HOMEOSTASIS IS THE KEY. LONGEVITY IS THE RESULT.

💡 **Summary**

The maintenance of homeostasis represents the central organizing principle of life, while its progressive disruption forms the biological basis of aging and age-related disease.

🏙️ **CELL CITY + LIBRARIAN MODEL**

🧠 ***"How the Body Works Like a City"***

🏙️ **CELL CITY**

🧠 EPIGENOME (LIBRARIAN)
Reads signals, controls gene expression

↓

CONTROL TOWER (Hormones & Signals)
Cortisol | Insulin | Growth Signals

↓

⚡ **POWER PLANT (Mitochondria)**	🧬 **REPAIR CENTER (DNA Repair)**	🧹 **CLEANING UNIT (Autophagy)**
ATP Production	**Fix DNA Damage**	**Remove Waste**

↓

⚖️ HOMEOSTASIS
(Balanced City Function)

If Breakdown:
→ Energy Failure
→ Repair Failure
→ Waste Accumulation
→ Aging & Disease

👉 **"Longevity is not about activating one gene—**
it is about maintaining homeostasis between growth, repair, and stress response pathways."

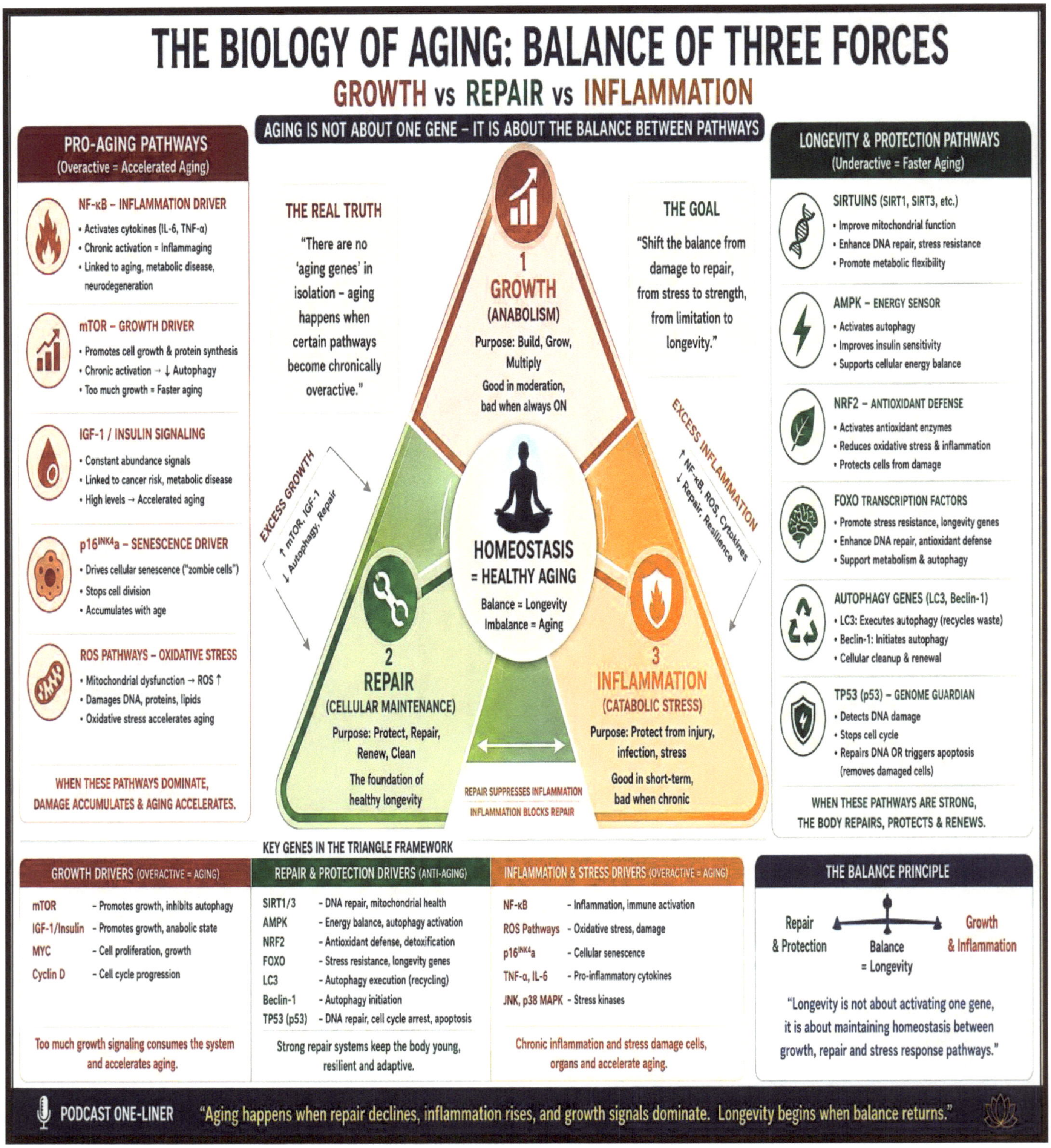
THE BIOLOGY OF AGING: BALANCE OF THREE FORCES
GROWTH vs REPAIR vs INFLAMMATION
AGING IS NOT ABOUT ONE GENE – IT IS ABOUT THE BALANCE BETWEEN PATHWAYS
PRO-AGING PATHWAYS
(Overactive = Accelerated Aging)
NF-κB – INFLAMMATION DRIVER
• Activates cytokines (IL-6, TNF-α)
• Chronic activation = Inflammaging
• Linked to aging, metabolic disease, neurodegeneration
mTOR – GROWTH DRIVER
• Promotes cell growth & protein synthesis
• Chronic activation → ↓ Autophagy
• Too much growth = Faster aging
IGF-1 / INSULIN SIGNALING
• Constant abundance signals
• Linked to cancer risk, metabolic disease
• High levels → Accelerated aging
p16INK4a – SENESCENCE DRIVER
• Drives cellular senescence ("zombie cells")
• Stops cell division
• Accumulates with age
ROS PATHWAYS – OXIDATIVE STRESS
• Mitochondrial dysfunction → ROS ↑
• Damages DNA, proteins, lipids
• Oxidative stress accelerates aging
WHEN THESE PATHWAYS DOMINATE, DAMAGE ACCUMULATES & AGING ACCELERATES.
THE REAL TRUTH
"There are no 'aging genes' in isolation – aging happens when certain pathways become chronically overactive."
1
GROWTH
(ANABOLISM)
Purpose: Build, Grow, Multiply
Good in moderation, bad when always ON
THE GOAL
"Shift the balance from damage to repair, from stress to strength, from limitation to longevity."
EXCESS GROWTH
↑ mTOR, IGF-1
↓ Autophagy, Repair
EXCESS INFLAMMATION
↑ NF-κB, ROS, Cytokines
↓ Repair, Resilience
HOMEOSTASIS
= HEALTHY AGING
Balance = Longevity
Imbalance = Aging
2
REPAIR
(CELLULAR MAINTENANCE)
Purpose: Protect, Repair, Renew, Clean
The foundation of healthy longevity
3
INFLAMMATION
(CATABOLIC STRESS)
Purpose: Protect from injury, infection, stress
Good in short-term, bad when chronic
REPAIR SUPPRESSES INFLAMMATION
INFLAMMATION BLOCKS REPAIR
LONGEVITY & PROTECTION PATHWAYS
(Underactive = Faster Aging)
SIRTUINS (SIRT1, SIRT3, etc.)
• Improve mitochondrial function
• Enhance DNA repair, stress resistance
• Promote metabolic flexibility
AMPK – ENERGY SENSOR
• Activates autophagy
• Improves insulin sensitivity
• Supports cellular energy balance
NRF2 – ANTIOXIDANT DEFENSE
• Activates antioxidant enzymes
• Reduces oxidative stress & inflammation
• Protects cells from damage
FOXO TRANSCRIPTION FACTORS
• Promote stress resistance, longevity genes
• Enhance DNA repair, antioxidant defense
• Support metabolism & autophagy
AUTOPHAGY GENES (LC3, Beclin-1)
• LC3: Executes autophagy (recycles waste)
• Beclin-1: Initiates autophagy
• Cellular cleanup & renewal
TP53 (p53) – GENOME GUARDIAN
• Detects DNA damage
• Stops cell cycle
• Repairs DNA OR triggers apoptosis (removes damaged cells)
WHEN THESE PATHWAYS ARE STRONG, THE BODY REPAIRS, PROTECTS & RENEWS.
KEY GENES IN THE TRIANGLE FRAMEWORK
GROWTH DRIVERS (OVERACTIVE = AGING)
mTOR - Promotes growth, inhibits autophagy
IGF-1/Insulin - Promotes growth, anabolic state
MYC - Cell proliferation, growth
Cyclin D - Cell cycle progression
Too much growth signaling consumes the system and accelerates aging.
REPAIR & PROTECTION DRIVERS (ANTI-AGING)
SIRT1/3 - DNA repair, mitochondrial health
AMPK - Energy balance, autophagy activation
NRF2 - Antioxidant defense, detoxification
FOXO - Stress resistance, longevity genes
LC3 - Autophagy execution (recycling)
Beclin-1 - Autophagy initiation
TP53 (p53) - DNA repair, cell cycle arrest, apoptosis
Strong repair systems keep the body young, resilient and adaptive.
INFLAMMATION & STRESS DRIVERS (OVERACTIVE = AGING)
NF-κB - Inflammation, immune activation
ROS Pathways - Oxidative stress, damage
p16INK4a - Cellular senescence
TNF-α, IL-6 - Pro-inflammatory cytokines
JNK, p38 MAPK - Stress kinases
Chronic inflammation and stress damage cells, organs and accelerate aging.
THE BALANCE PRINCIPLE
Repair & Protection
Balance = Longevity
Growth & Inflammation
"Longevity is not about activating one gene, it is about maintaining homeostasis between growth, repair and stress response pathways."
PODCAST ONE-LINER "Aging happens when repair declines, inflammation rises, and growth signals dominate. Longevity begins when balance returns."

👉 There are no strict "aging genes" vs "anti-aging genes" in a binary sense.
👉 It's about pathways being overactive vs underactive.

🧬 **Therefore:**

- Sirtuins (SIRT1, SIRT3, etc.) ✅ → Longevity-associated regulators
- PNC1 ⚠️ → Mainly studied in yeast (NAD^+ salvage pathway), not directly used in human clinical framing

👉 "Sirtuins and NAD^+ pathways support healthy aging."

🧬 Key "Aging/Pro-Aging" Pathways

1️⃣ NF-κB (Inflammation driver)

👉 Chronic activation = inflammaging

- Promotes cytokines (IL-6, TNF-α)
- Linked to:
  - aging
  - metabolic disease
  - neurodegeneration

👉 "Excess inflammation accelerates aging."

2️⃣ mTOR (Growth pathway)

👉 Great for growth, bad when always ON

- Promotes cell growth & protein synthesis
- Chronic activation → ↓ autophagy

👉 "Too much growth = faster aging."

3️⃣ IGF-1/Insulin signaling (overactivation)

👉 **Nutrient sensing pathway**

- High levels → accelerated aging (seen in multiple models)
- Linked to:
  - cancer risk
  - metabolic disease

👉 "Constant abundance signals shorten lifespan."

4️⃣ p16INK4a (Cellular senescence marker)

👉 Drives "zombie cells"

- Stops cell division
- Accumulates with age

👉 "More senescent cells = more aging tissue."

🛡️ "Anti-Aging/Longevity" Pathways (For Contrast)

Pathway	Role
Sirtuins (SIRT1, SIRT3)	**DNA repair, mitochondrial function**
AMPK	**Energy sensing, activates autophagy**
NRF2	**Antioxidant defence**
FOXO	**Stress resistance, longevity genes**
Autophagy genes (LC3, Beclin-1)	**Cellular cleanup**

⚖️ The REAL TRUTH

👉 It's NOT:

- "Good genes vs bad genes"

👉 It IS:

- Balance between pathways

**"There are no 'aging genes' in isolation—
aging happens when certain pathways become chronically overactive."**

- Inflammation (NF-κB) goes up
- Growth signaling (mTOR) stays constantly on
- Damaged cells accumulate (senescence pathways)

At the same time:

- Repair systems (Sirtuins, NRF2) decline

👉 **Aging is a shift in balance—from repair to damage.**

- SIRT/AMPK/NRF2 → Repair & protection 🛠️
- NF-κB/mTOR/IGF-1 → Growth & stress ⚡

👉 **When repair < damage → aging accelerates**

🔺 **The Triangle Model of Aging**

🟧 **A. Growth Pathways (Anabolism)**

Essential for development and reproduction, but harmful when chronically activated.

Key pathways:

- mTOR → Promotes protein synthesis, inhibits autophagy
- IGF-1/Insulin signaling → Nutrient abundance signaling
- Cyclins/MYC → Cell proliferation

Pathological effect when overactive:

- Reduced autophagy
- Increased cellular burden
- Accelerated aging and cancer risk

💥 Clinical Insight:

"Excess growth without repair leads to accumulation of damage."

🟩 **B. Repair & Longevity Pathways**

These maintain cellular integrity, promote resilience, and extend health span.

Key pathways:

- Sirtuins (SIRT1, SIRT3) → NAD^+-dependent DNA repair, mitochondrial regulation
- AMPK → Energy sensing, activates autophagy
- NRF2 → Antioxidant defence
- FOXO transcription factors → Stress resistance, longevity gene expression
- Autophagy genes (LC3, Beclin-1) → Cellular cleanup and recycling
- TP53 (p53) → Genome guardian (DNA repair or apoptosis)

Role:

- Maintain proteostasis
- Remove damaged organelles
- Enhance stress adaptation

💥 Clinical Insight:

"Longevity depends on efficient repair, not absence of damage."

🟧 C. Inflammation & Stress Pathways

Necessary for acute survival, but detrimental when chronically activated.

Key pathways:

- NF-κB → Master regulator of inflammation
- ROS pathways → Oxidative stress generation
- p16INK4a → Cellular senescence (irreversible growth arrest)
- Pro-inflammatory cytokines (IL-6, TNF-α)

Pathological effect:

- Chronic low-grade inflammation ("inflammaging")
- Tissue dysfunction
- Immune dysregulation

💥 Clinical Insight:

"Persistent inflammation transforms protective mechanisms into drivers of aging."

⚖️ Integrated Systems View

Aging is characterized by:

Pathway	Age-related Change
Growth	**↑ Chronic activation**
Repair	**↓ Efficiency**
Inflammation	**↑ Persistent activation**

👉 **This creates a self-amplifying loop:**

- **Increased damage → reduced repair → more inflammation → further damage**

🧠 Molecular Interpretation of Aging

🔺 Pro-Aging Drivers (When Overactive)

- NF-κB → chronic inflammation
- mTOR/IGF-1 → excessive growth
- ROS pathways → oxidative damage
- p16INK4a → senescence accumulation

🛡️ Longevity Regulators (When Active)

- Sirtuins (SIRT1/3) → repair & metabolic control
- AMPK → energy balance
- NRF2 → antioxidant defence
- FOXO → stress resistance
- LC3/Beclin-1 → autophagy
- TP53 → genomic integrity

🧬 Clinical Implications

🩺 Aging is not a single disease—but a network failure

- Metabolic syndrome
- Neurodegeneration
- Cardiovascular disease
- Cancer

👉 **All arise from:**

- **Chronic inflammation**
- **Impaired repair**
- **Dysregulated growth**

🎯 **Final Conceptual Model (High-Yield for Exams)**

👉 **Three Forces of Aging:**

- Growth (mTOR, IGF-1)
- Repair (SIRT, AMPK, NRF2, FOXO, p53, Autophagy)
- Inflammation (NF-κB, ROS, senescence)

👉 **Outcome:**

- Balance → Healthy aging
- Imbalance → Accelerated aging

🔥 **Final Take-Home Message**

"Aging is not driven by specific genes, but by the progressive imbalance between growth, repair, and inflammation pathways. Longevity is achieved not by activating a single pathway, but by maintaining homeostasis across this network."

🧠 **Ultra-Simplified Memory Model**

- **Growth ↑ + Inflammation ↑ + Repair ↓ = Aging**
- **Balanced Growth + Strong Repair + Controlled Inflammation = Longevity**

📚 **Scientific References**

1. **López-Otín C, Blasco MA, Partridge L, Serrano M, Kroemer G. The hallmarks of aging. *Cell*. 2013;153(6):1194–1217.**

   http://pubmed.ncbi.nlm.nih.gov/23746838/

2. **McEwen BS. Protective and damaging effects of stress mediators. *N Engl J Med*. 1998;338(3):171–179.**

   http://pubmed.ncbi.nlm.nih.gov/9624000/

3. **Ristow M, Schmeisser S. Mitohormesis. *Cell Metab*. 2014;19(5):759–767.**

   http://pubmed.ncbi.nlm.nih.gov/24506876/

4. **Revollo JR, Grimm AA, Imai S. The NAD biosynthesis pathway mediated by NAMPT. *Circ Res*. 2007.**

   http://pubmed.ncbi.nlm.nih.gov/17673663/

5. **Anderson RM, Bitterman KJ, Wood JG, et al. Nicotinamide and PNC1 regulate lifespan. *Nature*. 2003.**

   http://pubmed.ncbi.nlm.nih.gov/12646908/

🛡️ **REPAIR/LONGEVITY PATHWAYS**

Sirtuins/NAD$^+$

👉 https://doi.org/10.1038/nrm2230
👉 https://doi.org/10.1016/j.cmet.2018.03.008

AMPK

👉 https://doi.org/10.1038/nrm3318

NRF2

👉 https://doi.org/10.1016/j.freeradbiomed.2016.09.006

FOXO

👉 https://doi.org/10.1038/nrg2520

Autophagy (LC3, Beclin-1)

👉 https://doi.org/10.1038/nature11838

p53

👉 https://doi.org/10.1038/nrc1922

⚡ **PRO-AGING PATHWAYS**

NF-κB

👉 https://doi.org/10.1038/nri.2017.10

mTOR

👉 https://doi.org/10.1016/j.cell.2009.10.029

IGF-1/Insulin

👉 https://doi.org/10.1038/nature05916

Senescence (p16INK4a)

👉 https://doi.org/10.1038/nrm2233

ROS/Oxidative Stress

👉 https://doi.org/10.1152/physrev.00040.2014

🔺 **SYSTEMS/INTEGRATION**

Systems Biology of Aging

👉 https://doi.org/10.1038/nrg.2016.110

Inflammaging

👉 https://doi.org/10.1016/j.arr.2014.03.002

Aging as Network Disease

👉 https://doi.org/10.1038/nm.4007

👉

Hallmarks → doi:10.1016/j.cell.2013.05.039
mTOR → doi:10.1016/j.cell.2009.10.029
NF-κB → doi:10.1038/nri.2017.10
SIRT → doi:10.1038/nrm2230
AMPK → doi:10.1038/nrm3318

The Metabolic Factory — Cholesterol Transport, Hormone Production, Aging & The Sugar Overload Effect

🎨 **LEGEND (How to Read This Chapter)**

- 🧱 **Raw Material** → Cholesterol
- 🚚 **Transport** → LDL/HDL
- 🏭 **Factories** → Organs/Cells
- 🍞 **High Sugar Load** → Excess carbohydrate → high glucose/insulin
- 🔥 **Damage Signal** → Oxidative stress/inflammation
- ⚙️ **System Failure** → Aging processes

1. 🌍 Introduction: The Body as a Metabolic Supply Chain

Human metabolism is not random chemistry—it is a **highly coordinated factory system** involving:

➡️ Production → Transport → Conversion → Recycling

At its core:

🧠 **Cholesterol = Raw material | LDL/HDL = Transport | Organs = Factories**

But in the modern world, a new disruptor has entered the system:

⚠️ **Chronic high sugar (from excess carbohydrates) = System overload signal**

This framework bridges **biochemistry + systems biology + hallmarks of aging**.

2. 🧠 The Metabolic Headquarters: Liver

The liver is the **central command center** of the factory.

Key roles:

- 🧱 Produces cholesterol
- 🍞 Regulates blood sugar (glycogen storage/release)
- 🛢️ Processes fats (triglycerides, lipoproteins)
- 🍗 Handles protein metabolism (urea cycle)
- ☀️ Activates Vitamin D

🎯 **If one organ runs the factory—it's the liver**

⚠️ **High sugar impact:**

- 🍞 Excess glucose → converted to fat (de novo lipogenesis)
- 🛢️ ↑ triglycerides, ↑ VLDL, ↑ LDL
- 🔥 Fatty liver risk

3. 🚚 Cholesterol Transport System

🔄 **The Supply Chain Flow**

1. 🧱 **Production (Liver)**
2. 🚚 **Delivery (LDL)**
3. 🏭 **Conversion (Organs)**
4. ♻️ **Recycling (HDL)**

🏭 **Factories (Where real work happens)**

- 🧠 Adrenal → cortisol
- ⚧ Gonads → testosterone, estrogen
- ☀️ Skin → Vitamin D
- 🧠 Brain/Liver → structural roles

❗ LDL/HDL don't produce anything—they only transport

4. 🍞 Carbohydrates: The Hidden System Driver

Carbohydrates control the **energy traffic of the factory**.

- 🧠 Pancreas → insulin control
- 🏭 Liver → storage/release
- 💪 Muscles → usage

⚠️ **When sugar is chronically high:**

- 🍞 ↑ glucose → ↑ insulin
- 🔁 constant "fed state"

- ⚙️ metabolic inflexibility
- 🔥 glycation damage (AGEs)

5. ⚙️ The Two Modes of the Factory

🔧 **Growth Mode (mTOR ON)**

- 🍽️ Trigger: excess food (especially sugar + protein)
- 🏗️ Build, store, grow

🔍 **Repair Mode (AMPK ON)**

- ⏳ Trigger: fasting, exercise
- 🧹 Repair, clean, recycle

⚖️ **Health = switching between modes**

⚠️ **High sugar effect:**

- 🍞 keeps mTOR constantly ON
- ❌ suppresses AMPK
- → no repair time

🧬 **6. Aging = Breakdown of the Factory (Now with Sugar Overload)**

🟠 **6.1 Deregulated Nutrient Sensing**

- 🍞 High sugar → chronic insulin spikes
- 🔁 mTOR always ON

👉 Impact:

- 🛢️ ↑ triglycerides
- 🚚 ↑ LDL/ApoB
- ⚙️ insulin resistance

🔋 **6.2 Mitochondrial Dysfunction**

- 🍞 Excess glucose overloads mitochondria
- 🔥 ↑ ROS (oxidative stress)

👉 Impact:

- ⚡ ↓ ATP
- 🏭 factories lose efficiency
- ❌ poor hormone synthesis

🧬 **6.3 Genomic Instability**

- 🍞 High glucose → glycation (AGEs)
- 🔥 DNA damage increases

👉 Impact:

- ⚠️ hormone-producing cells damaged
- ↓ testosterone, estrogen

🧩 **6.4 Loss of Proteostasis**

- 🍞 Sugar modifies proteins (glycation)
- 🔧 enzymes malfunction

👉 Impact:

- ❌ poor cholesterol → hormone conversion
- 🏭 defective outputs

🧱 6.5 Cellular Senescence

- 🍞 chronic metabolic stress → early aging cells

👉 Impact:

- 🏭 factories stop working
- 🔥 release inflammatory signals

🔥 6.6 Chronic Inflammation (Inflammaging)

- 🍞 high sugar → pro-inflammatory state

👉 Impact:

- 🛢 ↑ triglycerides
- 🚚 LDL becomes more harmful
- ♻️ HDL function ↓

📡 6.7 Altered Intercellular Communication

- 🍞 insulin resistance disrupts signaling

👉 Impact:

- 📡 poor coordination between organs
- 🧠 confused metabolic signals

🧬 6.8 Stem Cell Exhaustion

- 🍞 chronic glucose stress → stem cell damage

👉 Impact:

- 🏭 fewer new cells
- ☀️ ↓ vitamin D production
- 🔧 ↓ repair capacity

➕ 🔬 EXTENSION: (Advanced Hallmarks Connection)

High sugar also contributes to:

- 🧬 Epigenetic alterations
- 🦠 Microbiome imbalance
- 🔁 Impaired autophagy

7. 🧪 Blood Tests = Factory Inspection Reports

System	Marker	What it Shows
🍞 Energy	Glucose, HbA1c	Sugar handling
🚚 Transport	LDL, HDL, TG	Lipid flow
🧱 Protein	Albumin, Urea	Building status
🚽 Waste	Creatinine	Disposal

🎯 **Tests measure performance, not intake**

8. ⚖️ Young vs Aging Factory

✅ **Young System:**

- Smooth transport 🚚
- Efficient factories 🏭
- Balanced signals ⚙️

❌ **Aging System:**

- 🍞 sugar overload
- 🚚 transport congestion
- 🏭 factory decline

9. 💡 Final Insight

[illegible]ging is not just damage—it is system overload + loss of coordination

[illegible]ne-Line Truth

[illegible]ol is the raw material, LDL delivers it, HDL recycles it—but excess sugar silently disrupts every step of [illegible]

[illegible]losing Message

[illegible]s not:

[illegible]d

It is:

✅ **A well-managed metabolic factory that balances fuel, repair, and resilience**

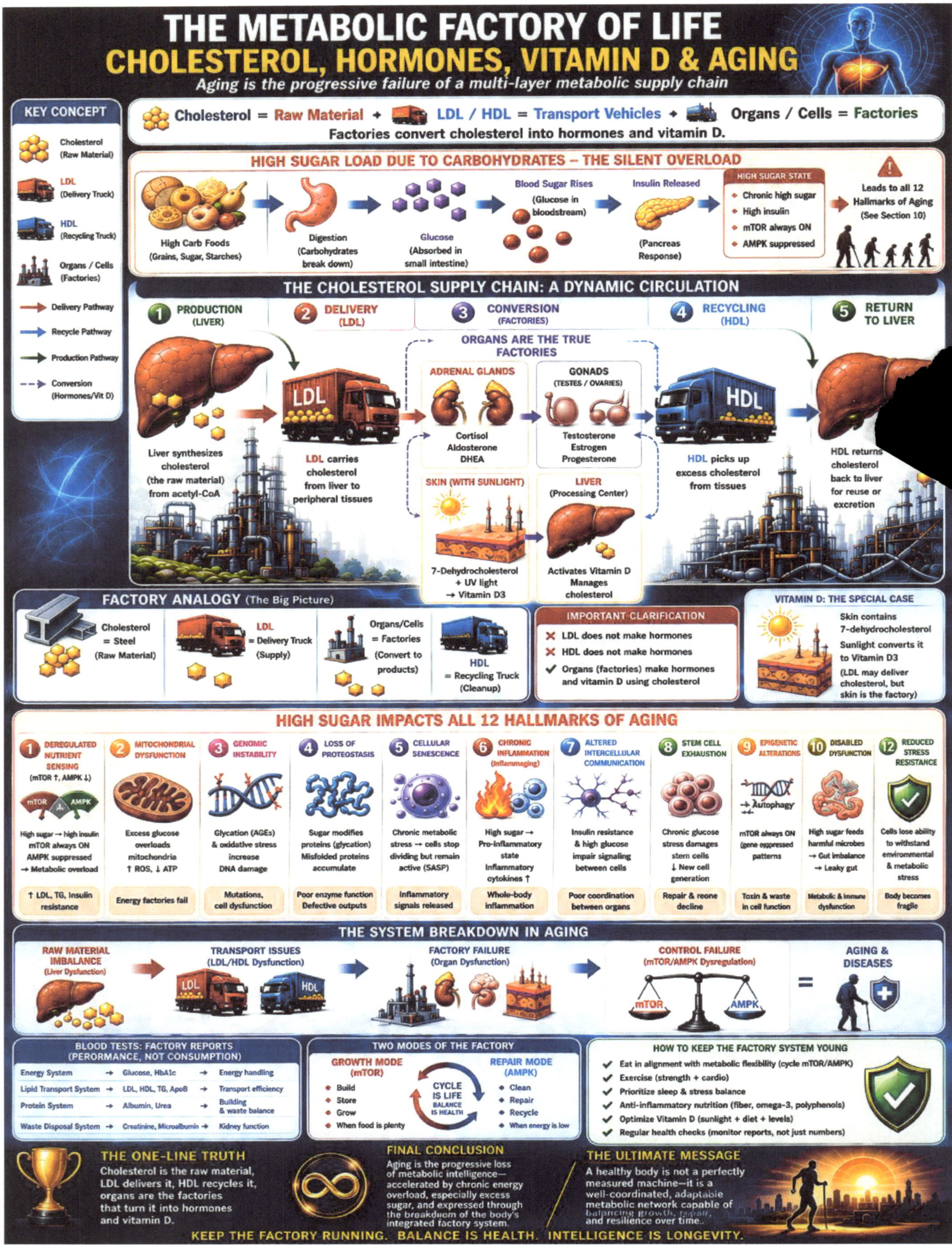
THE METABOLIC FACTORY OF LIFE
CHOLESTEROL, HORMONES, VITAMIN D & AGING
Aging is the progressive failure of a multi-layer metabolic supply chain
KEY CONCEPT
Cholesterol (Raw Material)
LDL (Delivery Truck)
HDL (Recycling Truck)
Organs / Cells (Factories)
Delivery Pathway
Recycle Pathway
Production Pathway
Conversion (Hormones/Vit D)
Cholesterol = Raw Material + LDL / HDL = Transport Vehicles + Organs / Cells = Factories
Factories convert cholesterol into hormones and vitamin D.
HIGH SUGAR LOAD DUE TO CARBOHYDRATES – THE SILENT OVERLOAD
High Carb Foods (Grains, Sugar, Starches)
Digestion (Carbohydrates break down)
Glucose (Absorbed in small intestine)
Blood Sugar Rises (Glucose in bloodstream)
Insulin Released (Pancreas Response)
HIGH SUGAR STATE
Chronic high sugar
High insulin
mTOR always ON
AMPK suppressed
Leads to all 12 Hallmarks of Aging (See Section 10)
THE CHOLESTEROL SUPPLY CHAIN: A DYNAMIC CIRCULATION
1 PRODUCTION (LIVER)
2 DELIVERY (LDL)
3 CONVERSION (FACTORIES)
4 RECYCLING (HDL)
5 RETURN TO LIVER
Liver synthesizes cholesterol (the raw material) from acetyl-CoA
LDL carries cholesterol from liver to peripheral tissues
ORGANS ARE THE TRUE FACTORIES
ADRENAL GLANDS
Cortisol
Aldosterone
DHEA
GONADS (TESTES / OVARIES)
Testosterone
Estrogen
Progesterone
SKIN (WITH SUNLIGHT)
7-Dehydrocholesterol + UV light → Vitamin D3
LIVER (Processing Center)
Activates Vitamin D
Manages cholesterol
HDL picks up excess cholesterol from tissues
HDL returns cholesterol back to liver for reuse or excretion
FACTORY ANALOGY (The Big Picture)
Cholesterol = Steel (Raw Material)
LDL = Delivery Truck (Supply)
Organs/Cells = Factories (Convert to products)
HDL = Recycling Truck (Cleanup)
IMPORTANT CLARIFICATION
LDL does not make hormones
HDL does not make hormones
Organs (factories) make hormones and vitamin D using cholesterol
VITAMIN D: THE SPECIAL CASE
Skin contains 7-dehydrocholesterol
Sunlight converts it to Vitamin D3
(LDL may deliver cholesterol, but skin is the factory)
HIGH SUGAR IMPACTS ALL 12 HALLMARKS OF AGING
1 DEREGULATED NUTRIENT SENSING (mTOR ↑, AMPK ↓)
High sugar → high insulin mTOR always ON AMPK suppressed → Metabolic overload
↑ LDL, TG, Insulin resistance
2 MITOCHONDRIAL DYSFUNCTION
Excess glucose overloads mitochondria ↑ ROS, ↓ ATP
Energy factories fail
3 GENOMIC INSTABILITY
Glycation (AGEs) & oxidative stress increase DNA damage
Mutations, cell dysfunction
4 LOSS OF PROTEOSTASIS
Sugar modifies proteins (glycation) Misfolded proteins accumulate
Poor enzyme function Defective outputs
5 CELLULAR SENESCENCE
Chronic metabolic stress → cells stop dividing but remain active (SASP)
Inflammatory signals released
6 CHRONIC INFLAMMATION (Inflammaging)
High sugar → Pro-inflammatory state Inflammatory cytokines ↑
Whole-body inflammation
7 ALTERED INTERCELLULAR COMMUNICATION
Insulin resistance & high glucose impair signaling between cells
Poor coordination between organs
8 STEM CELL EXHAUSTION
Chronic glucose stress damages stem cells ↓ New cell generation
Repair & reone decline
9 EPIGENETIC ALTERATIONS
Autophagy
mTOR always ON (gene expressed patterns
Toxin & waste in cell function
10 DISABLED DYSFUNCTION
High sugar feeds harmful microbes → Gut imbalance → Leaky gut
Metabolic & immune dysfunction
12 REDUCED STRESS RESISTANCE
Cells lose ability to withstand environmental & metabolic stress
Body becomes fragile
THE SYSTEM BREAKDOWN IN AGING
RAW MATERIAL IMBALANCE (Liver Dysfunction)
TRANSPORT ISSUES (LDL/HDL Dysfunction)
FACTORY FAILURE (Organ Dysfunction)
CONTROL FAILURE (mTOR/AMPK Dysregulation)
= AGING & DISEASES
BLOOD TESTS: FACTORY REPORTS (PERFORMANCE, NOT CONSUMPTION)
Energy System → Glucose, HbA1c → Energy handling
Lipid Transport System → LDL, HDL, TG, ApoB → Transport efficiency
Protein System → Albumin, Urea → Building & waste balance
Waste Disposal System → Creatinine, Microalbumin → Kidney function
TWO MODES OF THE FACTORY
GROWTH MODE (mTOR)
Build
Store
Grow
When food is plenty
CYCLE IS LIFE BALANCE IS HEALTH
REPAIR MODE (AMPK)
Clean
Repair
Recycle
When energy is low
HOW TO KEEP THE FACTORY SYSTEM YOUNG
Eat in alignment with metabolic flexibility (cycle mTOR/AMPK)
Exercise (strength + cardio)
Prioritize sleep & stress balance
Anti-inflammatory nutrition (fiber, omega-3, polyphenols)
Optimize Vitamin D (sunlight + diet + levels)
Regular health checks (monitor reports, not just numbers)
THE ONE-LINE TRUTH
Cholesterol is the raw material, LDL delivers it, HDL recycles it, organs are the factories that turn it into hormones and vitamin D.
FINAL CONCLUSION
Aging is the progressive loss of metabolic intelligence—accelerated by chronic energy overload, especially excess sugar, and expressed through the breakdown of the body's integrated factory system.
THE ULTIMATE MESSAGE
A healthy body is not a perfectly measured machine—it is a well-coordinated, adaptable metabolic network capable of balancing growth, repair, and resilience over time.
KEEP THE FACTORY RUNNING. BALANCE IS HEALTH. INTELLIGENCE IS LONGEVITY.

Final Conclusion: The True Driver of Aging

Aging is not caused by a single molecule—not cholesterol, not glucose, not protein, and not any isolated biomarker.

Instead, aging reflects the progressive breakdown of metabolic intelligence—the body's ability to sense, process, distribute, and adapt to energy and nutrients in a coordinated way.

At its core, the human body functions as an integrated metabolic network, not a single pathway:

- The liver regulates and produces key metabolic substrates
- Carbohydrates (glucose) provide immediate energy and signaling input
- Fats (lipids, cholesterol) provide structure, storage, and long-term fuel
- Proteins (amino acids) support repair, enzymes, and signaling pathways
- Energy molecules (ATP, NAD^+) power cellular processes
- Hormonal systems (insulin, glucagon, mTOR, AMPK) coordinate responses
- Transport systems (lipoproteins, circulation) distribute resources
- Cells and organs act as functional units, converting inputs into energy, structure, and signaling outputs

Health depends not on any one component—but on how well all of these systems communicate and adapt together.

Where the Breakdown Begins

With time—and more importantly, under modern lifestyle conditions—this coordination begins to fail.

One of the most powerful accelerators of this failure is:

Chronic energy overload—especially persistent high sugar exposure from excess refined carbohydrates.

This creates a cascade:

- Constant **insulin signaling**
- Persistent **mTOR activation (growth mode stuck ON)**
- Suppressed **AMPK (repair mode OFF)**
- Reduced **metabolic flexibility**

At the same time:

- **Protein signaling becomes imbalanced** (impaired repair vs excess growth signals)
- **Lipid handling becomes dysregulated** (not just LDL/HDL, but overall trafficking)
- **NAD^+ and mitochondrial efficiency decline**
- **Cellular energy sensing becomes inaccurate**

How This Drives All 12 Hallmarks of Aging

This imbalance does not stay isolated—it spreads across the entire biological system:

- **Deregulated nutrient sensing** → chronic insulin + mTOR dominance
- **Mitochondrial dysfunction** → inefficient energy production
- **Genomic instability** → damage accumulation
- **Loss of proteostasis** → faulty protein handling
- **Cellular senescence** → non-functional but inflammatory cells
- **Chronic inflammation** → system-wide stress (inflammaging)
- **Altered intercellular communication** → signaling breakdown
- **Stem cell exhaustion** → reduced regeneration

Scientific References

https://medlineplus.gov/cholesterol.html?utm_source=chatgpt.com

https://www.ncbi.nlm.nih.gov/books/NBK535438/?utm_source=chatgpt.com

https://pmc.ncbi.nlm.nih.gov/articles/PMC3704564/?utm_source=chatgpt.com

The Digital Blueprint of Aging: From Centenarians to Algorithms

🧬 What Scientists Have Found About Centenarians (People Living 100+ Years)

Centenarians are one of the most studied groups in aging research because they represent successful aging—not just long life, but often delayed disease and better function.

🧠 1. They Don't Avoid Aging — They Delay It

👉 **Key finding:**

Centenarians do not escape aging… they age slower and develop diseases much later.

- heart disease, diabetes, cancer → occur 10–20 years later
- many remain independent into their 90s

🧬 2. Unique Genetic Profile (But Not Everything)

Scientists found:

- only 20–30% longevity is genetic
- remaining 70–80% = lifestyle + environment

Key genes studied:

- FOXO3 (longevity gene)
- IGF-1 pathway genes
- APOE variants

👉 **Important:**

They don't have "perfect genes", they have better regulation of genes.

🔁 3. Lower IGF-1/Growth Signaling

Insulin-like Growth Factor 1

👉 **Many centenarians show:**

- lower IGF-1 activity
- reduced mTOR signaling

💥 **Meaning:**

- less constant "growth mode"
- more repair + maintenance mode

🧹 4. Better Cellular Cleanup (Autophagy)

- higher autophagy efficiency
- better removal of damaged proteins

👉 **Result:**

- less accumulation of cellular waste
- slower aging process

🔥 5. Low Chronic Inflammation

👉 **Called:**
"Inflammaging" (inflammation + aging)

Centenarians:

- have lower baseline inflammation
- better immune regulation

🔋 **6. Strong Mitochondrial Function**

- better energy efficiency
- less oxidative stress

👉 **They produce energy with:**

- less damage

🧠 **7. Resilient Brain & Nervous System**

- delayed cognitive decline
- better stress adaptation

👉 Not zero stress—but better handling of stress

🧘 **8. Lifestyle Patterns (Blue Zone Insights)**

Common habits:

- moderate calorie intake
- lower animal protein (in many populations)
- natural movement (not gym-based)
- strong social bonds
- sense of purpose

⚖️ **9. Metabolic Balance (Not Extreme)**

- stable blood sugar
- good insulin sensitivity
- not extreme diets

👉 **Key:**

Consistency > intensity

🧬 **10. Stem Cell Preservation**

- slower depletion of stem cells
- better repair capacity

🔁 **11. Delayed Senescence (Zombie Cells)**

- fewer senescent cells
- better immune clearance

📌 **Summary**

Centenarians typically have:

- balanced (often lower) IGF-1
- strong repair systems (autophagy)
- low inflammation
- efficient energy systems
- stable metabolism
- supportive lifestyle

👉 **Important truth first:**

❗ Scientists do NOT rely on a single blood test to conclude things like "stem cell preservation" or "autophagy." These conclusions come from a combination of blood tests + genetic tests + tissue studies + indirect biomarkers.

Let's break this down 👇

🧬 **1. IGF-1 Pathway (Direct Blood Test ✅)**

🧪 Test Used:

- Serum IGF-1 level
- Growth Hormone (GH)

👉 **Measured directly from blood**

📊 **What scientists observe in centenarians:**

- often lower or well-regulated IGF-1

🧬 **2. FOXO3, APOE, SIRT Genes (Genetic Testing 🧬)**

These are NOT blood level tests
👉 **These are DNA-based tests**

🧪 Test Used:

- Whole genome sequencing
- SNP genotyping

Genes:

- FOXO3 (longevity gene)
- APOE (lipid metabolism, Alzheimer's risk)
- SIRT1–SIRT7 (longevity regulators)

👉 **Sample source:**

- blood OR saliva (for DNA extraction)

💡 **Conclusion:**

Scientists look at gene variants, not "levels"

🔋 **3. Mitochondrial Function (Indirect Blood Markers ⚠️)**

You cannot directly measure mitochondria in blood easily.

🧪 **Tests Used (Indirect):**

- Lactate levels
- Pyruvate levels
- ATP production assays (research labs)
- Mitochondrial DNA (mtDNA copy number)

In research:

- muscle biopsy (more accurate)

👉 **What they conclude:**

- better energy efficiency
- less oxidative stress

🧹 **4. Autophagy (Very Important – NOT Directly Measurable ❗)**

There is no routine blood test for autophagy

🧪 **Research Markers:**

- LC3-II protein
- Beclin-1
- p62 (SQSTM1)

👉 **These are measured via:**

- tissue biopsy
- lab assays (not routine clinical tests)

Indirect blood clues:

- insulin sensitivity

- lower inflammation
- metabolic flexibility

🧟 **5. Cellular Senescence (Zombie Cells)**

🧪 **Markers Used:**

- p16INK4a
- p21
- SA-β-gal (lab test)

👉 **Mostly from:**

- tissue samples
- specialized research labs

🧬 **6. Stem Cell Preservation (Indirect Measurement)**

No simple blood test says:
👉 **"Your stem cells are preserved"**

🧪 **What scientists use:**

- CD34+ stem cell count (blood marker)
- bone marrow studies
- regenerative capacity tests

👉 **Interpretation:**

- higher regenerative markers → better stem cell function

🔥 **7. Inflammation (VERY IMPORTANT – Blood Test ✅)**

🧪 **Tests:**

- CRP (C-reactive protein)
- IL-6
- TNF-alpha

👉 **Centenarians:**

- **usually low chronic inflammation**

⚡ **8. NAD$^+$ Levels (Advanced but Measurable)**

🧪 **Test:**

- NAD$^+$/NADH ratio (specialized labs)

👉 **Not routine, but used in:**

- **longevity research**

⚖️ **9. mTOR/Nutrient Signaling (Indirect)**

No direct test for mTOR in clinic.

🧪 **Indirect markers:**

- insulin levels
- IGF-1
- amino acid profile

"Longevity science does not rely on a single biomarker. It is a systems-level interpretation derived from genetic, metabolic, inflammatory, and cellular signals."

Can AI Predict and Delay Aging? The Science of Personalized Longevity

For decades, scientists studied centenarians to understand longevity. Today, artificial intelligence is helping us decode those patterns—not just to study aging, but to predict and delay it.

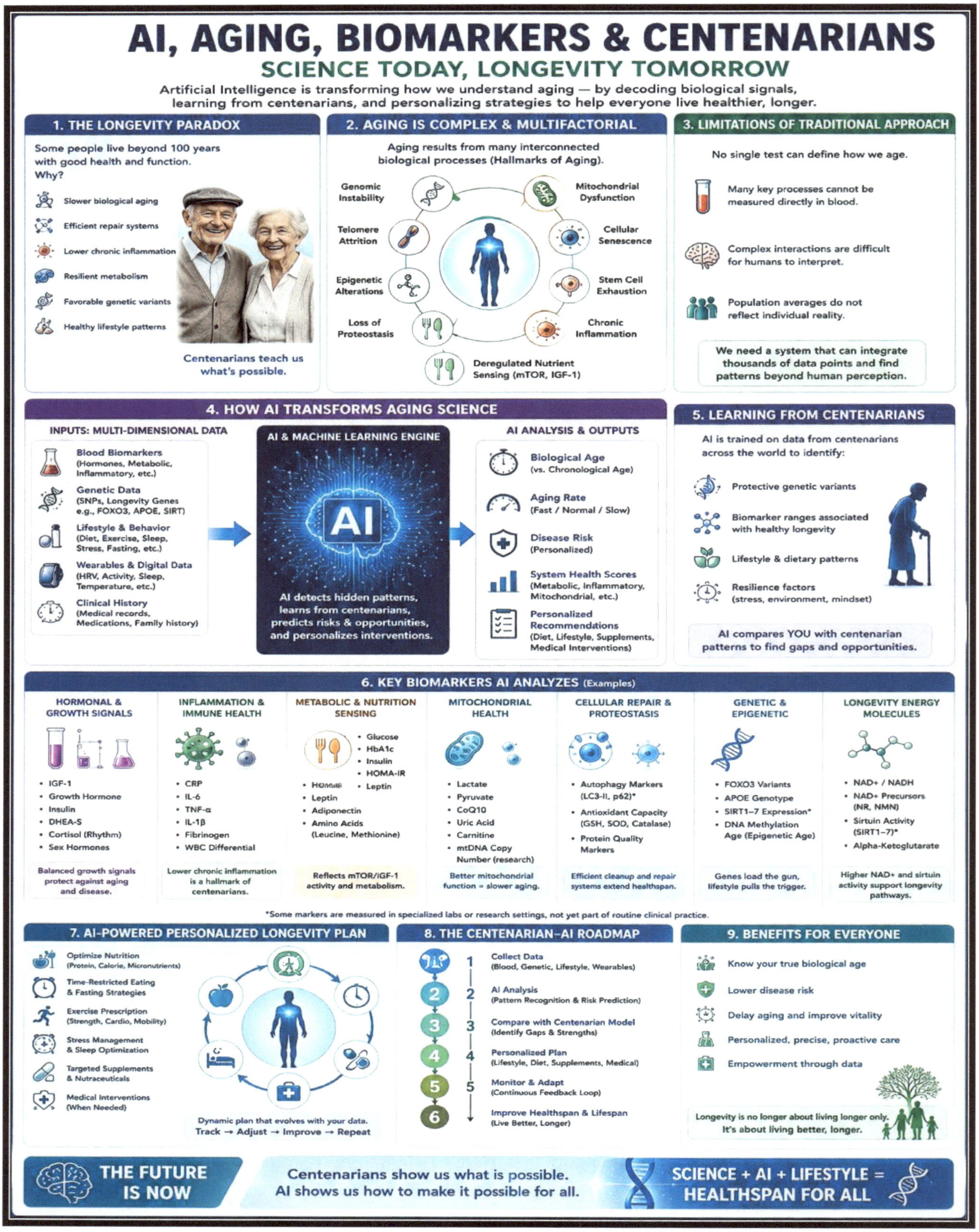

🧬 The Limitation of Traditional Testing

As we discussed:

- No single blood test defines aging
- Many processes (autophagy, stem cells, mitochondrial health) are not directly measurable

👉 **Doctors rely on:**

- partial biomarkers
- clinical judgment

💥 **Limitation:**

"Human interpretation is limited when dealing with complex biological networks."

🤖 3. Where AI Enters the Picture

AI does not create new biology—
👉 **it connects hidden patterns across systems**

AI can analyse:

- blood tests
- genetic data
- lifestyle inputs
- wearable data (sleep, HRV, activity)

👉 **and detect patterns humans cannot easily see**

🧠 What AI Can Actually Measure (Indirectly)

AI does NOT directly measure:

- autophagy
- stem cells
- mitochondrial efficiency

👉 **But it infers them using patterns**

🧪 **Example:**

Hidden Process	AI Uses These Inputs
Autophagy	**insulin, glucose, fasting pattern**
Mitochondria	**lactate, activity, fatigue**
Inflammation	**CRP, HRV, sleep**
Biological age	**multi-marker integration**

🧬 AI + Centenarian Data

Scientists feed AI with:

- genetic data of centenarians
- biomarker patterns
- lifestyle habits

👉 **AI learns:**

"What patterns are associated with long life?"

🧠 **AI then compares:**

👉 YOUR vs CENTENARIAN PROFILE

Example:

- IGF-1 too high → flagged
- inflammation slightly elevated → flagged
- sleep poor → flagged

👉 **AI gives:**
risk + recommendations

📊 **AI-Driven Longevity Scoring**

AI platforms now generate:

- Biological age
- Aging speed
- Disease risk

👉 **Based on:**

- 20–100+ biomarkers

💡 **Real Concept:**

"Chronological age = how many years you lived
Biological age = how your body actually behaves"

🧬 **7. Tools Available Today (For Common People)**

🧪 **Blood-based platforms:**

- multi-biomarker panels

🧬 **Genetic testing:**

- SNP analysis
- longevity genes

⌚ **Wearables:**

- heart rate variability (HRV)
- sleep tracking
- stress

👉 **AI integrates all:**

"From fragmented data → to one health story"

⚠️ **Limitations of AI (Very Important for Academic Honesty)**

AI is powerful but not perfect:

- depends on data quality
- cannot fully measure deep biology
- predictions ≠ certainty

👉 Important line:

"AI predicts probability, not destiny."

🔁 Translating Science into Action

AI helps in:

- optimizing diet
- adjusting protein intake (IGF-1 balance)
- improving sleep
- reducing inflammation
- tracking progress

🎯 **Example:**

If IGF-1 is high:

- reduce excess protein
- adjust fasting
- improve metabolic flexibility

🧬 The Bridge: Centenarians → Common People

Earlier:

- centenarians = rare case studies

Now:

- AI → brings those patterns to everyone

💥 **Meaning:**

"Longevity is no longer luck—it can become a strategy."

🧠 The Future of Medicine

Medicine is shifting from:

- disease treatment ❌
  👉 to
- predictive prevention ✅

🔮 **Future Possibilities:**

- AI predicting disease before symptoms
- personalized anti-aging plans
- real-time aging tracking

🎯 Final Integration

👉 **Combine everything:**

- Biology → signals
- AI → pattern recognition
- Lifestyle → intervention

🔥 Final Summary

"Centenarians showed us what is possible. Artificial intelligence is showing us how to get there."

Machine Learning in Aging Biology: From Pathway Networks to Predictive Longevity Modeling

In medicine, machine learning analyses large amounts of health data (blood tests, genetics, lifestyle) to find hidden patterns and predict disease or aging risk.

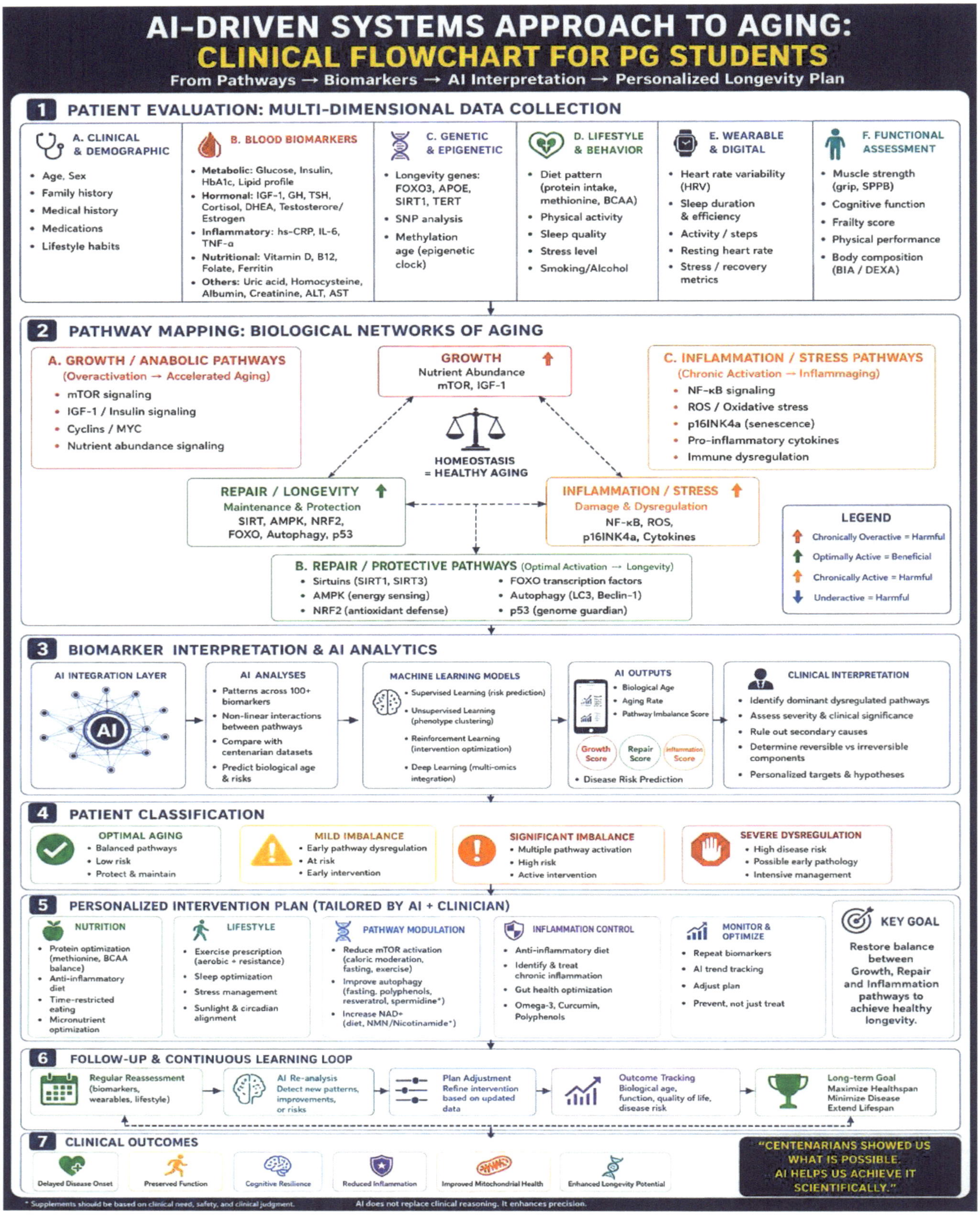

🌐 1. The Shift from Linear Biology to Network Biology

Machine Learning is a method of teaching computers to learn from data, recognize patterns, and make decisions—without being explicitly programmed—by analysing large amounts of biological and health data such as blood biomarkers, genetic information, and lifestyle factors to predict disease risk, assess biological age, and understand the processes of human aging.

🔬 Conceptual Integration

In the context of aging biology:

👉 Machine learning acts as a **pattern-recognition engine** that connects multiple systems:

- 🧬 Genetic signals (FOXO3, IGF-1 pathways, APOE variants)
- 🧪 Biomarkers (CRP, glucose, IGF-1, lipid profile)
- 🔋 Metabolic indicators (mitochondrial function, insulin sensitivity)
- ⌚ Lifestyle inputs (sleep, activity, stress)

👉 It integrates these into a **single interpretable model of aging risk and longevity potential.**

For decades, aging was studied as a collection of isolated processes—genes, hormones, or pathways acting independently. However, modern science has revealed a more complex reality:

Aging is not driven by single genes, but by dynamic interactions between growth, repair, and stress-response pathways.

These include:

- **Growth pathways → mTOR signaling pathway, Insulin-like Growth Factor 1**
- **Repair pathways → Sirtuins, AMPK, NRF2, FOXO**
- **Inflammation pathways → NF-κB, ROS, senescence markers**

This creates a multi-dimensional biological network, not a linear system.

💥 **Limitation:**

Traditional medicine struggles to interpret this complexity because:

- No single biomarker defines aging
- Many processes (autophagy, mitochondrial efficiency) are not directly measurable
- Interactions between pathways are non-linear and dynamic

🤖 2. Why Machine Learning is Needed in Aging Science

Machine learning (ML) is not replacing biology—it is augmenting our ability to understand it.

"Machine learning detects patterns across biological systems that are too complex for human interpretation alone."

ML becomes essential because:

- Aging involves hundreds of interacting variables
- Data comes from multiple layers:
    - blood biomarkers
    - genetic data
    - lifestyle inputs
    - wearable sensors

👉 Human analysis = limited pattern recognition
👉 ML = high-dimensional pattern detection

🧬 3. Translating Your Pathway Model into AI Language

Your biological framework maps perfectly into an ML model.

🔺 The Triangle Model → AI Feature Space

Biological Axis	Pathways	ML Interpretation
🔴 **Growth**	**mTOR, IGF-1**	**Anabolic signaling score**
🟢 **Repair**	**SIRT, AMPK, NRF2**	**Repair efficiency score**
🟠 **Inflammation**	**NF-κB, ROS**	**Inflammatory burden score**

👉 Machine learning converts biology into:

Quantifiable features → Predictive outputs

🧪 4. What AI Actually "Sees" (Very Important Concept)

AI does NOT directly measure hidden processes like:

- Autophagy
- Stem cell function
- Mitochondrial efficiency

Instead, it infers them indirectly.

Example Mapping:

Hidden Process	AI Uses These Inputs
Autophagy	insulin, glucose, fasting patterns
Mitochondria	lactate, fatigue, activity
Inflammation	CRP, IL-6, sleep, HRV
Biological Age	multi-marker integration

💡 **Key Insight:**

"AI infers biology—it does not directly measure it."

Scientific observations show:

- Lower IGF-1 and reduced mTOR signaling
- Better autophagy and cellular cleanup
- Lower chronic inflammation
- Efficient mitochondrial function
- Stable metabolic systems

In AI terms:

Centenarians = "ground truth dataset"

👉 Machine learning models are trained to learn:

"What biological patterns are associated with long life?"

📊 6. AI-Based Longevity Modelling

AI integrates multiple inputs to generate predictions.

Inputs:

- Blood biomarkers (IGF-1, glucose, CRP, lipids)
- Genetic data (FOXO3, APOE variants)
- Lifestyle (diet, sleep, activity)
- Wearables (HRV, stress, movement)

Outputs:

- Biological age
- Aging rate
- Disease risk prediction
- Personalized recommendations

⚙️ 7. Example: AI Interpreting Your Pathway Imbalance

Case:

- IGF-1 → high
- CRP → mildly elevated
- Sleep → poor

AI Interpretation:

- Growth pathway ↑
- Inflammation ↑
- Repair efficiency ↓

Output:

👉 **Accelerated aging risk**

Recommendation:

- Adjust protein intake
- Improve sleep quality
- Increase metabolic flexibility

⚠️ 8. Limitations of Machine Learning (Critical for Academic Rigor)

Machine learning is powerful but not absolute.

Limitations include:

- Dependent on data quality
- Cannot fully measure deep cellular processes
- Predictions are probabilistic, not deterministic

"AI predicts probability—not destiny."

🔄 9. From Biology to Action: The New Medical Model

Medicine is shifting from:

❌ **Reactive (treat disease after onset)**
➡️
✅ **Predictive (identify risk before disease)**

AI enables:

- Early detection of imbalance
- Continuous monitoring
- Personalized intervention strategies

🌍 10. The Bridge: From Centenarians to Common People

Previously:

- Longevity insights = observational (centenarians only)

Now:

- AI translates those patterns into actionable insights

"What was once rare biology is now becoming accessible intelligence."

🔬 FINAL INTEGRATION MODEL

🔺 The Aging Equation

- Growth ↑ (mTOR, IGF-1)
- Inflammation ↑ (NF-κB, ROS)
- Repair ↓ (SIRT, AMPK, NRF2)

👉 Result = Aging acceleration

🤖 AI Layer

- Detects imbalance
- Predicts outcomes
- Suggests correction

🔥 FINAL SUMMARY

"Longevity is not about activating one gene—it is about maintaining balance across biological systems. Machine learning does not change this biology—it allows us to measure, predict, and optimize it."

"Centenarians showed us what healthy aging looks like—machine learning is teaching us how to achieve it."

www.ingramcontent.com/pod-product-compliance
Lightning Source LLC
LaVergne TN
LVHW070944210926
848482LV00002B/90